Participatory Visual Methodologies in Global Public Health

T0199657

Participatory Visual Methodologies in Global Public Health focuses on the use of participatory visual methodologies such as photovoice, participatory video (including cellphilming or the use of cell phones to make videos), drawing and mapping in public health research. These approaches are modes of inquiry that can engage participants and communities, eliciting evidence about their own health and well-being, as well as modes of representation and modes of production in the co-creation of knowledge, and modes of dissemination in relation to knowledge translation and mobilization. Thus, the production by a group of girls or young women of a set of photos or videos from their own visual perspective can offer new evidence on how, for example, they see sexual violence. Unlike other data such as those collected through surveys or even conventional interviews, the images they have produced not only inform the empirical evidence, but also do not need to remain in a laboratory or the office of a researcher. They can, through exhibitions and screenings, reach various audiences: school or health personnel, parents and community members, and perhaps also policy-makers. This collection offers a critical overview for students, practitioners, researchers and policy-makers working in or concerned with the use of participatory methodologies in public health around the globe. This book was originally published as a special issue of *Global Public Health*.

Claudia Mitchell is a James McGill Professor in the Faculty of Education and Director of the Institute for Human Development and Well-Being at McGill University, Montreal, Canada. Her research cuts across visual and other participatory methodologies in relation to youth, gender and sexuality, girls' education, teacher identity and critical areas of international development linked to gender and HIV and AIDS.

Marni Sommer is an Associate Professor of Sociomedical Sciences in the Mailman School of Public Health, Columbia University, New York, USA. She is also the Executive Editor of the *Global Public Health* journal. Her research includes the use of participatory methodologies to explore how gender, sexuality and the transition through puberty intersect with education among young people in low-income countries.

Participatory Visual Methodologies in Global Public Health

Edited by
Claudia Mitchell and Marni Sommer

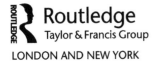

LONDON AND NEW YORK

First published 2017 by Routledge

2 Park Square, Milton Park, Abingdon, Oxfordshire OX14 4RN
52 Vanderbilt Avenue, New York, NY 10017

Routledge is an imprint of the Taylor & Francis Group, an informa business

First issued in paperback 2018

Copyright © 2017 Taylor & Francis

All rights reserved. No part of this book may be reprinted or reproduced or utilised in any form or by any electronic, mechanical, or other means, now known or hereafter invented, including photocopying and recording, or in any information storage or retrieval system, without permission in writing from the publishers.

Notice:
Product or corporate names may be trademarks or registered trademarks, and are used only for identification and explanation without intent to infringe.

British Library Cataloguing in Publication Data
A catalogue record for this book is available from the British Library

ISBN 13: 978-1-138-72426-6 (hbk)
ISBN 13: 978-0-367-14323-7 (pbk)

Typeset in MinionPro
by diacriTech, Chennai

Publisher's Note
The publisher accepts responsibility for any inconsistencies that may have arisen during the conversion of this book from journal articles to book chapters, namely the possible inclusion of journal terminology.

Disclaimer
Every effort has been made to contact copyright holders for their permission to reprint material in this book. The publishers would be grateful to hear from any copyright holder who is not here acknowledged and will undertake to rectify any errors or omissions in future editions of this book.

Contents

CONTENTS

Citation Information

The chapters in this book were originally published in *Global Public Health*, volume 11, issues 5–6 (May–July 2016). When citing this material, please use the original page numbering for each article, as follows:

Chapter 5

Exploring social inclusion strategies for public health research and practice: The use of participatory visual methods to counter stigmas surrounding street-based substance abuse in Colombia
Amy E. Ritterbusch
Global Public Health, volume 11, issues 5–6 (May–July 2016) pp. 600–617

Chapter 6

Bodies as evidence: Mapping new terrain for teen pregnancy and parenting
Aline C. Gubrium, Alice Fiddian-Green, Kasey Jernigan and Elizabeth L. Krause
Global Public Health, volume 11, issues 5–6 (May–July 2016) pp. 618–635

Chapter 7

From informed consent to dissemination: Using participatory visual methods with young people with long-term conditions at different stages of research
Cecilia Vindrola-Padros, Ana Martins, Imelda Coyne, Gemma Bryan and Faith Gibson
Global Public Health, volume 11, issues 5–6 (May–July 2016) pp. 636–650

Chapter 8

Beyond engagement in working with children in eight Nairobi slums to address safety, security, and housing: Digital tools for policy and community dialogue
Claudia Mitchell, Fatuma Chege, Lucy Maina and Margot Rothman
Global Public Health, volume 11, issues 5–6 (May–July 2016) pp. 651–665

Chapter 9

'People like me don't make things like that': Participatory video as a method for reducing leprosy-related stigma
R. M. H. Peters, M. B. M. Zweekhorst, W. H. van Brakel, J. F. G. Bunders and Irwanto
Global Public Health, volume 11, issues 5–6 (May–July 2016) pp. 666–682

Chapter 10

Supporting youth and community capacity through photovoice: Reflections on participatory research on maternal health in Wakiso district, Uganda
David Musoke, Rawlance Ndejjo, Elizabeth Ekirapa-Kiracho and Asha S. George
Global Public Health, volume 11, issues 5–6 (May–July 2016) pp. 683–698

Chapter 11

Using participant-empowered visual relationship timelines in a qualitative study of sexual behaviour
Tamar Goldenberg, Catherine Finneran, Karen L. Andes and Rob Stephenson
Global Public Health, volume 11, issues 5–6 (May–July 2016) pp. 699–718

For any permission-related enquiries please visit:
http://www.tandfonline.com/page/help/permissions

Notes on Contributors

Bree Akesson is an Assistant Professor at the Lyle S. Hallman Faculty of Social Work, Wilfrid Laurier University, Kitchener, Canada.

Miranda D'Amico is a Professor at the Department of Education, Concordia University, Montreal, Canada.

Karen L. Andes is an Assistant Professor at the Hubert Department of Global Health, Rollins School of Public Health, Emory University, Atlanta, USA.

W. H. van Brakel is the Head of Technical Department, Netherlands Leprosy Relief, Amsterdam, the Netherlands.

Sherryl Broverman is an Associate Professor at Duke Global Health Institute, Trinity College of Arts and Sciences, Durham, USA.

Gemma Bryan is based at the Department of Children's Nursing, London South Bank University, UK.

J. F. G. Bunders is a Professor at the Athena Institute, Faculty of Earth and Life Sciences, VU University Amsterdam, the Netherlands.

Fatuma Chege is a Professor at the Department of Educational Foundations, Kenyatta University, Nairobi, Kenya.

Imelda Coyne is a Professor of Children's Nursing at Research at the School of Nursing and Midwifery, Trinity College Dublin, Ireland.

Naydene de Lange is HIV and AIDS Education Research Chair at Nelson Mandela Metropolitan University, Port Elizabeth, South Africa.

Myriam Denov is a Professor and Canada Research Chair at the School of Social Work, McGill University, Montreal, Canada.

Elizabeth Ekirapa-Kiracho is a staff member at the Department of Health Policy, Planning and Management, Makerere University College of Health Sciences, Kampala, Uganda.

Alice Fiddian-Green is a Teaching Associate at the School of Public Health and Health Sciences, University of Massachusetts Amherst, USA.

NOTES ON CONTRIBUTORS

Maria Elena Figueroa is an Associate Scientist at the Department of Health, Behavior and Society, Johns Hopkins Bloomberg School of Public Health, USA.

Catherine Finneran is the Senior Public Health Program Associate at Rollins School of Public Health, Emory University, Atlanta, USA.

Asha S. George is an Assistant Professor at the Johns Hopkins Bloomberg School of Public Health, Baltimore, USA.

Faith Gibson is a Clinical Professor of Children's and Young People's Cancer Care at Great Ormond Street Hospital NHS Foundation Trust, London, UK.

Tamar Goldenberg is a doctoral student at the Center for Sexuality and Health Disparities, University of Michigan, Ann Arbor, USA.

Eric P. Green is an Assistant Professor of the Practice of Global Health, Duke Global Health Institute, Durham, USA.

Aline C. Gubrium is an Associate Professor and Program Head at the School of Public Health and Health Sciences, University of Massachusetts Amherst, USA.

Vu Song Ha is based at the Center for Creative Initiatives in Health and Population, Hanoi, Vietnam.

Catherine K. Harbour is manager of the Children's Investment Fund Foundation, London, UK.

Jennifer S. Hirsch is a Professor in the Department of Sociomedical Sciences, Mailman School of Public Health, Columbia University, New York, USA.

Emily S. Holman is a student at the Department of Health, Behavior and Society, Johns Hopkins Bloomberg School of Public Health, Baltimore, USA.

Irwanto is based at the Centre for Disability Studies, Faculty of Social and Political Sciences, Universitas Indonesia, Depok, Indonesia.

Kasey Jernigan is a PhD student at the Department of Anthropology, University of Massachusetts Amherst, USA.

Gloria Johnston is based at the Department of Sociology, University of New Brunswick, Fredericton, Canada.

Fatima Khan is a graduate student at the Department of Integrated Studies in Education, McGill University, Canada.

Elizabeth L. Krause is based at the Department of Anthropology, University of Massachusetts Amherst, USA.

Warren Linds is an Associate Professor at the Department of Applied Human Sciences, Concordia University, Montreal, Canada.

M. Brinton Lykes is a Professor at the Department of Counseling, Developmental and Educational Psychology, Center for Human Rights and International Justice, Boston College, Chestnut Hill, USA.

NOTES ON CONTRIBUTORS

Lucy Maina is a Senior Lecturer and Director of the Institute of Peace and Security Studies, Kenyatta University, Nairobi, Kenya.

Ana Martins is based at the Department of Children's Nursing, London South Bank University, UK.

Claudia Mitchell is a James McGill Professor in the Faculty of Education, Director of the Institute for Human Development and Well-Being, McGill University, Montreal, Canada.

David Musoke is based at the Department of Disease Control and Environmental Health, School of Public Health, College of Health Sciences, Makerere University, Kampala, Uganda.

Rawlance Ndejjo is a Research Associate at the Department of Disease Control and Environmental Health, School of Public Health, Makerere University, Kampala, Uganda.

Benson Ogwang is based at the Women's Institute for Secondary Education and Research, Muhuru Bay, Kenya.

R. M. H. Peters is based at the Athena Institute, Faculty of Earth and Life Sciences, VU University Amsterdam, the Netherland.

Morgan M. Philbin is a Postdoctoral Research Fellow at the HIV Center for Clinical and Behavioral Studies, New York State Psychiatric Institute and Columbia University, New York, USA.

Eve S. Puffer is an Assistant Professor in Psychology and Neuroscience and Global Health at Duke Global Health Institute, Durham, USA.

Amy E. Ritterbusch is an Associate Professor at the School of Government, Universidad de los Andes, Bogotá, Colombia.

Margot Rothman is based at the Groupe-conseil INTERALIA, Montreal, Canada.

Mónica Ruiz-Casares, PhD, is an Assistant Professor in the Department of Psychiatry and at the Centre for Research on Children and Families, McGill University, Montreal, Canada.

Rosa Valéria Azevedo Said is a Consultor at Johns Hopkins Center for Communication Programs, Johns Hopkins University, Baltimore, USA.

Holly Scheib is a Research Associate Professor at the Disaster Resilience Leadership Academy, School of Social Work, Tulane University, New Orleans, USA.

Marni Sommer is an Associate Professor of Sociomedical Sciences in the Mailman School of Public Health, Columbia University, New York, USA.

Rob Stephenson is a Professor and Vice Chair for Research at the Department of Health Behaviour and Biological Sciences, University of Michigan School of Nursing, Ann Arbor, USA.

NOTES ON CONTRIBUTORS

Cecelia Vindrola-Padros is a Research Associate in the Department of Applied Health Research at University College London, UK.

Virginia Rieck Warren is based at the Women's Institute for Secondary Education and Research, Muhuru Bay, Kenya.

Andrea Whittaker is an Associate Professor and ARC Future Fellow in Anthropology, School of Social Sciences, Monash University, Melbourne, Australia.

M. B. M. Zweekhorst is based at the Athena Institute, Faculty of Earth and Life Sciences, VU University Amsterdam, the Netherlands.

Participatory visual methodologies in global public health

Claudia M. Mitchell[a] and Marni Sommer[b]

[a]Department of Integrated Studies in Education, McGill University, Montréal, QC, Canada; [b]Department of Sociomedical Sciences, Mailman School of Public Health, Columbia University, New York, NY, USA

ABSTRACT

This Introduction serves to map out a range of participatory visual approaches, as well as critical issues related to the use of participatory visual methodologies in global health. In so doing, it offers both an overview of these innovative practices in global health and a consideration of some of the key questions that researchers might ask themselves in design and implementation.

This Special Issue of *Global Public Health* focuses on the use of participatory visual methodologies such as photovoice, participatory video (including cellphilming or the use of cell phones to make videos), drawing and mapping in public health research. These approaches are, in a sense, *modes of inquiry* that can engage participants and communities, eliciting evidence about their own health and well-being. At the same time, they are also *modes of representation* and *modes of production* in the co-creation of knowledge, as well as *modes of dissemination* in relation to knowledge translation and mobilisation. Thus, the production by a group of girls or young women of a set of photos or videos from their own visual perspective can offer new evidence on how, for example, they see sexual violence. Unlike other data such as that collected through surveys or even conventional interviews, the images they have produced not only inform the empirical evidence, but also do not need to remain in a laboratory or the office of a researcher. They can, through exhibitions and screenings, reach various audiences: school or health personnel, parents and community members, and perhaps also policy-makers. It was this type of research that Caroline Wang and colleagues pioneered in rural China in the early 1990s. Women working in the rice fields were given cameras to photograph what they saw as challenges in relation to child care and various healthcare issues (Wang, Burris, & Ping, 1996). The power of the visual to represent what is not easily put into words, especially by marginalised populations, is a key aspect of visual research. The idea of participant-generated data, and the power of participants to be in a position to create images, is also a significant feature of such approaches. Finally, the power of the images, as Sontag (2004) writes, to 'haunt' audiences, or, as Olins (2012) notes to 'touch' us, offers compelling arguments for the use of these emerging methodologies.

Although there is a great deal of enthusiasm for participatory visual methodologies when it comes to recognising the significance of shifting power imbalances between the researcher and the researched, and in relation to the meaningful engagement of various populations and patient groups, these methodologies remain contested with regard to their authority as 'evidence', as does their use in quantitative studies, particularly in relation to their relevance to randomised control trials. How might the evidence produced in participatory visual research complement other data? What would count as compelling evidence? At the same time, participatory visual research brings its own complexities and sometimes unresolved issues. What counts as meaningful participation, and when is participation tokenistic? What new ethical challenges arise when we work with visual data in relation to anonymity and confidentiality? Who owns the visual productions (photos, videos, drawings, and maps) in participatory visual research and how are issues of ethics and ownership negotiated? Many of these concerns are not unique to participatory visual research and, indeed, they are issues that are closely linked to patient rights, access to knowledge and other important aspects of global health research. Indeed, perhaps one of the greatest contributions of the use of participatory visual methodologies within research more broadly is the very visible reminder they provide of the significance of the participants and their rights in the research process.

When we issued the call for this Special Issue of *Global Public Health*, we had not anticipated the groundswell of interest we would receive. Clearly, there are many researchers working in health-related areas testing out these methods and seeking out platforms for reporting on this work. Early on in the process of vetting the many excellent submissions, it was clear that we would need to produce a double issue. There were, moreover, many ways of dividing up the articles accepted for this double issue based on the many different cross-cutting themes and issues that could guide the organisation of the Special Issue: (1) tools/methods used in participatory visual methodologies, (2) the actual populations and health-related issues for which these methodologies have been used, and (3) emerging themes in using participatory visual methodologies. In the end, we have opted to divide the articles according to the age of the participants (children and young people in Part 1 and adult populations in Part 2). In so doing, we acknowledge particular contextual issues in working with children and young people who are frequently left out of the consultation process when it comes to issues of health and well-being. Here, we are thinking especially of ethical issues, but also participation itself and the ways that children and young people are frequently tokenised in participatory research. At the same time, we are also mindful of the various age-related definitions attached to idea of children and childhood, very young adolescents, young people, and youth. We have chosen to put together work with children, young people, and youth up to the age of 24, recognising that the term 'youth' has in some definitions included participants up to the age of 29 or even 35.

In Part 1 of the Special Issue, we focus on participatory visual methodologies in work with children and young people. We start with an article by D'Amico, Denov, Khan, Linds, and Akesson who consider practical, theoretical, and ethical questions in relation to the use of various participatory visual methodologies in global health research with children and youth. Framing this work as 'research as intervention', they consider approaches such as photovoice, participatory video, drawing, digital storytelling and image theatre, and review literature to date addressing ethical concerns associated with these methodologies

– concerns that the papers in this special issue build on and deepen considerably through nuanced empirical cases and theory-driven discussion. In the next article, Song Ha and Whittaker consider the use of photovoice with a group of nine young people with Autism Spectrum Disorder. While the authors consider the challenges of interpreting the visual data, they highlight the significance of this approach as a means of mediating communication and participation. Next, Ruiz-Casares describes the use of photo-elicitation and community mapping with 7–11-year-old children in Lao People's Democratic Republic in order to study sources of risk and protection as identified by the children themselves. Extending the study of mapping as a participatory tool, Green describes the development of three innovative mapping tools for engaging rural youth in Kenya in community-based research related to such areas as food security and HIV prevention: 'dot map' focus groups, geocaching games, and satellite imagery-assisted daily activity logs. Ritterbusch's article with street youth in Bogota, Colombia, considers the ways that engaging youth through participatory video can contribute to the idea of a participatory forum to address *bazuco* and inhalant/glue consumption. Then, Gubrium, Fiddian-Green, Jernigan, and Krause in their article argue for the increased use of participatory visual methodologies – in this case body mapping – to complement traditional research methods in shifting notions of what counts as evidence in response to teen pregnancy and parenting and sexual health inequities. Like the article by Gubrium et al., the article by Vindrola-Padros, Martins, Coyne, Bryan, and Gibson interrogates the efficacy of participatory visual methodologies in engaging children and young people. In their work with hospitalised participants, they reflect on the use of photovoice and drawing with children and young people dealing with leukaemia, as tools relevant to informed assent/consent, data collection, and the dissemination of research findings. Part 1 ends with an article by Mitchell, Chege, Maina, and Rothman on ways of taking the products of participatory visual research (e.g. photos, videos, and drawings) into community and policy dialogue through digital media or, as the authors describe them 'digital dialogue tools'. Developing and using such tools can extend the life of the work of participants and offers innovative ways of engaging communities.

In Part 2, we shift our focus to the use of participatory visual methodologies in work conducted with adult populations. We start with an article by Peters, Zweekhorst, van Brakel, Bunders, and Irwanto who explore the use of participatory video as a method for both understanding the experience of living with leprosy and as a tool for reducing the stigma surrounding the disease of adults living in Indonesia. The authors highlight the importance of triangulation to validate the findings on leprosy, with participatory video methodology as one of six qualitative methods utilised in the study. Working on a maternal health project with 'older youth' (individuals between the ages of 18 and 29), Muoke, Ndejjo, Ekirapa-Kiracho, and George highlight the ways in which photovoice was used by participants to share through community dialogues knowledge and experiences of such issues as family planning. Next, Goldenberg, Finneran, Andes, and Stephenson extend the use of participatory visual methodologies to the innovative use of participant-empowered visual relationship timelines in a larger qualitative study aimed at understanding sexual behaviour among men who have sex with men in the Atlanta, Georgia metropolitan area in the USA. Visual methods, including a visual timeline made with labelled stickers, were built into the use of more traditional qualitative methods, such as interviews, to provide an alternative elicitation approach for understanding men's emotions and perceptions in relation to their sexual risk-taking and vulnerability to HIV. The use of participatory visual methodologies as part of the formative research process is presented by Holman, Harbour, Acevedo Said, and Figueroa, who describe using photo-based, projective techniques in Mozambique with adult men and women to explore content on HIV communication relevant to multiple sexual partnerships. The authors, in particular, emphasise initial concerns with the validity of using projective techniques that were subsequently allayed through analyses that indicated the robustness of such methods. Lykes and Scheib then provide a useful example of the resourcefulness of utilising visual methodologies while conducting participatory action research in a post-disaster context. The authors describe how visual techniques, including photo documentation and elicitation strategies, were particularly useful in working with vulnerable and diverse communities after Hurricane Katrina wrought devastation in New Orleans, Louisiana, in the USA. In examining the use of life history drawings as an important component of a larger ethnographic study in rural Mexico and among Mexican migrants living in Atlanta, Georgia in the USA, Hirsch and Philbin describe how the use of drawings with 13 pairs of women early in the research process significantly reoriented the planned research project. Highlighted, in particular, in this paper is the situating of participatory visual methodologies within the standards by which qualitative methods are traditionally deemed rigorous: reliability, validity, and triangulation. Then, DeLange and Mitchell examine the use of participatory visual methodologies with community health workers in South Africa, seeking to understand how the cultural productions created in media making (though photovoice and poster production) with community health workers might in turn contribute to mobilising social change around reducing experiences of gender-based violence in rural South Africa. Importantly, these authors explore, as others in the special issue do, what happens when the researchers depart and how the use of participatory visual methodologies can empower participants to continue their efforts beyond the study. Finally, Johnston discusses the rise in popularity of the application of photovoice methodology and whether its goal of reaching policy-makers or impacting policy change is in fact achieved in most applications of the methodology. The article raises important ethical questions about promises made to study participants in relation to expectations that they will become social change agents within their communities through participating, and whether the goal of policy change receives sufficient attention in most studies.

We end with three book reviews. The first by Jen Thompson is a review of Melvin Delgrado's book on the uses of photovoice with urban youth. The second, by Maureen Kendrick, reviews Gubrium et al.'s book *Participatory visual and digital research in action*. The issue ends with a review by Vanessa Oliver of *What is a cellphilm? Integrating mobile phone technology into participatory visual research and activism* (by MacEntee, Burkholder, and Schwab-Cartas) on the use of cellphilming as an emergent methodology with various populations ranging from sex workers, rural teachers, and young people, in Zapotec communities in rural Mexico.

Cross-cutting themes

Tools/methods

When we issued the call for papers, we were not certain how the tools would line up, although we expected there would be coverage of photovoice, digital storytelling, participatory video, cellphilming, drawing, and mapping. Photovoice and the use of photographs in photo-elicitation, photo documentation, and photo-based projection were the tools most frequently referenced. Various approaches to mapping (e.g. body mapping, geographic information system mapping) were used in several of the studies, along with life drawings in one article. Some methods, such as participatory video, are reported in only one study. While there are no articles specifically on digital storytelling, leading researchers such as Aline Gubrium working in this area nonetheless are represented in the Special Issue, and D'Amico et al.'s article in Part 1 offers a comprehensive account of a range of methods including digital storytelling with children and young people. Although cellphilming was not taken up directly in any of the articles, it is addressed in Vanessa Oliver's review of the edited book, *What's a cellphilm?* Perhaps one of the most important points to note about the various tools and methods is the significance of triangulation in so many of the articles by research teams who reported on the use of several methods in one study (e.g. photovoice and drawing; photovoice and poster production; photo-elicitation and mapping). It is also worth noting that several contributors refer to the triangulation of participatory visual methodologies with more traditional qualitative or quantitative methods. Importantly, our call for papers requested submissions that would not simply offer examples of these methods in action, but instead would approach these methods critically. Consequently, these are articles on method and methodology and should be read as such; authors present only briefly their empirical findings, focusing their attention instead on extended discussions of a broader set of theoretical and ethical implications these various tools bring to the fore.

Populations and health-related issues

As noted above, there was an almost even split between articles pertaining to work with children and young people and those working with adults. The actual health themes were varied, ranging from work with hospitalised children, to work on sexual and reproductive health, HIV, food security, substance abuse, teen pregnancy, and maternal health. Several of the articles taking up work with adults address issues of sexual health: men having sex with men, HIV communication with multiple partners, and addressing gender-based violence. Other health issues included leprosy and related stigma and disaster relief.

Emerging themes

The actual thematic areas that emerged in the use of participatory visual methodologies cut across the various articles in this double issue and shed light on critical themes in carrying out this work. At the heart of much of this work, for example, is the notion of *participation,* which in itself can be interrogated. What counts as participation? What does it mean to participate and why is it critical that citizens at whatever age have a say in the health and social conditions around them? There is one article in each section that looks more at the use of participatory visual methodologies in terms of helping to frame the actual design of the research, highlighting the significance of participation-driven research more broadly. Taken as a whole this double issue highlights the ways in which researchers across a spectrum of health-related issues are seeing the significance of participatory models.

A second thematic area relates to *ethics*. Indeed, this double issue as a whole, we think, can be read as a primer on visual ethics with contributors taking up a range of topics: how to assure a determined researcher or practitioner does not display the work of a child or youth who does not understand the concept of making artwork 'public' or does not have the power to say no, to determining who considers what 'good' visual research and artistic representation is. A number of the papers also offer practical solutions for negotiating application of these methods in the field of global public health, where ethical review boards may be less familiar with the use of such approaches than they are in other fields.

Another cross-cutting issue that arose was that of *policy dialogue and social change*; speaking to the topic of social change more broadly and especially the idea of 'why participatory visual methodologies, anyway'? While the article by Johnston makes this the central theme, numerous articles explore what social change and policy change might look like. These range from a consideration of the use of visual productions such as posters that could be used beyond the life of a project, to how the use of participatory videos to diminish stigma around a specific disease and how engagement by youth with the process of videotaping, editing, and screening can be a tool for social change, or how participatory processes can promote social inclusion.

Reflecting forward

Clearly, there is a great deal to celebrate with this double issue and for the future of participatory visual methodologies. Indeed, it is worth noting that the production of this Special Issue involved a much larger community of scholars with experience in participatory and visual research, those who served as scientific peer referees. This groundswell however points to new questions and new concerns. Perhaps the most obvious issue is the one of acceptance of these innovative research frameworks into the range of methodologies and approaches currently and increasingly utilised in health research. This is no small task and may require a re-thinking of not only what counts as evidence, but the significance of participant-driven agendas. With greater acceptance of these methodologies, there is likely to be a need to expand the discourse community in ways that facilitate discussions of codes of conduct and standards of practices for tools and methods.

As the editors of the *Handbook of participatory video* note in their Introduction: 'Now that there is an increase in the use of participatory video, it is imperative that as ethical, reflexive researchers we submit participatory video to a deeper analysis and do so through a more critical lens' (Milne, Mitchell, & De Lange, 2012, p. 10). In one of the chapters in that *Handbook*, Hugh, Singh, Petheram, and Nemes (2012) refer to PV-NET (2008) as a statement of practice for participatory video developed by a group of researchers in the UK. Gubrim and Harper (2013) in their book *Participatory visual and digital methods* include the Digital Storyteller's Bill of Rights produced by Amy Hill. At the same time, Gubrim and Harper (2013) also cite the work of Catherine Bateman who calls for our various professional organisations and academic bodies to develop guidelines, especially 'for considering PAR and public engaged work in the tenure and promotion process'. Such concerns also speak to the need for more support and resources for training in participatory visual methodologies. For example, units and centres such as the Participatory

Cultures Lab (participatorycultureslab.com) and Participatory Research at McGill (http://pram.mcgill.ca) both at McGill University in Montreal draw attention to the role of training for researchers in such areas as participatory analysis, visual ethics, and community-based research more broadly. Finally, we think that this Special Issue points to the question 'who are participatory visual methodologies for?' Many of the contributors have highlighted populations who are described as marginalised. Perhaps this suggests that we need to think more about what global public health would look like if we took seriously the place of all voices to drive health research.

Disclosure statement

No potential conflict of interest was reported by the authors.

References

Gubrim, A., & Harper, K. (2013). *Participatory visual and digital methods*. Walnut Creek, CA: Left Coast Press.

Hugh, C., Singh, N., Petheram, L., & Nemes, G. (2012). Defining participatory video from practice. In E.-J. Milne, C. Mitchell, & N. De Lange (Eds.), *Handbook of participatory video* (pp. 35–49). Lanham, MD: Altamira Press.

Milne, E.-J., Mitchell, C., & De Lange, N. (2012). *Handbook of participatory video*. Lanham, MD: Altamira Press.

Olins, M.R. (2012). *Touching photographs*. Chicago, MD: University of Chicago Press.

PV-NET. (2008, April). *The Walton Hall statement on participatory video in research*. Paper presented at the PV-NET closing conference, Walton Hall, UK.

Sontag, S. (2004). *Regarding the pain of others*. New York, NY: Picardor.

Wang, C., Burris, M., & Ping, X. (1996). Chinese women as visual anthropologists. A participatory approach to reaching policymakers. *Social Science & Medicine, 42*(10), 1391–1400.

Research as intervention? Exploring the health and well-being of children and youth facing global adversity through participatory visual methods

Miranda D'Amico[a], Myriam Denov[b], Fatima Khan[c], Warren Linds[d] and Bree Akesson[e]

[a]Department of Education, Concordia University, Montréal, Canada; [b]School of Social Work, McGill University, Montréal, Canada; [c]Department of Integrated Studies in Education, McGill University, Montréal, Canada; [d]Department of Applied Human Sciences, Concordia University, Montréal, Canada; [e]Lyle S. Hallman Faculty of Social Work, Wilfrid Laurier University, Kitchener, Canada

ABSTRACT

Global health research typically relies on the translation of knowledge (from health professionals to the community) and the dissemination of knowledge (from research results to the wider public). However, Greenhalgh and Wieringa [2011. Is it time to drop the 'knowledge translation' metaphor? A critical literature review. *Journal of the Royal Society of Medicine, 104*(12), 501–509. doi:10.1258/jrsm.2011.110285] suggest 'that while "translation" is a widely used metaphor in medicine, it constrains how we conceptualize and study the link between knowledge and practice' (p. 501). Often the knowledge garnered from such research projects comes from health professionals rather than reflecting the lived experiences of people and communities. Likewise, there has been a gap in 'translating' and 'disseminating' the results of participatory action research projects to policymakers and medical practitioners. This paper will look at how using participatory visual methodologies in global health research with children and youth facing global adversity incorporates the multiple functions of their lived realities so that research becomes a means of intervention. Drawing from a literature review of participatory visual methods as media, content and processes of global health research, this paper raises practical, theoretical, and ethical questions that arise from research as intervention. The paper concludes by exploring what lessons emerge when participatory visual methodologies are integrated into global health research with children and youth facing global adversity.

Introduction: marginalised youth and visual methods

Globally, many children and youth face challenges to their development and well-being through exposure to extreme adversity. Global adversity for children and youth can be broadly characterised to include structural conditions such as poverty and marginalisation, as well as life disruptions such as violence, disaster, and war. Children and youth living within these contexts of global adversity may be threatened not only with the potential for loss of life, but a myriad of long-term, adverse psychosocial issues (Betancourt & Khan, 2008; Pedersen, 2002; Pfefferbaum & North, 2013).

While practitioners have carried out numerous health interventions in conflict zones, there is a substantial gap between translating and disseminating research results at the policy and practitioner level. Participatory visual methodologies, which use visual and experiential art to understand, address, and engage with the lived experiences and realities of children and youth facing profound adversity, can be a form of research intervention that is 'collaborative, relevant, cost-effective, and generate[s] "innovations"' (Greenhalgh & Wieringa, 2011, p. 507).

Although research has begun to document the importance of using arts-based methodologies (Kanji & Cameron, 2010; Mitchell, De Lange, Moletsane, Stuart, & Buthelezi, 2005), information on their applicability with children and youth facing different forms of global adversity remains in its infancy. Nonetheless, emerging research has highlighted that arts-based methods may allow children and youth to represent their experiences in contexts of reduced stress (Harris, 2007), promote activism and empowerment (Moletsane et al., 2007), and be particularly successful with younger children who have limited vocabulary to verbalise their feelings (Gangi & Barowsky, 2009).

For the purposes of our discussion, we draw from Panter-Brick, Lende, and Kohrt (2012)'s definition of children facing global adversity as 'young people who face significant economic poverty, life disruption, violence, and social inequality within larger-scale processes of sociopolitical crises or rapid socioeconomic transformation demanding intervention' (p. 603). Further, for the purposes of our paper, we define children and youth affected by marginalisation, poverty, violence, disaster, and/or war as 'children and youth facing global adversity'. Based on this delineation, we ask:

- What is the role of these participatory visual methodologies in research as intervention with children and youth facing global adversity?
- Within the 'toolbox' of arts-based methods, what approaches are most appropriate to studying this population?
- What are the strengths and limitations of employing arts-based methods?
- What ethical, practical, and theoretical questions arise when research is also a form of intervention?

To answer these questions, we first interpret the notion of research as intervention. We then examine methods such as photovoice, participatory video (PV), drawing, Image theatre, and digital storytelling, and their potential to enhance the quality of data collected and to engage and empower child and youth participants. After reviewing these approaches, we provide a discussion on the strengths and limitations of employing arts-based methods, as well as the conceptual, ethical and practical questions that arise when research is also a form of intervention.

Research as intervention?

In reviewing research on promoting heart health, Haalboom, Robinson, Elliott, Cameron, and Eyles (2006) suggest that research can also contribute to capacity building in health promotion: 'Research as intervention entails purposefully using aspects of a research process and results feedback to contribute to desired changes in knowledge and practice of research participants and stakeholders' (p. 292). Research then becomes not only a means to gather data, but also a potential health intervention.

McNamee (1988) examined research as intervention in a systems context. Here, research is focused on facilitating change, not just observing or accounting for how change occurs. This requires an understanding and application of systems theory, termed 'systemic epistemology' (Bateson, 1972). McNamee underlines that if we look at research as a *social* intervention, the role of the researcher-as-intervener becomes complicated. When the process of researching as an intervention in the system being studied is at the centre, the researcher's active participation in the system is emphasised, which subsequently allows us to think that a researcher can stand outside of another social system and observe it objectively. Systems theory, coined and developed by cyberneticist Norbet Wiener (1948), is particularly relevant here. The emphasis in a systems perspective is on how the whole arises from the interrelations among the parts. Minute changes, operating in *feedback loops*, evoke systemic changes. Arts-based research as intervention is an example of a feedback loop evoking systemic change through art.

How might this play out in real communities with real health issues? Barndt (2009) writes that, when talking about community arts as research and intervention, '[t]he researcher/artist may structure processes to engage participants in creative inquiry, but if the process is to draw on the knowledge, skills and visions of community members, there must be space for this to happen' (p. 360). Put more simply, research using the arts can facilitate change while at the same time provide evidence of such changes. Participatory visual methodologies engage participants by producing a representation of their experiences of health and well-being, while also exploring what these representations mean and how they may contribute to change. In this way, the arts in general and participatory visual methods in particular become both the medium and the representation through which to investigate health and well-being.

Arts-based research with children and youth

Advances in research methodologies with children and youth call for innovative and adapted research techniques while emphasising their competence. Given the myriad ethical issues involved in conducting research with children and youth affected by global adversity, employing suitable methodologies to meet their diverse needs is vital (Boyden & de Berry, 2004). Historically, methodological approaches to research with children have tended to view children in largely passive ways as merely 'objects of research' or as 'vulnerable' and 'incompetent' (Clark, 2010). Drawing on a rights-based approach, which recognises children and youth as capable of making sense of and affecting the world around them, this paper seeks to examine research methodologies that seek to both empower and actively engage children and youth in the research process through participatory and arts-based methods. More specifically, we trace the potential of photovoice, PV, drawing, Image theatre, and digital storytelling as both method and intervention.

Photovoice: enabling empowerment, healing, and group cohesion

The use of photography in research has become recognised as a means of empowerment among marginalised youth and 'groups of people who do not normally get to speak' (Mitchell, 2011, p. 51). Within the toolbox of photographic methods, photovoice has emerged as an important methodological and community empowerment tool. Photovoice is a community-based participatory research method that combines photography, community awareness building, group discussions, and social action (Wang & Burris, 1994, 1997). First developed and implemented by Wang and Burris in research with women villagers in rural China, the method draws on 'community photography' (Spence, 1995), a way in which ordinary people photograph each other and their social environment.

Photovoice has three main objectives. First, participants receive training to become community researchers and ethically conscious photographers. In these new roles, they document, through photos images, issues of personal and community concern. Therefore, it seeks to enable individuals and groups, particularly those who face marginalisation and disempowerment, to record and reflect upon their community's strengths and challenges through photography. Second, using group discussions of participants' photographs, written photo narratives or captions of the photos, photovoice aims to promote critical dialogue and knowledge about important community issues. Through the ongoing data collection process, via photography, participants come together as a group to discuss and analyse what they have documented and to support each other. Finally, through the dissemination of their photographs to the wider community, and through such practices as exhibitions of the photographs, photovoice seeks to reach policy-makers who have the power to implement changes within that community (Wang & Burris, 1997).

De Lange, Mitchell and Stuart (2007) position photovoice within the broader category of 'visual methodologies for social change' and document the transformative possibilities of the process as photographs help people to 'reflect on their own lived experiences ... framing their ideas for change' (as cited in Burke, 2008, p. 26). Photovoice has been documented as a powerful research tool to engage communities and enable a deeper understanding of the lives of marginalised youth (Burke, 2008). Photovoice may also hold powerful 'intervention' capacities with marginalised youth. First, it has the capacity to serve as a platform from which youth are able to develop skills such as photography techniques, team building, cooperation, leadership, and critical thinking skills (Wang & Burris, 1997). Second, given its emphasis on group work and team building, photovoice offers a format that can alleviate the sense of isolation often associated with social marginalisation (Denov, Doucet, & Kamara, 2012). Through group meetings and discussions inherent to the photovoice process, youth participants can begin to develop and nurture a sense of belonging and collective identity and foster a sense of empowerment within the project. Third, photovoice, and arts-based projects in general, can provide a venue to deal with emotions rarely addressed in conventional research methods, such as shame, guilt and feelings of accountability (Harris, 2010). Moreover, sensitive issues may be easier to address through the lens of a camera, allowing as much proximity or distance from the topic as necessary. Finally, photovoice allows participants to create and establish the research agenda, ensuring greater control over the methodological process (Burke, 2008).

The intervention capacity and potential of photovoice has also been highlighted by various researchers. Denov et al. (2012), for example, conducted a photovoice project with a group of former child soldiers in Sierra Leone living in an urban settlement community, who reported experiencing various forms of rejection, stigma and marginalisation in the post-war period. The study highlighted the post-conflict lives of former child soldiers and their complex experience of reintegration into mainstream society. Denov et al. noted that at the end of the project, all participants reported that the project fostered a gradual change in community members' perception of them. They reported that community members began referring to them as 'professional photographers', which instilled pride and confidence. Other participants noted that prior to the project, they did not have 'good reputations' in the community; the photovoice process helped to show sceptical community members the positive potential of participants, thereby challenging preconceived views. Blackman and Fairey (2007) argue that photovoice holds much promise in terms of intervention. They maintain that participants in photovoice projects gain confidence in their ability to assert ideas and engage in self-advocacy, have improved self-esteem from skill building, and offer an opportunity to influence decisions that affect their lives.

Since its original use with women in rural China, photovoice has since been adapted to a range of communities. While the focus in much of the literature has been on the method's inherent ability to capture the lived realities of complex individuals, communities, and contexts, photovoice also appears to hold 'therapeutic' capacities, enabling empowerment, healing and group cohesion.

PV: developing skills and illuminating experience

The use of PV has increasingly emerged as a 'unique empowering process that enhances the political capabilities of grassroots communities to influence those with power over them' (Colom, 2010, p. 1). PV, as defined by Lunch and Lunch (2006) is:

> a set of techniques to involve a group or community in shaping and creating their own film. The idea behind this is that making a video is easy and accessible, and is a great way of bringing people together to explore issues, voice concerns or simply to be creative and tell stories. (p. 10)

In using PV to understand violence and how people respond to it, Wheeler (2009, 2011) emphasises how PV is a process that encompasses the construction of knowledge from those who participate, 'expanding boundaries of knowledge, from the self to the group to the community, to beyond' (Wheeler, 2011, p. 53).

Like photovoice, PV participants are provided with access to, and training in, the use of video recording equipment (Jewitt, 2012). PV is used to delve into individual's lives and according to Jewitt (2012) generates three kinds of data: '1) the video "as product", 2) the process of its production – which itself is often video recorded, and 3) the process of video editing' (p. 3). These forms of data become the focus of further exploration and study, although some PV research prioritises one over the other or may emphasise the interaction between them (Jewitt, 2012).

The PV process gives power to, and provides a group with, the opportunity to elucidate their own difficulties and to communicate their needs and ideas to others, such as decision-makers or other groups and communities (Lunch & Lunch, 2006). Likewise, Lunch and Lunch (2010) advocate for a rights-based approach to PV that can be an effective tool to engage and mobilise marginalised people and to help them implement their own forms of sustainable development based on local needs. In other words:

> by asserting the right to self determination, rights-based approaches demand that the power-ful (duty-bearers) seek out and listen to less powerful people (rights-holders) and incorporate their needs and values, their 'home-known' rights into policy. This obligation also asks decision-makers to make room for the feedback and contribution of those less powerful at their decision-making table. (p. 35)

Furthermore, PV permits working with children and youth as research partners rather than research subjects, and serves as a way to address the 'over-didactic, centrally con-trolled and one-way information flow approach commonly found in traditional health education/promotion practice' (Chiu, 2009, p. 14). With participants in control of the process, PV provides children and youth with an opportunity to freely record what they see through their own eyes, presenting a child-based representation of knowledge that is grounded in their community (Pink, 2001; Sandercock & Attili, 2010). PV is also seen as an 'equalizing' tool, minimising reliance on literacy skills and communicating a message without a reliance on writing or reading (Okahashi, 2000).

In this way, the process of videotaping, editing and screening can be an effective tool for social change (Sandercock & Attili, 2010). PV can provide children and youth – especially those who have experienced various forms of global adversity – with a voice. PV can empower children and youth who previously may have had no control over what is reported about them and their experiences (Garrett, 2011; Sandercock & Attili, 2010). Fur-thermore, encouraging children and youth in research and encouraging their right to have a voice, 'has long term implications for participatory citizenship' (Pascal & Bertram, 2009, p. 249).

In a longitudinal study on the use of PV to build an archive of children's and youth's experiences of growing up in a disadvantaged neighbourhood, PV was used to challenge 'preferred identities, aspirations and passion', thus allowing the participants to highlight their characteristics, individualities and personalities while illuminating other parts of themselves not always present in their relationships with adults, especially those in pos-itions of authority (Luttrell, Restler, & Fontaine, 2012, p. 164). Recognising the importance of listening to the perspectives of children and youth and supporting their meaningful par-ticipation through methodologies such as PV can lead to action and social awareness, which has the potential to help children and youth feel empowered, to think and act on the conditions that shape their lives, and ultimately contribute to greater agency and well-being (Pascal & Bertram, 2009).

Drawing, painting, and mapmaking: alternative and therapeutic means of collecting data

As described above, the trend in visual research has emphasised pictorial representation, particularly through photographs (such as photovoice) and video (such as PV) (Banks, 2001; Pink, 2007; Prosser, 1998). But visual research can also include non-photographic illustrations. This section considers non-photographic illustrations such as drawings, paintings, maps as a specific form of visual evidence within the wider category of visual material, and reviews the literature on how this form of visual research method can be a means of intervention for children and youth affected by global adversity.

Non-photographic methods such as drawing, painting, and mapmaking are increasingly being used with children and youth affected by global adversity in order to better understand their experiences and worldviews. Their capabilities can be made more readily accessible by the use of visual image-making than by sole reliance on typical methods of information-gathering, such as interviews, surveys, and questionnaires (Leitch, 2008; Veale, 2005). Whereas these methods focus on verbal or written data, younger children (Thong, 2007) or children who have experienced distressing events may not be able to communicate in this manner. Therefore, drawing, painting, and mapmaking are alternative ways to effectively gain meaningful participation of these children and youth. Furthermore, these visual tools create an environment where they may be more at ease, where they feel more able to express themselves freely, and where they do not feel as much of a risk of giving a 'wrong' answer. Coates (2004) suggests that the care and concentration which children give to their illustrated representations indicates that the content has a real significance. Therefore, it can be viewed as an intentional practice and an important part of their understanding of his or her own experience. Leitch (2008) notes that these visual representations, used sensitively in combination with methodologies that elicit some contextualising narrative, have the potential to help children and youth effectively convey aspects of their lived experience.

These methods have also been effective in addressing children's emotional well-being (Hamilton & Moore, 2004). Traditionally, drawing, painting, and mapmaking has been used in clinical and diagnostic research such as art therapy (Linesch, 1994) or to better understand children's knowledge and experience in contexts of global adversity due to protracted political violence (see e.g. Akesson, 2014, 2015; Boğaç, 2009; Marshall, 2013) . Nevertheless, no evaluations have demonstrated that expression of emotion in art is therapeutic for children and youth (Thomas & Silk, 1990). Furthermore, despite the relevance of using drawing, painting, and mapmaking in research with children and youth, especially those who have experienced global adversity, there are few studies that address this type of visual representation as an intervention that can improve health and well-being. For example, Miles (2000) conducted a study with 60 unaccompanied refugee children (ages 9–16 years) in southeast Asia. The study integrated drawing accompanied with writing in order to learn more about children's understandings of their futures. Nevertheless, the research did not include an element to determine the therapeutic impact of art-making. Arts-based research studies examining the psychosocial experiences of children affected by global adversity are more likely to include drawing, painting, or mapmaking as actual interventions, rather than conceptualising them as research *as* intervention. For example, Gupta and Zimmer (2008) describe the Rapid-Ed intervention for war-affected children in Sierra Leone, including trauma healing activities such as storytelling, drawing, small group discussions, writing essays about their experiences, role-playing, singing and performing, and music-making. Ironically, and despite such rich arts-based intervention, the authors still use a verbal and written research methodology, administering pre- and post-test surveys to the child-participants in order to evaluate the arts-based intervention.

There is much written about the value of integrating drawing, painting and mapmaking into research processes with children and youth (Miles, 2000; Theron, Mitchell, Smith, &

Stuart, 2011), especially those who have experienced global adversity. Yet data on the value of using drawings and maps in research as a therapeutic process is anecdotal. One example comes from Volker and Kellogg (as cited in Junge, Alvarez, Kellogg, & Volker, 1993) who conducted research with refugee families from Central America who had migrated to Los Angeles. The researchers found that the drawings helped the research participants 'to explore the uprooting, the migration, and the relocation' and 'the opportunity to address their traumas and to integrate them' (p. 153). Even though it is implied, this research did not explicitly connect the expression of these drawings as being therapeutic for the research participants. Similarly, one study conducted with a third-grade class of first- and second-generation immigrant and refugee children (Rousseau & Heusch, 2000) used drawing combined with storytelling to help children work through emotions. Through the rich visual data, the authors found children used the drawings and stories to 'make sense of traumatic experiences and dislocation to devise their own culturally accep-table adaptive strategies' (p. 39).

Based on the above studies and others, it is likely that arts-based methods such as drawing, painting, and mapmaking can not only serve as a data point, but also as a poten-tial means of intervention for research participants. For example, in Akesson's (2014) research with Palestinian children and families affected by political violence in the West Bank and East Jerusalem, parents expressed gratitude to the research team for encouraging their children to create art as a part of the research process, noting that it helped their chil-dren express their feelings and included them in the research process. Nonetheless, we need more than anecdotal evidence and the positive feedback from adult research partici-pants to support this assertion.

Image theatre: embodied imagery as catalysts for research

Image theatre (Boal, 1979; Linds & Vettraino, 2008) enables participants to use their bodies as a particular visual language to convey their lived experience.[1] One method involves an individual telling a story with others silently using their bodies to visually rep-resent a key moment in the story. Once the image (also known as tableau) emerges it can be manipulated in many ways through, for example, fast-forwarding to the future or rewinding to events in the past. This enables a manipulation of time and space.

Images created through Image theatre can 'offer a screen onto which a group can project a variety of ideas and interpretations' (Boal as cited in Jackson, 1992, p. 174), invit-ing both the individual and the collective to problem-solve. If a group has varying levels of verbal or linguistic ability, Image theatre levels difference and becomes a common visual language.

Kuftinec (2009, 2011) has effectively used Image theatre in research with youth in the conflict situations of Afghanistan, Israel, and Macedonia. In Kabul, Kuftinec's work centred on transforming a culture of violence, a common concern among Afghan youth, while also developing strategies to address this. One strategy focused on the core conflict in the image, discussing precipitating factors, subsequent events, and potential means to transform the situation to avoid future conflict. Kuftinec found that the 'image-making provided the youth with a way to both create distance from and illuminate the ethos of violence in which they are steeped' (2011, p. 114), enabling an exploration of possibilities for change from, and through, the embodied image. This is what Boal (quoted in Jackson, 1992) calls a 'rehearsal for reality' (p. xxi), activating the youths' imagination of a world without violence and how to get there.

In Jerusalem, images 'clarified the competing paradigms through which Israeli and Palestinian youth understood the conflict situation in their own communities' (Kuftinec, 2011, p. 110). Alon, Kuftinec, and Turkiyye (2010) and Viewpoints Theatre used Image theatre with children and youth to develop ways of communicating between groups who have historically been in conflict. Their method used images to make concrete the differences in perception between two groups. Once a group defined an identity category that divided the whole group in half, each group made an image of how they see them-selves and how they thought the other group sees them. Then, the groups engaged in dia-logue about the perceptions of themselves and of the other group.

Kuftinec (2009) shares a similar process from a workshop with a group of Macdeonian, Albanian, Kosovar Albanian, Kosovo Serb, and Roma youth in Macedonia in 2004. Cul-tural mapping groups were formed based on particular categories: for example, non-national identity, self-selecting relationships, and month of birth. Participants made a map of the room based on where they were born and where they now lived (or where they felt comfortable). Each group then silently created an embodied image of their situ-ation. Articulating 'a violent trauma beyond language' (p. 240), the groups illustrated the tensions in the Balkans, still present years after the war, followed by intense discussion of the realities of war and inter-ethnic tension in the region. Group discussion of the image revealed as much about those outside the particular image as those inside it as it focused on the aesthetic space of the image and the process of talking about it. Therefore, Image theatre slowed down the conversation and directed it away from a heated discussion.

Relevant to research on the health and well-being of children and youth affected by global adversity, the interpretation of the embodied image comes from those watching, thereby becoming another data point. When there are multiple and competing worldviews like in Israel or Macedonia, asking the storytellers to explain their image is also helpful as 'decodings [interpretations] serve as projections rather than authoritative definitions; par-ticipants put more energy into interpretation and reflection than argumentation' (p. 238).

Sloane and Wallin (2013) worked with families and youth affected by global adversity who had fled zones of war and conflict to create a 'theatre of the commons' where image formed the basis of plays about the participants' lives after immigration. Photo elicitation processes identified significant illuminative moments (Stringer, 2008), which became prompts for interviews about what enabled participants to have a voice. Participants named what they struggled with, analysed the power relationships in their experiences, and generated individual and collective actions to overcome what they were facing.

As we have noted, embodied storytelling through Image theatre enables the acquisition of understanding through both psychological and kinaesthetic processes as 'stories show what is possible in impossible situations' (Frank, 2013, p. 133). As a form of research as intervention, Image theatre becomes a process of articulating and transforming 'dominant ideologies at the level of communities and individual bodies' (Perry, 2012, p. 103).

Digital storytelling: a safe space to express marginalised voices

With the advent of increasingly available multimedia tools and a wide array of social network platforms, children and youth have greater opportunities to share their narratives by using their own voices through digital storytelling. According to Burgess (2006), '[d]igital storytelling is a workshop-based process by which "ordinary people" create their own short autobiographical films that can be streamed on the Web or broadcast on television' (p. 207).

Over the last two decades, this method has gained prominence in the fields of education and public health by encouraging children and youth to express themselves creatively and fostering a sense of individuality, agency, and ownership over their creations. Digital humanist Jason Ohler, asserts 'digital storytelling helps students develop *creatical thinking skills*, merging creativity and critical thinking, to solve important problems in imaginative, thoughtful ways' (2013, p. 13). Children's narratives, based on their own interpretations and perspectives, are expressed using a combination of methods such as drawings, images, music, videos, and voice to create a three to five minute digital story (Alexander, 2011; Rossiter & Garcia, 2010). This multimodal, child-led production can be a transformative experience due to its potential for their meaningful engagement with their topic and engagement in deeper learning, critical reflection, meaning-making, self-expression, and effective communication.

Digital storytelling grew as a phenomenon in the 1980s based on the works of Dana Atchley (who coined the term) and Joe Lambert, which led to the creation of the *Center for Digital Storytelling* (CDS) (Rebmann, 2012). The CDS proposed seven elements essential to digital storytelling (Kajder, Bull, & Albaugh, 2005; Lambert, 2013; Robin, 2006) including: point of view, dramatic question, emotional content, gift of voice, power of soundtrack, economy, and pacing. Following the production of the digital story with these elements, there are numerous options for dissemination such as social networking sites (Facebook, Twitter, YouTube), television outlets, collaborative community projects (Life Stories of Montrealers Displaced by War, Genocide, and Other Human Rights Violations),[2] websites (Mapping Memories: Experiences of Refugee Youth),[3] and workshops (Learn-Récit).[4] For underrepresented and marginalised digital storytellers, such as children and youth facing global adversity, this form of dissemination can contribute to their 'empowerment, voice, and dialogue' (Garcia & Rossiter, 2010).

Though highlighted as an effective arts-based method for intervention with children and youth in public health (Guse et al., 2013; Sawyer & Willis, 2011), the capacity of digital storytelling to serve as intervention for youth affected by global adversity, specifically as a tool for peacebuilding, is gradually being realised. Hanebrink and Smith (2013) note that participatory methods such as digital storytelling 'can enable transformation, both individually and communally, of their realities from the wreckage of war towards acceptance and a construction of peace that includes social rehabilitation and conflict prevention' (p. 195). This concept of peace education through digital storytelling is further explored in *Voices Beyond Walls*, a series of digital storytelling workshops conducted with children and youth (aged 10–16 years) in 6 refugee camps in the West Bank, East Jerusalem, and Jordan. Due to the availability and accessibility of digital tools, young Palestinians in the West Bank have used participatory arts-based methods, such as digital storytelling, to produce short videos on their day-to-day experiences. The *Voices Beyond Walls* workshops conducted from 2006 to 2008 had four objectives: first, to enable youth to conceptualise personal narratives through storytelling; second, to create storyboards and scripts for digital media projects; third, to learn digital media production techniques; and fourth, to produce media projects in the field (Voices Beyond Walls,

2006). In a span of 3 years, 60 digital stories were produced and 16 were showcased through the project's website.[5] Norman (2009) asserts that such media involve 'amplifying young people's voices on issues of importance to them' (p. 251). As a form of intervention, the digital storytelling workshops empowered youth to explore and express their emotions as well as their hopes and aspirations on a wide range of issues, from education and water shortages to tensions between Israelis and Palestinians in their communities. Buckner and Kim (2012) argue that digital storytelling, as a form of peace education,

> allows children to not only bear witness to the experience of childhood amidst conflict and develop an awareness of life on the other side of the conflict, but also helps build international awareness of the realities of conflict generally and the Israeli–Palestinian conflict specifically. (p. 12)

Similar workshops have been conducted in different parts of the globe, such as the student-led peace project, *Voices of Kashmir*.[6] Such examples of digital storytelling illustrate how participatory arts-based methods are effective in attempting to understand the lived experiences of children and youth facing global adversity, creating a safe space for young people to express their marginalised voices and ideas, interact with each other, and engage in a critically reflective process.

Implications: raising conceptual, ethical, and practical issues

As we have previously stated, children and youth who grow up within environments where they experience global adversity through experiences of marginalisation and exposure to poverty, violence, disaster and/or war, may be threatened not only with the potential for loss of life, but with numerous long-term mental health issues (Betancourt & Khan, 2008). In examining a number of participatory arts-based methodologies that seek to both empower and actively engage children and youth in the research process, we have emphasised that these methods allow the representation of the lived realities of children and youth by incorporating the multiple functions of translation and dissemination and in turn, that research becomes a means of intervention.

Additionally, in an era of increased awareness of human rights in response to the multiple forms of adversity that continue to affect children and youth, there is also increased attention to the specific ethical concerns raised when working with marginalised children and youth. Those who are often denied basic human rights are the very children and youth whose voices should be heard in programming and research. However, there are often complex conceptual, ethical, and practical issues that arise because of the nature of working with visual methods with marginalised children and youth.

Conceptual issues

Drawing from Western conceptions of childhood and its association with vulnerability and the need for protection, much of the theoretical and conceptual literature on children and youth affected by global adversity has tended to construct them as dependent, helpless, and as objects of assistance rather than agents of their own welfare (Honwana & de Boeck, 2005). While victimisation invariably characterises the experiences of these children and youth, failing to explore their rights and capacity to overcome adversity provides a skewed picture of their reality. Participatory visual research methods, such as those described in this paper, aim to promote more egalitarian methods whereby children and youth can participate in research, thereby returning a sense of control to the child. Participatory approaches turn upside down the traditional research paradigm by transforming participants from passive objects of research, into active agents, enabling a research environment in which children are at ease, are able to express themselves freely, and do not feel the risk of giving a wrong answer (De Lay, 2003). Visual methods capitalise on children's and youth's strengths: their local knowledge of their contexts and environments, their attention to detail, and their visual and verbal communication skills. However, using participatory visual research methods can challenge traditional adultist assumptions about children's and youth's experience in the context of global adversity. In particular, embarking on participatory approaches and visual methods require researchers to relinquish their roles as unequivocal controllers, owners, and knowledge constructors, requiring a fundamental conceptual shift in approach. Moreover, because children and youth have much of their lives dominated by adults, they may anticipate adults' power over them. In this sense, children and youth are not used to being treated as equals by adults, particularly in the context of research. In line with the shifting paradigm of participatory approaches, it is thus critical that children and youth are provided space to feel accepted and able to tell their story through arts-based methods such as photovoice, PV, drawing, Image theatre, or through digital storytelling.

Ethical and practical realities

Within participatory, visual approaches there may be complex ethical dimensions that have not yet been contemplated. For example, how do researchers ensure sensitivity? How do we stop the zealous researcher or practitioner from immediately displaying the work when the child who produced the drawing or photo or the story through Image theatre may have no idea of what 'making public' means and has no power to say no? What are the ethical implications when meaningful transformation is, at best, challenging or, at worst, an impossibility? In such cases, participatory research can have potential adverse and detrimental effects. Ethical issues, therefore, hold an important and vital place throughout the research process.

We have previously (Akesson et al., 2014) identified four critical ethical issues that represent specific challenges in relation to using visual methods with children and youth affected by war:

(1) *informed consent* whereby researchers need to develop specific approaches that ensure children understand the benefit of participating voluntarily in research and that consent is informed and an ongoing process;
(2) *truth, interpretation, and representation*, which acknowledges that the arts-based research process uncovers multiple truths whereby children and youth become co-constructors of knowledge, and its interpretations, with adult-researchers;
(3) *dangerous emotional terrain*, which asks us to consider the implications of portraying and/or embodying experiences, for both the child-participant and those watching, which are both critical to ensure participant safety; and

(4) *aesthetics*, which raises questions of what is 'good research' (and who decides this) when you are dealing with artistic representation.

We suggest that researchers should consider these elements when assessing the risks and benefits of children's and youth's participation and to develop specific ethical protocols and safeguards to ensure that participants understand the benefit of participating in research, that the participation is voluntary, and that the informed consent process (which can be presented visually to children and youth (see e.g. Ruiz-Casares & Thompson, 2014)) is ongoing.

A goal for participatory arts-based methods is often to reach policy-makers who have the power to implement systemic change within communities. What are the ethical implications of employing methods that seek transformation where such transformation can in no way be guaranteed? This means being transparent in voicing these limitations with participants. Researchers should be conscientious that in actively engaging participants in a research project – whereby disclosing of an issue or topic can lead to isolation and/or distrust and suspicion on the part of the other community members – that this might be a possible consequence in participating. That is, in some instances, because of the type of disclosure, it may lead to sanctions rather than systemic change or social justice. As Bergold and Thomas (2012) have stated:

> this gives rise to the dilemma of having to choose whether to defer the publication of problems that are in urgent need of public discussion or to publish them for that very reason. If the latter option is chosen, counter-strategies must be developed with the research partners. (p. 109)

Boydell et al. (2012) suggest that 'determining the goodness of art in terms of its role in research is even more complex, requiring attention to the aims of the research and the context in which the research is being conducted' (p. 12). By examining the ethics of any use of visual methodologies a complex inter-relationship of aesthetics, context, and purpose emerges that needs to be taken into account. For example, the use of youth participants' smart phones to photograph the results of a particular visual process might be ethically appropriate in one way, but in another way, if the ramifications of the use of the data (e.g. the easy capability of being shared on social networks) are not discussed in light of purpose and context, an ethical challenge has arisen.

The above-noted realities underscore that when working with their visual representations of their experiences, children and youth must be allowed to provide insight into the representation part of the process – essentially becoming co-constructors of knowledge with adult researchers. Furthermore, the research process should allow child and youth participants to challenge the researcher's interpretation. In our desire to document their experiences, we should ensure that children's and youth's agency and voice and the diversity of their lived experiences is rightly noted and represented.

As we have previously highlighted, as researchers we require 'tools for reflection' (Akesson et al., 2014, p. 85) so that we may think about how we work collaboratively with these tools and how these tools have an impact on children facing global adversity in terms of power and participation. In other words, ethical issues are not something to consider after designing research, but rather are an intrinsic and ongoing part of the design and implementation processes.

Conclusion

In this paper, we reviewed multiple forms of participatory visual research methods with children and youth affected by global adversity. Honouring means and methods of knowledge production that are suited to children and youth can lead to better ways of knowing and understanding them and their experiences. In this sense, children and youth are social actors in their own right, and they should be recognised as active participants rather than objects in the research process (Pascal & Bertram, 2009). In addition to gathering rich and valuable data, using visual research methodologies in research with children and youth affected by global adversity has the potential to make a positive difference in the research participants' lives. In other words, arts-based methods can serve as data points, but also as potential means of intervention for research participants. Use of these methods – photovoice, PV, drawing, painting, and mapmaking, Image theatre, and digital storytelling – offers a potential opportunity to engage in *both* research *and* intervention to ultimately improve the health and well-being of children and youth affected by global adversity.

Notes

1. We use the capitalised Image theatre to indicate the concept of using the bodies to tell a story, and image to indicate the representation of the story itself.
2. http://www.lifestoriesmontreal.ca/en/experiences-of-refugee-youth.
3. http://www.mappingmemories.ca/.
4. http://www.learnquebec.ca/en/content/professional_development/workshops/.
5. http://voicesbeyondwalls.org/.
6. http://voicesofkashmir.com.

Disclosure statement

No potential conflict of interest was reported by the authors.

Funding

This work was supported by Fonds Québécois de la recherche sur la société et la culture.

References

Akesson, B. (2014). *Contradictions in place: Everyday geographies of Palestinian children and families living under occupation* (PhD dissertation). McGill University, Montréal, QC.

Akesson, B. (2015). Using mapmaking to study the personal geographies of young children affected by political violence. In N. Worth, I. Hardill, & S. Lucas (Eds.), *Researching the lifecourse: Critical reflections from the social sciences* (pp. 123–141). Bristol: Policy Press.

Akesson, B., D'Amico, M., Denov, M., Khan, F., Linds, W., & Mitchell, C. (2014). 'Stepping back' as researchers: How are we addressing ethics in arts-based approaches to working with war-affected children in school and community settings. *Educational Research for Social Change, 3*(1), 75–89.

Alexander, B. (2011). *The new digital storytelling: Creating narratives with new media*. Santa Barbara, CA: ABC-CLIO.

Alon, C., Kuftinec, S., & Turkiyye, I. (2010). Viewpoints on Israeli-Palestinian theatrical encounters. In P. Duffy & E. Vettraino (Eds.), *Youth and theatre of the oppressed* (pp. 83–96). New York, NY: Palgrave MacMillan.

Banks, M. (2001). *Visual methods in social research.* London: Sage.

Barndt, D. (2009). Touching minds and hearts: Community arts. In G. J. Knowles & A. Cole (Eds.), *Handbook of the arts in qualitative research* (pp. 351–362). Thousand Oaks, CA: Sage.

Bateson, G. (1972). *Steps to an ecology of mind.* New York, NY: Ballantine Books.

Bergold, J., & Thomas, S. (2012). Participatory research methods: A methodological approach in motion. *Forum Qualitative Sozialforschung/Forum: Qualitative Social Research, 13*(1), 191–222. Retrieved from http://www.qualitative-research.net/index.php/fqs/article/view/1801/3334

Betancourt, T. S., & Khan, K. T. (2008). The mental health of children affected by armed conflict: Protective processes and pathways to resilience. *International Review of Psychiatry, 20,* 317–328. doi:10.1080/09540260802090363

Blackman, A., & Fairey, T. (2007). *The photovoice manual: A guide to designing and running participatory photography projects.* London: Photovoice.

Boal, A. (1979). *Theatre of the oppressed.* (C. A. McBride & M.-O. L. McBride, Trans.). London: Pluto Press.

Boğaç, C. (2009). Place attachment in a foreign settlement. *Journal of Environmental Psychology, 29,* 267–278. doi:10.1016/j.jenvp.2009.01.001

Boydell, K. M., Volpe, T., Cox, S., Katz, A., Dow, R., Brunger, F., … Wong, L. (2012). Ethical challenges in arts-based health research. *The International Journal of the Creative Arts in Interdisciplinary Practice, 11*(Spring), Art. 56. Retrieved from http://www.ijcaip.com/archives/IJCAIP-11-paper1.html

Boyden, J., & de Berry, J. (2004). *Children and youth on the front line.* Oxford: Berghan Books.

Buckner, E., & Kim, P. (2012). Storytelling among Israeli and Palestinian children in the era of mobile innovation. In M. Orey, S. A. Jones, & R. M. Branch (Eds.), *Educational media and technology yearbook: Volume 36* (pp. 7–22). New York, NY: Springer.

Burgess, J. (2006). Hearing ordinary voices: Cultural studies, vernacular creativity and digital storytelling. *Continuum: Journal of Media & Cultural Studies, 20,* 201–214. doi:10.1080/10304310600641737

Burke, C. (2008). Play in focus: Children's visual voice in participative research. In P. Thomson (Ed.), *Doing visual research with children and young people* (pp. 23–36). London: Routledge.

Chiu, L. F. (2009). Culturally competent health promotion: The potential of participatory video for empowering migrant and minority ethnic communities. *International Journal of Migration, Health and Social Care, 5*(1), 5–14. doi:10.1108/17479894200900002

Clark, C. D. (2010). *In a younger voice: Doing children's qualitative research.* New York, NY: Oxford University Press.

Coates, E. (2004). "I forgot the sky!" Children's stories contained within their drawings. In V. Lewis, M. Kellett, C. Robinson, S. Fraser, & S. Ding (Eds.), *The reality of research with children and young people* (pp. 5–21). London: Sage.

Colom, A. (2010). *Participatory video and empowerment.* Retrieved from http://www.powercube.net/wp-content/uploads/2010/03/Pv-and-empowerment.pdf

De Lange, N., Mitchell, C., & Stuart, J. (2007). An introduction to putting people in the picture: Visual methodologies for social change. In N. de Lange, C. Mitchell, & J. Stuart (Eds.), *Putting people in the picture: Visual methodologies for social change* (pp. 1–9). Rotterdam: Sense.

De Lay, B. (2003). *Mobility mapping and flow diagrams: Tools for family tracing and social reintegration work with separated children.* New York, NY: International Rescue Committee.

Denov, M., Doucet, D., & Kamara, A. (2012). Engaging war-affected youth through photography: Photovoice with former child soldiers in Sierra Leone. *Intervention: The International Journal of Mental Health, Psychosocial Work and Counselling in Areas of Armed Conflict, 10,* 117–133. doi:10.1097/WTF.0b013e328355ed82

Frank, À. W. (2013). *The wounded storyteller: Body, illness and ethics* (2nd ed.). Chicago, IL: University of Chicago Press.

Gangi, J. M., & Barowsky, E. (2009). Listening to children's voices: Literature and the arts as means of responding to the effects of war, terrorism, and disaster. *Childhood Education, 85,* 357–363. doi:10.1080/00094056.2009.10521401

Garcia, P., & Rossiter, M. (2010). Digital storytelling as narrative pedagogy. In D. Gibson & B. Dodge (Eds.), *Proceedings of society for information technology & teacher education international conference 2010* (pp. 1091–1097). Chesapeake, VA: AACE.

Garrett, B. L. (2011). Videographic geographies: Using digital video for geographic research. *Progress in Human Geography, 35,* 521–541. doi:10.1177/0309132510388337

Greenhalgh, T., & Wieringa, S. (2011). Is it time to drop the 'knowledge translation' metaphor? A critical literature review. *Journal of the Royal Society of Medicine, 104,* 501–509. doi:10.1258/jrsm. 2011.110285

Gupta, L., & Zimmer, C. (2008). Psychosocial intervention for war-affected children in Sierra Leone. *The British Journal of Psychiatry, 192,* 212–216. doi:10.1192/bjp.bp.107.038182

Guse, K., Spagat, A., Hill, A., Lira, A., Heathcock, S., & Gilliam, M. (2013). Digital storytelling: A novel methodology for sexual health promotion. *American Journal of Sexuality Education, 8,* 213–227. doi:10.1080/15546128.2013.838504

Haalboom, B. J., Robinson, K. L., Elliott, S. J., Cameron, R., & Eyles, J. D. (2006). Research as intervention in heart health promotion. *Canadian Journal of Public Health, 91,* 291–295.

Hamilton, R., & Moore, D. (2004). *Educational interventions for refugee children: Theoretical perspectives and implementing best practice.* New York, NY: Routledge Falmer.

Hanebrink, J. R., & Smith, A. J. (2013). The art of peace in northern Uganda. *African Conflict and Peacebuilding Review, 3,* 195–218.

Harris, D. A. (2007). Pathways to embodied empathy and reconciliation after atrocity: Former boy soldiers in a dance/movement therapy group in Sierra Leone. *Intervention, 5,* 203–231. doi:10. 1097/WTF.0b013e3282f211c8

Harris, D. A. (2010). When child soldiers reconcile: Accountability, restorative justice, and the renewal of empathy. *Journal of Human Rights Practice, 2,* 334–354.

Honwana, A., & De Boeck, F. (2005). *Makers and breakers: Children and youth in postcolonial Africa.* Oxford: James Currey.

Jackson, A. (1992). *Games for actors and non-actors* (Translator's introduction to A. Boal). New York, NY: Routledge.

Jewitt, C. (2012). *An introduction to using video for research.* National centre for research methods working paper (unpublished). Retrieved from http://eprints.ncrm.ac.uk/2259/4/NCRM_ workingpaper_0312.pdf

Junge, M. B., Alvarez, J. F., Kellogg, A., & Volker, C. (1993). The art therapist as social activist: Reflections and visions. *Art Therapy: Journal of the American Art Therapy Association, 10*(3), 148–155.

Kajder, S., Bull, G., & Albaugh, S. (2005). Constructing digital stories. *Learning & Leading with Technology, 32*(5), 40–42.

Kanji, Z., & Cameron, B. L. (2010). Exploring the experiences of resilience in Muslim Afghan refugee children. *Journal of Muslim Mental Health, 5*(1), 22–40. doi:10.1080/ 15564901003620973

Kuftinec, S. (2009). Violent reformations: Image theatre with youth in conflict regions. In P. Anderson & J. Menon (Eds.), *Violence performed. Local roots and global routes of conflict* (pp. 223–243). New York, NY: Palgrave Macmillan.

Kuftinec, S. (2011). Rehearsing for dramatic change in Kabul. In T. Emert & E. Friedland (Eds.), *Come closer: Critical perspectives on Theatre of the oppressed* (pp. 109–116). New York: Peter Lang.

Lambert, J. (2013). *Digital storytelling: Capturing lives, creating community.* New York, NY: Routledge.

Leitch, R. (2008). Creatively researching children's narratives through images and drawings. In P. Thomson (Ed.), *Doing visual research with children and young people* (pp. 37–58). London: Routledge.

Linds, W., & Vettraino, E. (2008). Collective imagining: Collaborative story telling through image theater. *Forum Qualitative Sozialforschung/Forum: Qualitative Social Research, 9*(2). Retrieved from http://nbn-resolving.de/urn:nbn:de:0114-fqs0802568

Linesch, D. (1994). Interpretation in art therapy research and practice: The hermeneutic circle. *The Arts in Psychotherapy, 21*, 185–195. doi:10.1016/0197-4556(94)90048-5

Lunch, N., & Lunch, C. (2006). *Insights into participatory video: A handbook for the field.* Oxford: Insight. Retrieved from http://insightshare.org/resources/pv-handbook

Lunch, N., & Lunch, C. (2010). *A rights-based approach to participatory video: Toolkit.* Oxford: Insight.

Luttrell, W., Restler, V., & Fontaine, C. (2012). Youth video-making: Selves and identities in dialogue. In E.-J. Milne, C. Mitchell, & N. de Lange (Eds.), *Handbook of participatory video* (pp. 164–177). Lanham, MD: AltaMira Press.

Marshall, D. J. (2013). *A children's geography of occupation: Imaginary, emotional, and everyday spaces of Palestinian childhood* (Doctoral dissertation). University of Kentucky, Lexington, KY.

McNamee, S. (1988). Accepting research as social intervention: Implications of a systemic epistemology. *Communication Quarterly, 36*(1), 50–68. doi:10.1080/01463378809369707

Miles, G. M. (2000). Drawing together hope: 'Listening' to militarised children. *Journal of Child Health Care, 4*, 137–142. doi:10.1177/136749350000400401

Mitchell, C. (2011). *Doing visual research.* London: Sage.

Mitchell, C., De Lange, N., Moletsane, R., Stuart, J., & Buthelezi, T. (2005). Giving a face to HIV and AIDS: On the uses of photo-voice by teachers and community health care workers working with youth in rural South Africa. *Qualitative Research in Psychology, 2*, 257–270. doi:10.1191/1478088705qp042oa

Moletsane, R., De Lange, N., Mitchell, C., Stuart, J., Buthelezi, T., & Taylor, M. (2007). Photo-voice as a tool for analysis and activism in response to HIV and AIDS stigmatisation in a rural KwaZulu-Natal school. *Journal of Child and Adolescent Mental Health, 19*(1), 19–28. doi:10.2989/17280580709486632

Norman, J. M. (2009). Creative activism: Youth media in Palestine. *Middle East Journal of Culture and Communication, 2*, 251–274. doi:10.1163/187398509X12476683126464

Ohler, J. (2013). *Digital storytelling in the classroom: New media pathways to literacy, learning, and creativity.* Thousand Oaks, CA: Corwin Press.

Okahashi, P. (2000). The potential of participatory video. *Rehabilitation Review, 11*(1), 1–4. Retrieved from wwwmcc.murdoch.edu.au/ReadingRoom/3.2/Tomaselli.html

Panter-Brick, C., Lende, D., & Kohrt, B. A. (2012). Children in global adversity: Physical, mental, behavioral, and symbolic dimensions of health. In V. Maholmes & R. B. King (Eds.), *The Oxford handbook of poverty and child development* (pp. 603–621). Oxford: Oxford University Press.

Pascal, C., & Bertram, T. (2009). Listening to young citizens: The struggle to make real a participatory paradigm in research with young children. *European Early Childhood Education Research Journal, 17*(2), 249–262. doi:10.1080/13502930902951486

Pedersen, D. (2002). Political violence, ethnic conflict, and contemporary wars: Broad implications for health and social well-being. *Social Science & Medicine, 55*(2), 175–190. doi:10.1016/S0277-9536(01)00261-1

Perry, A. J. (2012). A silent revolution: 'Image theatre' as a system of decolonisation. *Research in Drama Education: The Journal of Applied Theatre and Performance, 17*(1), 103–119. doi:10.1080/13569783.2012.648991

Pfefferbaum, B., & North, C. S. (2013). Assessing children's disaster reactions and mental health needs: Screening and clinical evaluation. *Canadian Journal of Psychiatry, 58*, 135–142.

Pink, S. (2001). *Doing visual ethnography.* London: Sage.

Pink, S. (2007). *Doing visual ethnography: Images, media, and representation in research* (2nd ed.). London: Sage.

Prosser, J. (1998). *Image-based research: A sourcebook for qualitative researchers.* London: Falmer Press.

Rebmann, K. (2012). Theory, practice, tools: Catching up with digital storytelling. *Teacher Librarian, 39*, 30–34.

Robin, B. (2006). *The educational uses of digital storytelling.* Retrieved from http://digitalliteracyintheclassroom.pbworks.com/f/Educ-Uses-DS.pdf

Rossiter, M., & Garcia, P. A. (2010). Digital storytelling: A new player on the narrative field. *New Directions for Adult and Continuing Education, 2010*(126), 37–48. doi:10.1002/ace.370

Rousseau, C., & Heusch, N. (2000). The trip: A creative expression project for refugee and immigrant children. *Art Therapy: Journal of the American Art Therapy Association, 17*(1), 31–40.

Ruiz-Casares, M., & Thompson, J. (2014). Obtaining meaningful informed consent: Preliminary results of a study to develop visual informed consent forms with children. *Children's Geographies, 14*, 35–45. doi:10.1080/14733285.2014.971713

Sandercock, L., & Attili, G. (2010). Digital ethnography as planning praxis: An experiment with film as social research, community engagement and policy dialogue. *Planning Theory and Practice, 11* (1), 23–45. doi:10.1080/14649350903538012

Sawyer, C. B., & Willis, J. M. (2011). Introducing digital storytelling to influence the behavior of children and adolescents. *Journal of Creativity in Mental Health, 6*, 274–283. doi:10.1080/ 15401383.2011.630308

Sloane, J. A., & Wallin, D. (2013). Theatre of the commons: A theatrical inquiry into the democratic engagement of former refugee families in Canadian public high school communities. *Educational Research, 55*, 454–472. doi:10.1080/00131881.2013.844948

Spence, J. (1995). *Culturing sniping: The art of transgression*. New York, NY: Routledge.

Stringer, E. (2008). *Action research in education* (2nd ed.). Don Mills: Pearson.

Theron, L., Mitchell, C., Smith, A., & Stuart, J. (2011). *Picturing research: Drawing as visual methodology*. Rotterdam: Sense.

Thomas, G. V., & Silk, A. M. J. (1990). *An introduction to the psychology of children's drawings*. Hertford: Harvester Wheatsheaf.

Thong, S. (2007). Redefining the tools of art therapy. *Art Therapy: The Journal of the American Art Therapy Association, 24*, 52–58. doi:10.1080/07421656.2007.10129583

Veale, A. (2005). Creative methodologies in participatory research with children. In S. Greene & D. Hogan (Eds.), *Researching children's experience: Approaches and methods* (pp. 253–272). London: Sage.

Voices Beyond Walls. (2006). *Digital storytelling workshops*. Retrieved from http:// voicesbeyondwalls.org/projects/digital_storytelling.html

Wang, C., & Burris, M. (1994). Empowerment through photo novella: Portraits of participation. *Health Education & Behavior, 21*, 171–186.

Wang, C., & Burris, M. A. (1997). Photovoice: Concept, methodology, and use for participatory needs assessment. *Health Education & Behavior, 24* , 369–387.

Wheeler, J. (2009). 'The life that we don't want': Using participatory video in researching violence. *IDS Bulletin, 40*(3), 10–18. doi:10.1111/j.1759-5436.2009.00033.x

Wheeler, J. (2011). Seeing like a citizen: Participatory video and action research for citizen action. In N. Shah & F. Jansen (Eds.), *Digital (alter)natives with cause? 2* (pp. 47–60). Retrieved from http:// issuu.com/hivos/docs/book_2_final_print_rev/1

Wiener, N. (1948). *Cybernetics, or control and communication in the animal and the machine*. Cambridge, MA: Technology Press.

'Closer to my world': Children with autism spectrum disorder tell their stories through photovoice

Vu Song Ha[a] and Andrea Whittaker[b]

[a]Center for Creative Initiatives in Health and Population, Hanoi, Vietnam; [b]Anthropology, School of Social Sciences, Monash University, Melbourne, Australia

ABSTRACT

One of the challenges in doing research with individuals with autism spectrum disorder (ASD) is the difficulty in communication. This study employed a modified form of photovoice with a group of young people with ASD in Hanoi, Vietnam, to provide a means of meaningful participation in research about their lives, experiences, and needs. We describe the process of conducting photovoice with nine children with ASD from June 2011 to May 2012, many of whom had limited verbal communication skills. More than 2100 photos were taken by children. Undertaking photovoice with children with ASD required some modification of the method. In particular we consider the difficulties in analysing and interpreting the photographs produced by children with ASD. Due to the ambiguities of the visual images produced we found content analysis of photographs alone was inadequate. There was a discrepancy between our initial interpretations of the photographs and our understandings derived from information from interviews with children, parents, carers, and our own observations. Our study points to the need to understand context through multiple methods and the potential of photovoice as a means to mediate communication and participation in research for groups with communication difficulties.

Introduction

A key challenge in public health research is the inclusion of disadvantaged and vulnerable groups as participants in research and interventions. This paper reports on the use of a modified form of photovoice with a group of young people with autism spectrum disorder (ASD) in Hanoi, Vietnam, to provide a means of meaningful participation in research about their lives, experience, and health needs. Within Vietnam, there is a lack of public awareness and education about ASD and considerable stigma and discrimination attached to developmental disabilities (Ha, Whittaker, Whittaker, & Rodger, 2014). Addressing the needs of families of children with ASD and other disabilities for appropriate support and interventions in Vietnam remains an important public health challenge.

Photovoice is a visual-based participatory method that has gained popularity in public health research including public health, community development, nursing, education, social work, and occupation therapy (Lal, Jarus, & Suto, 2012). It involves the use of photography by participants to document their daily lives and experiences so as '1) to enable research participants to record and reflect their community's strengths and concerns, 2) to promote critical dialogue and knowledge through group discussion of photographs, and 3) to reach policy makers' (Wang & Burris, 1997, p. 369). Literature suggests that photovoice is effective for engaging and allowing meaningful participation in research by people often underrepresented, including people with mobility limitations due to neurological conditions (Bishop, Robillard, & Moxley, 2013) and mental illnesses (Cabassa, Nicasio, & Whitley, 2013), as well as migrants, homeless people, people living with HIV, gender based violence survivors and people with chronic diseases (Catalani & Minkler, 2010; Hergenrather, Rhodes, Cowan, Bardhoshi, & Pula, 2009). As Povee, Bishop, and Roberts (2014) note on their work using photovoice with people with intellectual disabilities, participatory approaches to research such as photovoice allow greater meaningful participation and influence by people with intellectual disabilities in research as they become actively engaged partners or co-researchers. Since people with ASD have difficulty in communication (American Psychiatric Association [APA], 2013), visual support strategies and techniques are suggested as effective strategies in improving the understanding and communication with people with ASD (Hodgdon, 1995; Wong et al., 2014).

In this paper we describe the process and challenges posed in using photovoice with this group and the modifications to the technique that were necessary. In particular, we consider the difficulties in analysing and interpreting the photographs produced by children with ASD, many of whom have difficulties in verbally expressing themselves. We found that it was difficult to interpret the photographs produced through this technique when the participants had only limited verbal abilities. However, the collection of more contextual information on the children allowed us to see how they used the photographs as a means to communicate their experience and worldview and that this technique was a powerful and appropriate means of involving young people with ASD in the research process. The photographs demonstrate how important it is to acknowledge the voices of the participants in health research and not to impose our own categories of interpretation, whether these are from biomedicine or assumptions about participants' abilities.

Autism spectrum disorder

According to the latest *Diagnostic and statistical manual of mental disorders* (DSM-5), ASD is a developmental disability characterised by impairment in reciprocal social communication and social interaction, as well as restricted and repetitive patterns of behaviours (APA, 2013). It has profound lifelong effects upon the children affected and their families, including difficulties with education, neglect and rejection, stigma and social isolation, dependent living and health problems, high levels of physical and psychological exhaustion for parents, and significant economic costs (Altiere & von Kluge, 2009; Howlin, 2005).

ASD (*tự kỷ* in Vietnamese) has been recognised in Vietnam as a condition only since the late 1990s (Giang, 2012; Minh, 2011; Ying, Browne, Hutchinson, Cashin, & Binh, 2012). Although there is no official data, it is estimated that there are 160,000 people living with ASD in Vietnam (Vietnam Public Health Association cited in Ying et al., 2012). Statistics from the National Children's Hospital based in Hanoi show that the number of children diagnosed with autism each year has risen from 450 in 2008, 950 in 2009 and 1792 in 2010, respectively (Minh, 2011). Health service provision, education, and intervention services for children diagnosed with ASD in Hanoi are scarce and expensive and inaccessible for most poor families or those living in rural areas (Ha et al., 2014).

Photovoice studies with people with ASD

Although limited, research suggests the value of photovoice as a tool for engaging young people with ASD. One US-based study by Carnahan (2006) describes how photovoice improved the engagement of two young boys with ASD in education settings in a suburban school in Ohio. In another study, Obrusnikova and Cavalier (2011) focused on 12 boys and 2 girls with ASD, aged 8–14 years old, and utilised photovoice as part of a study of barriers to and facilitators of after-school participation in physical activities of children with ASD. Apart from published research, other reports of community projects engaging individuals with ASD in photovoice tend to be found within unpublished 'grey' literature, most notably the projects 'Life as it is with aspergers' from Toowoomba, Queensland (Photovoice Australia, 2012), and 'Picture that' for young people with ASD aged from 12 to 15 in London (Photovoice, 2012).

The method and process of analysing photographic data in photovoice projects is not well described in the literature. Wang, Yi, Tao, and Carovano (1998) argue that as a participatory methodology, photovoice does not aim to analyse the entire body of photographic data. Instead, photovoice requires an innovative framework in which participants can actively participate and drive the analysis in all three stages, from (1) selecting photographs, (2) contextualising or telling stories, to (3) codifying photographs (Wang & Burris, 1997). However, in their review, Hergenrather et al. (2009) suggest that although the majority of photovoice studies reviewed (26 of 31) report collaboration, its extent varies. In particular, in some projects participants were not involved in data analysis. Catalani and Minkler (2010) note that researchers tend to use transcripts from photo-elicited interviews as the main source of data rather than the photographs themselves and rarely describe how they generate findings from the photographs.

These challenges in photographic data analysis need more consideration in projects in which participants have limited verbal communication capacity. There are difficulties in eliciting in-depth discussions with people with cognitive disabilities or young children (Lal et al., 2012). In her research with people with intellectual disability, Jurkowski (2008) reported that non-verbal people would engage in photograph taking, but not in individual or group discussion, namely, the contextualising stage in analysis. Two published papers from projects with children with ASD did not describe in detail how they engaged children in selecting, contextualising and decoding photos nor on the challenges that they encountered (Carnahan, 2006; Obrusnikova & Cavalier, 2011).

Methods

The study was undertaken with a group of nine young people with ASD in Hanoi, Vietnam from early November 2011 until March 2012. Photovoice was used as part of a broader ethnographic study of the experiences, health, and well-being of children and families with ASD, which included participant observation, in-depth interviews with parents, caregivers, and health professionals, an online survey and a public exhibition, the results of which are published elsewhere (Ha et al., 2014).

Setting

Young people participating in photovoice activities were recruited through a community organisation, The Hanoi Club of Parents of Children with Autism (hereafter referred to as the Hanoi Club) and a parent-run school for children with ASD. Hanoi Club and the parent-led school were selected for recruitment of the sample as they provided ready access to a network of families of children with ASD.

Participants

Information sheets about the photovoice project were distributed to all families with children and young people considered to h ASD[1] at the parent-led school and Hanoi Club. Families who indicated they were willing to participate were contacted and given further information. The inclusion criteria for children included: being from 10 to 19 years old, being considered to have ASD, having parents' consent, and being willing to participate. In the beginning of the project 10 children were involved. However, after two weeks one child withdrew because he had difficulties in motor skills and was not interested in taking photographs. Thus, a total of 9 young people aged from 10 to 17 years old participated in the photovoice project. The verbal abilities of the children varied. One participating child could talk but generally did not have conversations with other people. Two children could answer questions with prompts but they preferred to talk about their own interests. Three children could have limited conversations for a short time, and three other children are able to initiate and maintain conversation for a while. Table 1 summarises the demographic characteristics of the young people participating in the photovoice project.

Ethical considerations

An important ethical consideration in this study was the need to obtain informed consent from parents of participating children and informed assent from the children. After informed consent was received from parents, the children were provided information sheets to confirm if they wanted to participate: one was written in simple language, and the other one was modified with pictures to help children easily understand. Permission

Table 1. Demographic characteristics of children with ASD who participated in photovoice.

Pseudonym	Age	Sex	Current school attendance
Anh	17	Male	Parent-run school
Minh	12	Male	Studying at home
Quỳnh	15	Female	Studying at centre for children with intellectual disabilities
Đào	13	Female	Parent-run school
Phuong	10	Male	Parent-run school
Thái	13	Male	Grade 6 in mainstream class
Son	11	Male	Parent-run school
Thuy	14	Male	Parent-run school
Linh	14	Male	Parent-run school

was also explicitly given for the display and use of any photographs eventually selected for the public exhibition and written permission obtained from any people represented in photographs or videos in accordance with the ethical protocols for this project.

Modifications to the photovoice process

Undertaking photovoice with children with ASD required a modification of the technique to suit their abilities, interests, and practical considerations. Figure 1 shows the process of training and repeated visits during the study. All children undertook training sessions on photovoice. An experienced photovoice practitioner who has used the technique in a number of different community settings and the first author planned and conducted the training at the school with support from some teachers. A simple introduction

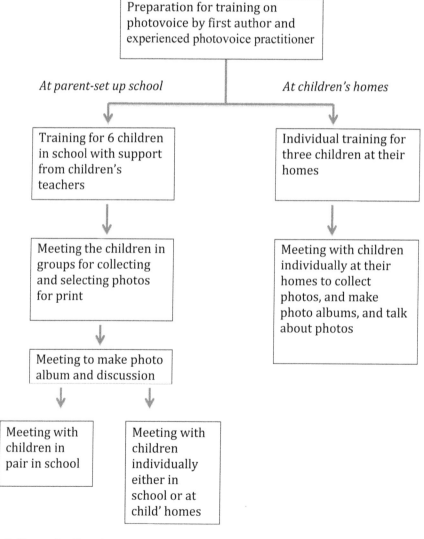

Figure 1. Photovoice flow chart.

about the cameras was given to the group of 6 children and then they took photos by themselves for about 20 minutes. A handout with simple language and pictures was also given to children. Every child was given a Canon A3200 digital camera with minimal zoom and good picture quality. This training was repeated with the three other children individually at home.

At fortnightly meetings with the children, they were asked to choose photos that they wanted to print as a means of engaging them. At the next meeting these selected photographs were given to children to make their own albums in combination with craft materials for decoration. As the children made their albums, they were asked about their photos. Although few of the children gave details verbally about their photographs, this process allowed them to indicate their preferences. Three of the children had more communication skills and were able to give more detailed explanations.

Descriptions of the photovoice technique suggest working with themes or topics to direct the participants in choosing their subject matter (Wang & Burris, 1997). Our initial instruction for children to photograph particular topics was not workable and instead children freely photographed whatever they wished. The authors originally planned to have children take their photographs each week by topics, such as: 'my family', 'my school', 'what I like', 'what I do not like', 'what makes me happy' but this was abandoned when it was clear that most of the children took photos according to their own interests. The photographs hence became documents of children's interests rather than structured by the researchers.

Asking consent to take photographs of other people was one of the most challenging aspects of conducting photovoice with children with ASD. Although this issue was stressed at the introductory training, and further reinforced whenever possible, the children rarely asked for consent when taking photos of other people. We ensured that the teachers at the school informed and asked oral consent from parents of other children at the school to allow the children participating in this project to take photos of their children for this research.

Analysis of visual material

In participatory action research in general and photovoice in particular, analysis is a process of engagement between researchers and research participants (Giacomini, 2010; Wang & Burris, 1997; Wang et al., 1998). However, the communication challenges related to ASD often made such analysis challenging. Contextualising or storytelling during discussions between participants and between participants and facilitator/ researcher is considered essential in photovoice analysis (Wang et al., 1998). However, the storytelling ability of children with ASD is limited. Likewise, focus group techniques were not appropriate for these children who can find groups stressful due to their limited verbal abilities and poor social skills. The realities of these communication difficulties resulted in a different analytic weight placed upon the photographs. In this study, the photographs became central sources of data as a record of children's daily lives. Therefore, in this study two approaches were used to analyse photos taken by children with ASD: a participatory action research approach and content analysis for visual images (Bell, 2001; Koch & Kralik, 2006; Wang et al., 1998).

Content analysis

Conceptualised as a technique for systematic, 'objective', and quantitative description of visual images, content analysis allows researchers to reduce the large number and the complexity of visual materials to a small number of codes (Bell, 2001; Bock, Isermann & Knieper, 2011). In addition, the researchers are able to consider what are presented in images through frequency analysis (Bock et al., 2011). In this case each photograph was coded according to: I. Focus, II. Location, and III. Distance. The 'Location' category referred to the place in which photos were taken. 'Focus' meant the object or subject at the centre of the photos, and 'Distance' referred to the distance from the child to the focus of the photo. In some cases a photograph could include elements from several sub-categories. Such categorizations, however, assume that the person taking the photograph has clear intent and the skill to compose the visual elements as they wish. This cannot always be assumed for these photographs and so an element of ambiguity remains. In some cases the focus of the photos could not be identified. These were coded as 'unknown' and were not coded in other categories. Table 2 is an example of the code book for category I, Focus.

Participatory analysis

Using a participatory action research approach, children with ASD were involved in the whole photovoice process as much as they could, and it was journey of learning from the children. The first author did not use the SHOWeD set of questions,[2] which are commonly used to elicit discussion about photographs in photovoice (Carnahan, 2006; Wang et al., 1998) since most children found these questions too abstract and hard to answer. Instead, children described whatever they wanted about their photos, and the first author used simple prompt questions, such as: 'Tell me about your photos?', 'What was in the photos?', 'Where did you take the photos?', 'Who was in the photo?', 'What was the person(s) in the photo doing'. Careful attention was paid to their reactions and feelings when they answered questions. This need for a more flexible and simple interview protocol speaks to the challenges in working with both young children and those with

Table 2. An example of the code book for content analysis of photographs, category I, 'Focus'.

Category/variable	Sub-categories/values	Sub-sub categories
Focus	People	II.1.2 Mother
		II.2.2 Father
		II.2.3 Sibling
		II.2.4 Other family members
		II.2.5 Friends
		II.2.6 Strangers
		II.2.7 Unknown
	Objects	II.3.1 Toys
		II.3.2 Their own stuff
		II.3.3 Family stuff
		II.3.4 Others
	Body	II.4.1 Their own body
		II.4.2 Other body
		II.4.3 Self photo
	Scenes	
	Activities	
	Other	
	Unknown	

communication difficulties. It draws attention to the difficulties in social science more generally where great analytic weight is placed upon verbal expression and less upon sensory experience and other forms of non-verbal communication. All encounters with children with ASD to discuss the photos were audio recorded or through notes and later transcribed verbatim. In addition, information obtained through interviews, observations, and parents' interviews were used to help contextualise photographs and situate them in the broader context of the children's and families' lives.

Findings

A total of 2142 photographs were used for analysis, and a public exhibition of photographs from the project took place between March and May 2012 (see YouTube videoclip available online as a supplementary file). Table 3 shows the number of photographs contributed by the participating children.

Table 4 provides a description of the focus of the photographs. There is a sampling bias due to the different numbers of photographs contributed by each child, hence the percentages should be treated with caution; however, content analysis does give some useful insights.

Content analysis of photographs

Objects and other items

Photographs with objects as the focus accounted for 30% of the total number of photographs. These included photos of toys, dolls, pen cases, backpacks, books, food, and family furniture. Advertisements and film trailers appeared in more than 10% of children's photos. In addition, children photographed various images that displayed their interests, including film trailers, cars, computer games, dolls, or foods. Some children with ASD also expressed special interests demonstrated through a large number of photographs about the same topic. For example, Son, an 11-year-old boy was very interested in advertisements and cartoon programmes. Among his 189 photos, 177 photos were of advertisements and Disney channel images. He could repeat precisely the catch phrases in all the advertisements.

The 'Other' category included photographs capturing lights, walls, trees, an altar, and space between objects. Combining objects, advertisements, and other category, the percentage of these reached about 50%.

People

Content analysis data, however, challenges the stereotype that people with ASD are only interested in objects, not in people. Twenty-five per cent of children's photos focused on people, typically family members and significant others including their siblings, mothers, friends, and teachers. The 'group activities' category included photos of people gathering

Table 3. Numbers of photographs contributed by each participating child.

Pseudonym	Minh	Phuong	Anh	Thuy	Linh	Quỳnh	Son	Đào	Thái	Total
Number of photos	168	54	12	56	517	232	189	808	106	2142

Table 4. Frequency of the focus of the photographs taken by children with ASD.

Focus of the photos	Number of photos	Percentage*
Objects	645	30%
People	530	25%
Advertisement, film trailer, computer games	281	13%
Myself	253	12%
Scenes	218	10%
Group activities	88	4%
Others	111	5%
Unknown	56	3%

*The total percentage of photo focus is more than 100% since some photos were coded in two codes: scenes and people.

for social activities such as a birthday parties, dancing, or singing at a Christmas party. The combination of the two categories 'people' and 'group activities' applied to nearly 30% of the photographs. Siblings appeared most often in children's photos, about a third of photos in the 'people' category, suggesting that siblings have a significant role in the daily life of children with ASD and that they share a lot of time together. Friends, mothers, and other extended family members such as grandparents, aunts, and nephews featured in 16–18% of photographs. Children captured different images of their mothers from looking and smiling, talking on the telephone, doing housework, resting in beds, and even turning away to avoid being photographed. In contrast, fathers were almost invisible, and not as visible as domestic helpers in children's photos. The images of the children's fathers accounted for less than 5% of photos in the category 'people'. This suggests that fathers are less likely to be caring for their children (with little opportunity to be photographed) and possibly do not have as close a relationship with their children as mothers and domestic helpers.

The self

More than 10% of children's photos were in the category 'myself' – the category included images of children taking photos of themselves via mirrors, or as they posed for their own portrait, or parts of their bodies. For example, Đào, a 13-year-old girl, took 101 photos of her hands. She took photos of her hands in different positions, under different lighting, from a range of distances and in different times during the three-month photovoice project (see Figure 2). Of the total 253 photos that children took about themselves, two thirds of these (63%) involved exploration of their own bodies including a series of photos about their hands, eyes, mouths, and legs. About one third (94 photos) of these photos involved self-portraits using mirrors.

Content analysis alone provides only limited insight into the photographs. The following case studies show how in-depth contextual information from interviews with children, parents and carers, combined with our observations helped in the interpretation of visual images.

Case studies

Quỳnh

Quỳnh is a good example to illustrate that the more time we spent talking and getting to know children, the more we were able to understand what they wished to convey.

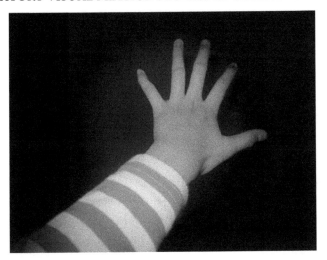

Figure 2. Photograph 1: Đào's hand.

When we initially saw Quỳnh's photograph we wondered what the focus was. Drawing upon our knowledge of autism, we supposed that she might be interested in the space between objects, or the pattern on the floor as some children with autism are known to fixate on repeated visual patterns. However, when the first author met with Quỳnh and asked her about her photograph, she said 'It is my shoe. I love these shoes, but it has a small hole in my shoe, and my mom does not know about it' (Figure 3).

Likewise, Figure 4 is difficult to interpret without having more contextual information. Quỳnh took numerous photographs of this scene, and both her mother and the first author were not sure what attracted her interest. When asked for a title during the preparation for exhibition, we brought back the photo to her and she gave the title for this photo 'Vắng vẻ' (Emptiness). Later we learned that this photo was taken at the end of

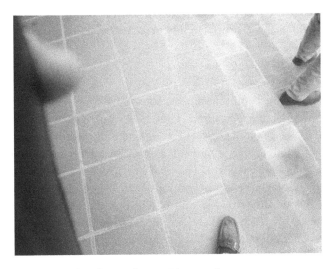

Figure 3. Photograph 2: Quynh's photo: what could we see?

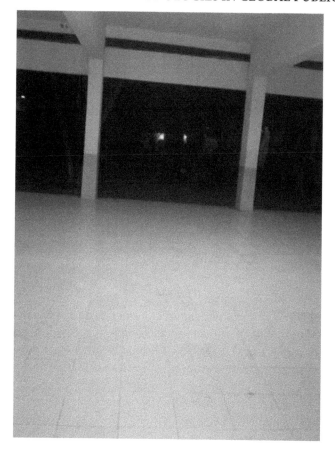

Figure 4. Photograph 3: Emptiness.

the party organised by Hanoi Club in a public school. During the party, there were many people, and Quỳnh captured the moment when most people went home, giving the school back to the emptiness. Quỳnh's photographs taught us not to impose our own categories of interpretation whether these are from biomedicine or assumptions about children's abilities.

Thuy

Quỳnh was able to verbally communicate, but some other children had more limited communication skills. Thuy is a one example. Thuy took relatively few photographs, 56 in all. Among these, he took two photographs of a dog and a number of photos about lights in different contexts, including, decoration lights on a tree, light from a car moving at night, and computer modem lights at night. Thuy did not answer questions when asked about the dog and light photographs. Conversations with his mother and teachers revealed that the dog was his neighbour's dog, and he did not like the dog's barking. Later, we learned from one of his teachers that Thuy was highly sensitive to sounds. He calms down with some selected sounds but will run away immediately when therapists try other sounds. His teachers informed me that in the past he did not allow the school to play any music for a year. He is also very interested in lights, which calm him down and make him smile. In this case, perhaps Thuy was showing us what he liked (different kinds of lights) and what he did not like (dogs barking).

Thái

Thái also surprised us with his photographs. He is 13 years old, studies in a mainstream class with some other peers with special needs and communicates using verbal language. Around 50% of photographs taken by Thái were of his body. He took 28 photos about his hand and 18 photos of his eyes, throat, and teeth. On one level such repetitive interest in the relationship between parts of the body is symptomatic of autism, yet his explanations also revealed his photographs as explorations of the world. One series of photos had red and some dark lines and then a couple of photos with red and a white spot (see Figure 5). When we asked Thái, he told us that he put the lens camera inside his hand to take photographs of the sun. Thái smiled when he showed the photo that had a white spot and named this photograph, 'Tia sáng trong mặt trời' ('Light inside the sun').

Minh

Another set of photographs by Minh led to us understanding his experience of social isolation. Figure 6 was taken by Minh. His brother played bubbles with a neighbour's boy in the small path in front of Minh's house. When asked about this photo, he explained briefly 'My little brother played bubbles with a friend', and quickly moved onto another photo of his mother standing outside of their house gate. When asked, he said, 'Mum was looking for me'. His mother explained:

> Minh liked blowing bubbles and wanted to play with his brother and the neighbour. But the neighbour did not want Minh to play. He said Minh did not know how. So I was outside to keep an eye out for them.

This photo and story illustrates how Minh was excluded by other children in their play. Minh wished to be included, but in this context he was relegated to status as outsider/

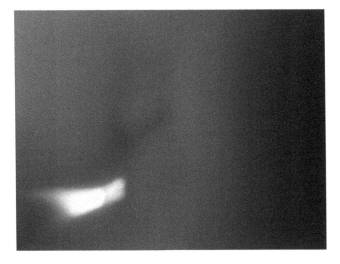

Figure 5. Photograph 4: Light inside the sun.

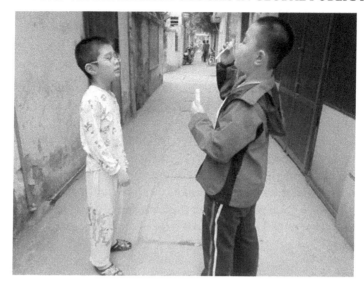

Figure 6. Photograph 5: Little brother played bubble with a friend.

observer. The subsequent photograph of his mother also reveals her concern for him and her felt need to supervise his interactions so he is not subjected to bullying. His photo also captures how there is very little outdoor space in Hanoi for children to play. These two boys played on the local path, which was used for pedestrians, bikes, and motorbikes.

Minh's photographs made us consider the barriers against engaging with the outside world posed for children with ASD. Most of the children' photos were taken within the domestic environment of the home and reveal something of the limited opportunities of these children to engage with the outside world. Seventy-two per cent of photographs were taken at the children's homes and another 6% at their grandparent's homes. A small number took photographs at their schools. Only 4% of photos were taken at events and places outside the home, usually at organised activities at the 'Friends' café' (for people with ASD) or a school Christmas party for children with ASD. Through their subject matter but also through their angles and distance, these photographs displayed children's social and physical exclusion from outside and the restricted environmental conditions that they grow up in.

Discussion

Photovoice provided rich research data and vivid insights into the experiences and lives of children with ASD but also provided benefits to the participants and their families. Employed within a participatory approach, photovoice empowered the children and their parents as active collaborators and shifted the power imbalance in the relationship between researcher and research participants. These photographs proved a valuable source of data in themselves, especially given that children with ASD have difficulties engaging in verbal modes of communication with other people. Much social science research assumes non-mediated communication and dialogue, sometimes problematic for people with certain forms of disability. Instead, the interactive process in the photovoice project required the researchers to spend more time to observe, engage with, listen to and experience the children's lives while also acknowledging our differences and accepting the limitations of our abilities to fully understand another's perspective and the inadequacies of our representations.

The importance of context in interpreting visual material

The difficulty of entering another person's worldview lies at the heart of anthropological research, especially when researching populations with different sensory experiences of the world. On one hand, such photographs could be dismissed as having no intent or as the result of inadequate skills of representation. On the other hand, one might interpret some photographs as the product of particular autistic fixations. But we learned not to make assumptions about the photographs. The intention with which these photographs were taken and their aesthetic values remind us that these are artistic expressions and forms of communication, not only photographs by children with autism or products of their disabilities. Children with ASD had their own perspectives and often surprised us with what they were trying to express. The challenge was how to give them opportunities to explain what they thought to us.

Analysis of the visual material posed challenges. Both content analysis and contextualised analysis using various forms of participation and observation had strengths and limitations. As discussed, the focus of photographs from a viewer's point of view sometimes differed markedly from what the children wanted to capture. In some cases, interpretations could be verified through conversations with the children. Content analysis alone proved very limited in helping to understand the visual data, other than at a descriptive level. Using forms of participatory analysis and combining this with the ongoing ethnographic observations and interviews with parents and caregivers enhanced the interpretation of the visual images from insiders' perspectives (Bock et al., 2011) rather than through a biomedical gaze.

A number of photographs defied initial interpretation. For these content analysis was inadequate and it was only through shared interpretation with the children and those closest to them that these photographs were discovered to carry a wealth of meaning for the children. The case studies we describe in this paper demonstrate the need for triangulation with observations and interviews with parents and others in the interpretation of the photographs providing greater understanding how and why children took and choose the images they did and through this the lived experience of ASD for children. Quỳnh's photographs demonstrate how important it is to acknowledge the voices of the children in interpreting these expressions of their world and not to impose our own categories of interpretation, whether these are from biomedicine or assumptions about children's abilities. Initially interpreting photographs of a shoe or empty space through a lens of autism, these images were later revealed to carry emotional importance to Quỳnh. Through his photographs Thuy was showing us what he liked and disliked. Likewise, Thái clearly enjoyed using his camera to explore the world around him. He experimented with creative images, using his camera to look at toys and objects close up and from unusual angles. These photographs reveal his aesthetic response to patterns, colour, and scale. Without the photovoice method, we would not have been given insight into Minh's everyday experience of isolation nor of the concerns of his mother.

Benefits for participants

For the children who participated, it was the first time they owned a camera themselves. They used cameras to take the photos that they wanted, entertained themselves with the cameras, and enjoyed sharing them. Parents also experienced benefits. Parents expressed their pride in their children's photographs and reported that participating in photovoice with their children helped them understand their children better. As one mother wrote:

> I always think that I am the person who understands most about you. I thought I could understand what you want through your eyes, your gestures. However, since you and I joined this group, I realize that you have so many things that I might not understand. Through your photos I know more about your world, and know why you say like this, laugh like this ... I criticize you less, and see your life having more fun and I know that you love me more.

Modifications to photovoice required

The use of photovoice posed several challenges and required a number of modifications. Photovoice with children with ASD required an enormous amount of flexibility and patience and was time-consuming. The level of participation and communication of children needed to be taken into consideration. Some children could communicate about their photos, yet some provided very little other information. This raises questions of who is able to participate in research and who has the right to interpret their photos. We used a variety of techniques such as simplified questions and asking children to choose photographs and develop albums in order to engage them. Caregivers also became involved in discussions about photographs.

Ethical protocols were also adapted for this research. Simple language, as well as modified forms with pictures, were used to communicate with children about the study purpose and informed consent. Even so, it was difficult to always be certain the children fully understood the nature of their participation, an issue also raised by Jurkowski (2008) in her photovoice project with individuals with intellectual disability. In addition, issues surrounding protecting anonymity and confidentiality in research involving images (Bell, 2010) was problematic, especially when they involved images of other people.

Study limitations

As a small urban sample recruited through a parent-led school and an advocacy organisation, this study has several limitations. The sample of children in this study represents a privileged group of children with ASD as they have access to education and limited forms of intervention. As schools catering to children with ASD are expensive, most average-income families in Hanoi cannot afford to send their children to private schools and such facilities do not exist outside of major cities. As such we make no claims about the representativeness of our sample. Further study is needed to understand the lives of children with ASD from less privileged backgrounds and in rural communities in Vietnam.

Conclusions

Photovoice proved a useful means of allowing children with ASD and their parents an opportunity to describe their lived experience and engage meaningfully with research.

The photographs mediated communication between the children and researchers and parents. As a result of their involvement, the Hanoi Club decided to hold a public exhibition of selected photographs from the project (reported elsewhere Ha, 2014) to provide education for members of the public and to advocate for the needs of children with ASD within a context in which there is limited public understanding of the condition, heavy social stigma, and very few health or intervention services.

The resultant photographs operate on multiple levels. They may be read simultaneously as artistic works reflecting the aesthetic choices of the photographers; as works which inform us of the unique views and sensory perceptions of people with ASD; but also as forms of communication, powerfully, and often poetically expressing the interests, significant people, and the experience of the children who took them. As health researchers, the use of photovoice allowed us to ensure the participation of an otherwise voiceless group of children in research concerning their needs and experiences. Our study suggests that photovoice and other visual and sensory methods may be valuable tools for researchers in determining the acceptability and social validity of interventions used for people with ASD in education, public health, and social policy.

Notes

1. Originally the criteria for inclusion of children with ASD in this study were those who received official diagnosis of ASD from paediatricians or psychologists. However, because the diagnosis of ASD only began in the early 2000s in Vietnam, many teenagers have never received a formal diagnosis of ASD by paediatricians. In our study, three teenagers had not received a formal diagnosis, but have been considered autistic by international experts who have come to Vietnam and met them, as well as by and their parents.
2. What do you See here? What is really Happening? How does this relate to Our lives? Why does this problem or strength exist? What can we Do about it?

Acknowledgements

We also thank Paul Zeter for his guidance on photovoice, colleagues at the Center for Creative Initiatives in Health and Population (CCIHP), and Hanoi Club of parents of children with ASD for their support during fieldwork, Maxine Whittaker and Sylvia Rodger for their advice and inputs. Most of all, we thank the children with ASD in Hanoi and their parents for their invaluable contribution in this project. The observations and conclusions herein are those of the authors and do not represent CCIHP, the University of Queensland or the Organization for Autism Research.

Disclosure statement

No potential conflict of interest was reported by the authors.

Funding

This research received support from the Australian government through International Postgraduate Research Scholarships, the University of Queensland through UQadvance, and the Organization for Autism Research through Graduate Student Grants.

References

Altiere, M. J., & von Kluge, S. (2009). Searching for acceptance: Challenges encountered while raising a child with autism. *Journal of Intellectual and Development Disability, 34*(2), 142–152. doi:10.1080/13668250902845202

American Psychiatric Association (APA). (2013). *Diagnostic and statistical manual of mental disorders* (5th ed.). Arlington, VA: Author.

Bell, P. (2001). Content analysis of visual images. In T. V. Leeuwen & C. Jewitt (Eds.), *Handbook of visual analysis* (pp. 10–34). London: Sage.

Bell, S. (2010). Visual methods for collecting and analysing data. In I. Bourgeault, R. Dingwall, & R. De Vries (Eds.), *The Sage handbook of qualitative methods in health research* (pp. 513–535). London: Sage.

Bishop, J., Robillard, L., & Moxley, D. (2013). Linda's story through photovoice: Achieving independent living with dignity and ingenuity in the face of environmental inequities. *Practice: Social Work in Action, 25*(5), 297–315. doi:10.1080/09503153.2013.860091

Bock, A., Isermann, H., & Knieper, T. (2011). Quantitative content analysis of the visual. In E. Margolis & L. Pauwels (Eds.), *The Sage handbook of visual research method* (pp. 265–282). London: Sage.

Cabassa, L., Nicasio, A., & Whitley, R. (2013). Picturing recovery: A photovoice exploration of recovery dimensions among people with serious mental illness. *Psychiatric Services, 64*(9), 837–842. doi:10.1176/appi.ps.201200503

Carnahan, C. R. (2006). Photovoice: Engaging children with autism and their teachers. *Teaching Exceptional Children, 39*(2), 44–50.

Catalani, C., & Minkler, M. (2010). Photovoice: A review of the literature in health and public health. *Health Education & Behavior, 37*(3), 424–451. doi:10.1177/1090198109342084

Giacomini, M. (2010). Theory matters in qualitative health research. In I. Bourgeault, R. Dingwall, & R. De Vries (Eds.), *The Sage handbook of qualitative methods in health research* (pp. 125–156). London: Sage.

Giang, N. H. (2012). *Study on screening autism by M-CHAT 23, epidemiological and clinical features of ASD, and early intervention for young children with ASD* (Unpublished doctoral dissertation). Hanoi Medical University, Hanoi, Vietnam.

Ha, V.S., 2014. *Understanding Autism spectrum disorder in Hanoi, Vietnam* (Doctoral Dissertation). The University of Queensland, Brisbane, Australia.

Ha, V. S., Whittaker, A., Whittaker, M., & Rodger, S. (2014). Living with of autism spectrum disorder in Hanoi, Vietnam. *Social Science & Medicine, 120,* 278–285. doi:10.1016/j.socscimed.2014.09.038

Hergenrather, K. C., Rhodes, S. D., Cowan, C. A., Bardhoshi, G., & Pula, S. (2009). Photovoice as community-based participatory research: A qualitative review. *American Journal of Health Behavior, 33*(6), 686–698. doi:10.5993/ajhb.33.6.6

Hodgdon, L. (1995). *Visual strategies for improving communication: Practical supports for school & home.* Troy, MI: Quirk Roberts.

Howlin, P. (2005). Outcomes in autism spectrum disorders. In F. R. Volkmar, R. Paul, A. Klin, & D. Cohen (Eds.), *Handbook of autism and pervasive developmental disorders* (pp. 201–220). Hoboken, NJ: John Wiley and Sons.

Jurkowski, J. (2008). Photovoice as participatory action research tool for engaging people with intellectual disabilities in research and program development. *Intellectual and Developmental Disabilties, 46*(1), 1–11. doi:10.1352/0047-6765(2008)46[1:PAPART]2.0.CO;2

Koch, T., & Kralik, D. (2006). *Participatory action research in health care.* Oxford: Blackwell.

Lal, S., Jarus, T., & Suto, M. J. (2012). A scoping review of the photovoice method: Implications for occupational therapy research. *Canadian Journal of Occupational Therapy, 79*(3), 181–190. doi:10.2182/cjot.2012.79.3.8

Minh, Q. T. (2011). *Activities of department of psychiatry, national hospital of pediatrics in assessment and treatment for children with ASD.* Training on ASD for staff of Department of Psychiatry. Hanoi: Khoa tâm bệnh.

Obrusnikova, I., & Cavalier, A. (2011). Perceived barriers and facilitators of participation in after-school physical activity by children with autism spectrum disorders. *Journal of Developmental and Physical Disabilities, 23*(3), 195–211. doi:10.1007/s10882-010-9215-z

Photovoice. (2012). *Picture that* [Blog]. Retrieved from http://www.photovoice.org/blog/article/bromley-workshop-working-with-young-people-with-autism-and-aspergers

Photovoice Australia. (2012). *Life as it is with aspergers* [Blog]. Retrieved from http://photovoiceaustralia.blogspot.com.au/

Povee, K., Bishop, B., & Roberts, L. (2014). The use of photovoice with people with intellectual disabilities: Reflections, challenges and opportunities. *Disability & Society, 29*(6). doi:10.1080/09687599.2013.874331

Wang, C., & Burris, M. (1997). Photovoice: Concept, methodology, and use for participatory needs assessment. *Health Education & Behavior, 24*(3), 369–387.

Wang, C., Yi, W. K., Tao, Z. W., & Carovano, K. (1998). Photovoice as a participatory health promotion strategy. *Health Promotion International, 13*(1), 75–86. doi:10.1093/heapro/13.1.75

Wong, C., Odom, S., Hume, L., Cox, K., Fettig, A. X., Kucharczyk, A., & Schultz, T. R. (2014). *Evidence-based practices for children, youth, and young adults with autism spectrum disorder.* Chapel Hill: University of North Carolina, Frank Porter Graham Child Development Institute: Autism Evidence-Based Practice Review Group.

Ying, K. C., Browne, G., Hutchinson, M., Cashin, A., & Binh, B. V. (2012). Autism in Vietnam: The case for the development and evaluation of an information book to be distributed at the time of diagnosis. *Issues in Mental Health Nursing, 33*(5), 288–292. doi:10.3109/01612840.2011.653039

Growing healthy children and communities: Children's insights in Lao People's Democratic Republic

Mónica Ruiz-Casares[a,b,c]

[a]Department of Psychiatry, McGill University, Montreal, Canada; [b]Centre for Research on Children and Families, McGill University, Montreal, Canada; [c]SHERPA-Institut Universitaire, Centre Intégré Universitaire de Santé et de Services Sociaux du Centre-Ouest-de-l'île-de-Montréal, Montreal, Canada

ABSTRACT

A diverse group of 103 children aged 7–11 years old living in family and residential care in rural and urban settings in two northern provinces in Lao People's Democratic Republic participated in group discussions using images and community mapping. Children's identified sources of risk and protection illustrate primary public health and protection concerns and resources. Young children worried about lack of hygiene, unintentional injuries, corporal punishment, and domestic violence. They also expressed concern about gambling and children sleeping in the streets, even if they had never seen any of the latter in their communities. In contrast, food and shelter; artistic, religious, and cultural practices; supportive interpersonal relationships; and schooling largely evoked feelings of safety and belonging. Images that prompted conflicting interpretations surfaced individual and contextual considerations that nuanced analysis. Researchers and decision-makers will benefit from using this developmentally appropriate, context-sensitive child-centred visual method to elicit young children's views of risk and protection. It may also serve as a tool for public health education. Involving young children in the initial selection of images would further enhance the efficiency of the method.

Introduction

Over the last 25 years, the Lao People's Democratic Republic (from now on 'Laos') has steadily improved in a number of human development indicators and also taken up the commitment to advance the well-being and interests of children by adopting the UN Convention on the Rights of the Child (UNCRC). Ratified by Laos in 1991, the UNCRC provides that children have the right to express their views and be involved in decision-making in matters that affect them, according to their own maturity (Art. 12). Not only may children's input improve the effectiveness of interventions (Aldiss, Horstman, O'Leary, Richardson, & Gibson, 2009; Cavet & Sloper, 2004; Davies & Wright, 2008), but it may also increase children's safety and well-being (Rampazzo & Twahirwa, 2010; Vis, Strandbu, Holtan, & Thomas, 2011). In the context of research more specifically, effective participation is needed to accurately understand how children perceive the world that surrounds them. Listening to children as an 'active process of communication' involving co-construction of meaning by means beyond the spoken word is 'a necessary stage in participation in daily routines as well as in wider decision-making processes' (Clark, 2005, p. 491). Researchers need to be aware, however, that children may chose not to participate in research and that a better understanding of children's perspectives may be used to further control children (Clark & Moss, 2001). Despite these potential pitfalls of listening, better understanding children's views can lead to increased support for children interests and well-being (Dockett & Perry, 2005).

Nonetheless, children's participation in service development and public decision-making is limited (Powell & Smith, 2009). This is often the case with young children (Aubrey & Dahl, 2006; Clark, 2005; Jacquez, Vaughn, & Wagner, 2013), despite children's frequent willingness to participate in research (Woolfson, Heffernan, Paul, & Brown, 2010). Involving children in research must be undertaken in ways that ensure ethical practice, facilitate communication, and balance power relations (Cousins & Milner, 2006; Ruiz-Casares & Thompson, 2014). Child-focused visual research methods hold the potential to adapt to a child's development level and to promote children's active involvement while also reducing adult–child power disparities and increasing the validity of findings (Clark-Ibáñez, 2004; Hunleth, 2011; Whiting, 2009). Images, for example, have been successfully used in interviews with young children (Aubrey & Dahl, 2006; Sharples, Davison, Thomas, & Rudman, 2003). To study risk and protective factors in a group setting in the Republic of Liberia, Ruiz-Casares, Rousseau, Morlu, and Browne (2013) developed a methodology consisting of children's iterative selection and discussion of locally relevant, pre-selected images by researchers. This facilitated the surfacing of divergent views and interpretations among and within participants. The present study adapted this methodology to the Northern Lao socio-economic and cultural context (see Methods section) and added a mapping component to engage with young children in the identification of factors affecting risk and well-being in their communities. Recruitment procedures differed across studies.

With a population of a little over 6.5 million people, Laos is a landlocked country in Southeast Asia with a largely rural (63.5%) population (UN, 2014). Over one-third (35%) of the population is under 15 years old and primary school enrolment and completion rates (96% and 95%, respectively) are high (UN, 2014; World Bank, 2014). The country is home to 49 distinct ethnic groups (Lao Statistics Bureau, 2005), and predominant Buddhism coexists with animism (Dommen, Lafont, Osborne, Silverstein, & Zasloff, 2013). Despite rapid economic and human development in the last two decades, the country ranks 138 out of 187 in the 2012 Human Development Index and 100 out of 148 countries in the 2012 Gender Inequality Index (UNDP, 2013). Widespread poverty and inequities still prevail (UNDP, 2007), thus accentuating health disparities and public health challenges (Chongsuvivatwong et al., 2011; WHO, 2014). Chronic child malnutrition particularly among ethnic minority groups (Annim & Imai, 2014; Kamiya, 2011; Sa et al., 2013), inadequate housing, and access to potable water and sanitation infrastructure (Desai, Sinclair, Rawson, & Gamboa, 2013; Haines et al., 2013), particularly in rural, mountainous areas, are among the main challenges that the population currently faces. Unexploded ordnance from the Second Indochina War (a.k.a. Vietnam War) (Durham & Hoy, 2013), unsafe road practices (Ichikawa, Nakahara, Phommachanh, Mayxay, &

Kimura, 2013), and violent discipline (Save the Children, 2012) have also been documented and contribute to the increasing burden of injuries and disability.

This manuscript describes empirical evidence gathered with primary school-going children within the context of a larger project focused on alternative care in two provinces in Northern Laos – Luang Prabang and Xayabury. Specifically, this study used images and maps to actively engage young children in the discussion of their daily routines and their perceptions of risk and protection in their communities. Young children's perspectives are often not elicited in programme planning and evaluation. Their voices are particularly absent in the academic literature from low- and middle-income settings. This study contributes to redressing that.

Methods

In order to gain a deeper understanding of young children's risk perceptions and to uncover the meanings that children attach to community features that may facilitate or hinder well-being, this study used two visual methods, namely photo-elicitation and community mapping. These were complemented with oral discussions about children's daily routines and sources of support. Photo-elicitation is a research method that incorporates images in the interview process to elicit participants' subjective explanations (Clark, 1999; Harper, 2002). The use of age-appropriate prompts and visual tools has gained recognition in research with children across a range of disciplines as a way to better capture children's attention, ease rapport and balance power differentials with adults, and facilitate sharing complex or emotionally difficult information (Clark-Ibáñez, 2004; Pyle, 2013; Zartler & Richter, 2014). Photo-elicitation also gives researchers 'privileged access to the child's world, as the child frames it' (Clark, 2011, p. 165), thus holding the potential for allowing hidden and non-normative perspectives to surface. Whether the images are pre-selected by the researchers (as in the current study) or generated by participants themselves, photo-elicitation is a method that allows for cultural sensitivity since visual prompts can be adapted to children's specific environments and settings (Ruiz-Casares et al., 2013).

Similarly, community mapping is a method to identify community-based needs and resources in a way that is sensitive to socio-cultural contexts (Ordoñez-Jasis & Jasis, 2011). Community mapping as a research method has been used by urban planners, sociologists, educators, and other professionals to gain a better understanding of community assets and needs, particularly when the experiences of community members are taken into consideration (Cadag & Gaillard, 2012; Ordoñez-Jasis & Myck-Wayne, 2012; Tindle, Leconte, Buchanan, & Taymans, 2005). Research has shown how child-made community maps provide valuable insights into children's everyday environments and can facilitate discussion within the context of a group (Hart, 1997; Wridt, 2010). Together, these methods advance an ecological understanding of children's lives.

Data collection procedures

Eleven group discussions were conducted in Luang Prabang and Xayabury provinces in January 2013. Overall, 103 children aged 7–11 years old ($\mu = 9$, range = 8–13 participants per group), including 49 boys and 54 girls participated. Three group discussions were conducted with children ($n = 33$) in residential settings (2 ethnic boarding schools (EBS) and 1 orphanage) situated in the provincial capital towns; the rest involved children ($n = 70$) living in family settings in a balanced number of rural and urban locations in each province. It was expected that risk and safety concerns would vary across these groups as a result of different geographical locations/surroundings, living conditions and mobility (e.g. residential care facilities were situated in urban/peri-urban settings; had separate kitchen, bathroom facilities, and covered wells; and set stricter limits to the mobility of children outside of the orphanage buildings and compound).

Village and neighbourhood authorities were approached to obtain approval for conducting the study in the community and to gain assistance with recruitment. The purpose of the study and the profile of participants that we aimed to recruit were explained in detail. Our goal was to convene a balanced group of boys and girls aged 7–11 years who represented the diversity of the community in terms of ethno-cultural background, levels of physical ability, and family composition, with preference for children from different households to maximise diversity of views and experiences. Village/neighbourhood authorities held a community meeting to advertise the study and identify willing participants (parents and children). Although the team was accompanied to each village/neighbourhood by a district government official, following government regulations, they were not present in any of the discussions with young children.

Group discussions were conducted in community centres and school premises during out-of-school time and lasted on average two hours. No teachers or other community adults were present. All group discussions took place in Lao and were managed by local research team members, who were male and female child protection professionals and university students experienced in working with young children (Krueger & Casey, 2009). Both facilitators and note takers (one of each per session) were trained in advance and Topic Guides were developed to facilitate discussion and note-taking. For data collection, this study adapted to the Lao context the method used by Ruiz-Casares et al. (2013) (i.e. discussion of daily routines followed by photo-elicitation) plus a community mapping exercise. After obtaining informed consent, participants introduced themselves and joined in a local game or song. The Topic Guide explored children's daily routines and identified people, places, and activities that facilitated or hindered healthy child development.

For the second activity, a total of 74 colour photographs and drawings representing positive and negative elements of the natural and social environment that Northern Lao children could easily relate to were used. They included settings and individuals across a range of ethnicities, age groups, sex, and wealth/living conditions. These images were obtained from websites that are open and available to the public, thus inferring that consent had been originally obtained from the individuals and places portrayed. No attempts were made to anonymise individuals or places; no names or text was attached to the images either (Wiles et al., 2008). Local and international research team members critically reviewed the selected images to ensure that they captured primary local public health and child welfare risks and that they were culturally appropriate. This dialogue was particularly important because both researchers and participants contribute to the construction of social reality, and there are many unconscious ways in which researchers may influence their selection of images (e.g. gender, ethnicity, or class) (Harper, 2004; Pink, 2003) and political, social, and cultural contexts may influence how data will be interpreted (Pink, 2013).

During the group discussions, all images were extended on a flat surface (table or floor mat) and children were first asked to select one that represented something that made them feel safe and, then later, unsafe. Including all images on both rounds allowed to surface conflicting interpretations of the same images. After each round, children showed and explained to the group their choices, thus allowing facilitators to validate interpretations among participants. All images were numbered in the back to facilitate note-taking.

After taking a short break, children were given a large white sheet of paper, colour markers, pencils, and paper clippings. All children in each group worked collaboratively to draw a map of their community, starting with roads and natural features and then identifying key buildings, family residences, and places where children like or dislike to go. They were free to use paper clippings or to draw features themselves – in fact, all maps contained a combination of both. Whereas some children were very forthcoming drawing different community features directly in the large sheet of paper, others preferred to colour paper clippings and later glue them to the map. Facilitators respected each child's preferred level of participation and followed up with probes to understand the meaning of these different locations and why children had selected to include them.

Daily research team meetings were held to reflectively debrief on and plan data collection activities and to identify emerging themes and patterns; notes were taken during those meetings. Children did not participate in these sessions, which usually took place in the evenings. Permission to access the communities was obtained from central and provincial government officials before approaching village/neighbourhood officials, families, and directors from residential institutions. Informed consent was obtained from parents/caregivers and children before all group discussions. The SC Child Safeguarding Policy was adopted by all research team members, although no incident was reported that required its use. Refreshments were provided during the group discussions. Permission to undertake the study was granted by the National University of Laos. Ethics approval was obtained from McGill University and the Centre de Santé et de Services Sociaux de la Montagne (Canada). An ad hoc Advisory Committee comprised of researchers and representatives from child-oriented organisations (UNICEF and international non-governmental organizations) was convened in Vientiane to ensure contextual appropriateness of research design and procedures.

Data analysis

All images were numbered before data collection and numbers noted to keep track of participants' comments. A table-type form developed for note-taking allowed ongoing analysis of results by documenting, for each selected image, individual children's comments as well agreement/disagreement in interpretation by other children in the group. An Excel database was used to keep track of participants and locations. Notes from group discussions were typed in a word processor and translated into English using a similar table, substituting photo-numbers with the actual images (embedded in the text) and brief descriptive captions to facilitate comparison of images with their corresponding verbal explanations. Notes taken at daily team meetings and memos written during fieldwork were included in the analysis. Reflective journaling was kept throughout data collection and analysis by the primary researcher. Content analysis was manually performed by one researcher at two points in time on all notes (Schreier, 2014). To surface the different meanings assigned by children to each image as a representation of risk or well-being, our analysis moved back and forth between each image and the commentaries that it evoked across all groups. Through comparing and contrasting, similar descriptions of images were grouped. These groupings were later combined into broader, conceptual public health categories. Special attention was paid to images and narrative data representing co-occurrence of both safe and unsafe categories (Miles, Huberman, & Saldaña, 2014). Illustrative notes from the group discussions are used to show children's representations of public health and child development themes.

Results

Children's image selections, drawn maps, and description of daily tasks illustrated the prominence of the following public health and child development issues and resources (Table 1).

Food and nutrition

Children were first invited to orally describe their daily routines and responsibilities. Upon waking up in the morning (sometime between 4:00 and 6:00 am), children in family-based care described going to find food with their parents and/or 'steaming sticky rice and

Table 1. Child-selected representations of public health and child development issues by domain and theme of visual tool.

Domain	Theme	Safe	Unsafe
Food and nutrition	Breastfeeding	✓	
	Animal husbandry	✓	✓
	Cultivation	✓	
	Cooked food	✓	
	Meal sharing		✓
Housing and environmental conditions	Dirt/garbage		✓
	Washing oneself (hands/body)	✓	
	Housing	✓	✓
Physical activity	Sports	✓	
	Games	✓	✓
	Chores/work	✓	✓
Culture, religion, and education practices	Alms giving ceremony	✓	
	Soukhouan or Baci ceremony	✓	
	'Traditional' clothing	✓	
	'Traditional' festival	✓	
	Music & dance	✓	
	Schooling	✓	
Relationships			
Supportive	Loving family	✓	✓
	Friends/Peers	✓	
Interpersonal violence	Domestic fights		✓
	Corporal punishment (home/school)		✓
Unintentional injuries	Road accidents	*	✓
	Fear of drowning in river		✓
	Sunburn	**	✓
Illicit behaviours	Video games & gambling		✓
	Child detention		✓
	Alcohol (ab)use		✓
	Waking up late		✓

Notes: List contains only images selected by participants and not the full set of images presented to them. Asterisks indicate confusion in the interpretation of images representing children living in the street (*) and one infant covering face with both arms (**).

feeding the duck and chicken' before washing up, having breakfast, and going to school. Fishing and harvesting vegetables was appreciated as 'fun' and something that can be done with friends, particularly in the EBSs. Indeed, children in EBSs explained how a rotation system allowed several students to earn some cash by cultivating a small plot of land or orchard on the school premises and selling the produce to the cooks of the institution, who in turn used it to feed all students. Female household members (grandmother, mother, sister, child herself if ≥10 years of age at home and teachers in EBSs) were described to do most of the cooking. There was variation in terms of cooking ingredients. According to children living with their families, breakfast usually included 'grilled fish, boiled chicken, and chilli sauce', 'coconut milk with sauce soup, condiments, and hard-boiled egg', or 'sauce, meat, vegetables, pork, and birds'. In the orphanage, children described having 'condiment and egg with sticky rice' for breakfast. Children in EBSs indicated not always having breakfast, but sometimes eating sticky rice cake or (donated) bread. For lunch (noon) and dinner (5:00–6:00 p.m.), however, they had vegetable soup, chicken, pork, or fish. Children in family-based care described having rice porridge, noodle soup, condiments, meat, and fish for lunch and dinner. At the orphanage, 'fried greens, meat, and fish' were provided for lunch and dinner 'but it might change to non-glutinous rice' for the latter.

Images, including several representing edible goods and eating behaviour, were next presented to children. Images of a woman breastfeeding a baby, an orchard, cultivation, and bowls containing cooked dishes unanimously evoked feelings of safety. 'I like eating', explained one child, 'because it makes me full and grow well and healthy'. Two other children, upon selecting one of the food images, indicated wanting to eat 'because at home we do not have food'. In contrast, an image of a cock generated a twofold interpretation – while for some it was as a positive source of 'food for people', for others it represented danger and concern 'because the chicken droppings in front of the house don't leave place for playing and dance'. The use of images representing animals and their environment paired with the iterative use of the same set of images to identify sources of risk and safety allowed surfacing dual, less normative interpretations such as this one. Another link of food and play occurred with the image of a water buffalo in a rice field – 'I like to do the rice field' and 'I love to ride the buffalo!' were expressions used by participants. An image of a group of children eating with their hands from the same pot was interpreted as a source of danger. Children in residential care made their selections out of concern for lack of 'unity' or of hygiene – '[They are] eating so dirty!' Thus, two public health issues (i.e. violence prevention and sanitation) were evoked.

Housing, hygiene, and environmental conditions

Consistently, through the description of daily activities and physical spaces as well as the selection of images and mapping of the community, children stated disliking garbage and bad smells. They also acknowledged having 'a lot of rubbish at home' – 'I don't like dirty [places]. It is easy to get a disease', said one child in Luang Prabang. In this line, children in family-based and residential care mentioned, among their daily early morning routines, taking a shower or bath, cleaning the dorm (EBS), and washing clothes, cups, and dishes. On their community maps (Figure 1), children also drew 'many trees and beautiful forest' surrounding their villages/neighbourhoods as well as other elements that

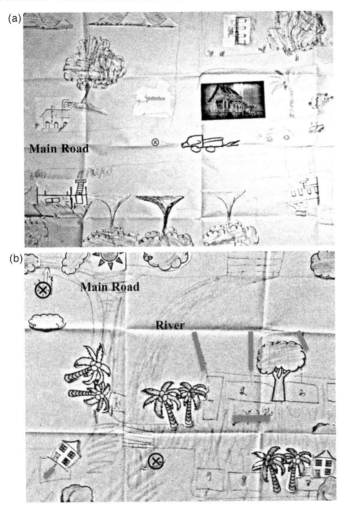

Figure 1. Children's maps indicating dangerous places in their communities (⊗).

contributed to making them feel safe. Among those, the provincial hospital and local clinics, primary and/or secondary schools, Buddhist temples, and safe recreational spaces.

During the initial discussion about daily routines and supports, children indicated how sleeping on mats and sharing sleeping quarters with parents, grandparents, and siblings or, in the case of EBSs, with up to 20 other children in the room, was common. Less frequently, a few children also described sleeping alone. In the orphanage, where there were about two to five boys or girls per bedroom, each child had a bed with a mattress and linen. To complement these descriptions, fear of falling from bunk beds (EBS) and overcrowding were expressed during photo-elicitation. For example, while describing why an image showing several children in bunk beds in the same bedroom represented risk, one child in Luang Prabang said that 'sleeping with many people is uncomfortable. I don't like to sleep with many people ... I breathe with difficulty'. Images of 'traditional' housing structures sometimes triggered feelings of homesickness for children living in residential care.

Physical activity

Football, volleyball, rattan ball, basketball, and dancing (including participation in community (dance) clubs) were common physical activities that children engaged in both EBSs and family-based settings. Gender differences were noted such as boys playing football and girls playing jumping rope, tamarind seed, or Lao dance; some boys were said to enjoy Lao dance, too. Play time was often a time to socialise with friends and the community, which triggered positive feelings in children. In the words of a participant in Luang Prabang: 'I like the dance image because [when we] go to dance to the city, it is joyful and there are many people. We dance on Teacher's Day.' Children were, nonetheless, aware of the risks involved in some games and sports. For example, one child explained not liking to play leapfrog[1] because of fear 'of [feeling] pain [or] getting hurt'.

Children in EBSs indicated exercising first thing in the morning, upon waking up. Some of them also engaged in cultivation activities, as mentioned earlier. Children living in family-based care described participating in household tasks such as going to fetch water or wood, feeding the animals, cooking, or cleaning up. 'What I love the most', said one participant in Luang Prabang, 'is to collect cane wood to sell'.[2] However, an image of children carrying a big load of firewood on their heads generated negative feelings among participants 'because it is heavy and [causes] pain'. This was a common practice in many communities, particularly among poorer families, and 'indirectly' stimulated some children 'to study hard for a good grade' so that they could improve their future prospects. The discussion that ensued also surfaced other risks when carrying out daily chores. For example, one child shared feeling afraid of an accident when 'children are sent to buy food', often linked to road traffic accidents (see below).

Culture, religion, and education practices

A number of local festivities, objects, and practices were mentioned among the things that contribute to children's well-being, including Baci ceremony, elephant festival, boat racing festival and Lao New Year, to name a few. Ethnic wear and customary practices were praised as 'beautiful' and familiar, even if on occasion they might trigger feelings of nostalgia. One child in an EBS, for example, selected as positive the image of the Lao wind instrument (Khen Hmong) 'because we always see it when we go back home'. As with games and sports, schooling, religious festivities, and community gatherings offered a space for social interaction with relatives and community members that children appreciated: 'I feel happy. It is beautiful to see, because I [too] gave alms with my mother.'[3]

Positive and negative relationships

Among the things that make children feel safe are caring relationships with grandparents and elderly people, other family members and friends. Images of multi-generational families and of adults hugging or showing affection to children were selected among the protective factors, even if one child indicated that an image of an elderly woman embracing young children made him unhappy 'because [he] saw older people sick'. Children in residential care described how teachers and children alike took care of each other, plus on occasion there was a nurse in the institution who cared for children when they were sick.

In contrast, parents yelling and hitting children was mentioned in one group as the thing they liked the least of their community. In children's words, not only can fighting between parents 'make children suffer' but also if each parent pulls the child in different directions 'it can break the arm [of the child]' or 'make the child to be orphan and once again be afraid of the child's pain'. In fact, the use of corporal punishment was widely reported. According to one of the participants: 'In my family, my parents teach me to be a good person. If I am not obedient or I am lazy, my father will hit me but they don't hit hard because they worry that I am in pain.' Other children, however, described some parents beating their children hard. Fighting among peers, particularly boys, was also identified as source of risk.

Unintentional injuries

Safety concerns were present in rural and urban areas, mostly around roads and water sources. Constantly, children marked the 'edge of the big road' on their maps as a place of danger. Reflecting on their drawings (Figure 1), children explained how 'children play close to the road, in the village/neighbourhood ground, in the patty field and near the river. The close road and deep river are dangerous locations for children'. Images of children running, playing, or sleeping on the road, were selected as representing risk – 'If I saw this [children sleeping in the street] I would be afraid because an accident can cause me to be disabled' or dead, commented children in Xayabury. For this reason, children in the orphanage explained how they were not allowed to go outside of the fence and when they did have to go out, they first needed to get permission from the orphanage staff.[4] Similarly, children in an EBS indicated that when they went into the forest to pick up fruits or to hunt birds, an adult would accompany a group of four to five children and that they had to 'be back in the dormitory at the right time because of safety'. It was not clear, though, whether children were also alluding to other risks. Several children living in family-based care indicated walking to school by themselves, or sometimes with friends, though they volunteered no safety incident.

Another dangerous space was around water. 'I do not like to play in the river. I am afraid I will fall from the boat. Some children have dropped in the river [in this community]', said a child in Xayabury upon selecting an image of children on a rowboat. Although some children enjoyed playing at the waterfront and admitted to sometimes going there by themselves if there was no 'adult to go with', fear of rivers and 'deep waters' was pervasive. Awareness of the danger of drowning was present in a child's description of frequent activities he liked to engage in, and which included 'playing near my house and (…) swimming with my friend and an adult'.

Children also showed awareness about sun safety. Children interpreted an image of an infant alone with his arms protecting his face as a sign of protection against sunburn and, to a lesser extent, against violence. In the words of participants from Xayabury, 'It [standing outdoors] is not good for health' and 'I feel afraid that someone will hit me because I am alone and I worry that I will be ill because I was standing under sunlight.'

Illicit activities

One last set of images selected by children to represent risk exemplified socially undesirable behaviours such as gambling, playing videogames during school hours, alcohol abuse, or child detention. Gambling was despised 'because it is illegal and causes debt'. One child in Xayabury further explained: 'I saw many people playing cards in the house where I was born. I am afraid of police arrest.' Fear of confronting the police in this context was shared in group discussions in Luang Prabang, as well. An image of children in school uniform playing videogames, a common occurrence in several communities, triggered negative reactions for a variety of reasons. According to children, not only did this behaviour interfere with children's school performance but it could also affect their eyesight and well-being. One child in Xayabury explained: 'I feel unhappy because I am afraid of electrical shock and I [also] worry that children are not going to school and so the learning is lost.' Alcohol use was also a matter of concern. As one child in residential care in Xayabury put it: 'drinking more to get drunk is not good for health and it is dangerous for driving. [It also] creates family disputes'. Finally, although children had not seen other children in detention, some nonetheless selected an image of a child behind bars as an illustration of risk because, as one of them eloquently explained, 'I am afraid not to see my parents [again].'

Discussion

Findings of this study show how children in Luang Prabang and Xayabury identified sources of risk and protection in their communities by means of selecting images, drawing community maps, and reflecting on the rationale for their choices. Overall, images depicting garbage or suggesting absence of hygiene, unintentional (fatal) injuries, violence, old age, and illicit behaviours were selected as representations of risk or illness. In contrast, artistic, religious, and cultural practices; supportive interpersonal relationships; and schooling were seen as safe. Finally, a few images elicited conflicting interpretations across children.

Children's concerns with lack of hygiene and road traffic accidents clearly illustrate public health's concern with injury and disease prevention in the home and daily lives. This is not surprising considering morbidity and mortality associated to infectious diseases and road traffic accidents in Laos (WHO, 2013, 2014). In 2011, for example, a high percentage of the rural population had no access to sanitation facilities (52%) or improved drinking-water sources (37%) (WHO, 2014). The selection of an image representing several children eating with their hands from the same dish as a source of risk contradicts 'traditional' eating practices in the country,[5] yet corroborates concern over inadequate hand-washing practices. Between 1990 and 2009, the number of crash fatalities increased sixfold, mostly as a result of head trauma of motorcycle riders (Global Road Safety Partnership, 2014). In consequence, disability prevention and rehabilitation with a focus on road traffic accidents and violence, prevention and control of communicable diseases, and access to safe water and sanitation are currently among the strategic priorities for cooperation between WHO and Laos (2014). Less frequently selected, yet still common among participants were concerns of violence and physical punishment, which children admitted occurred in their communities. Indeed, recent findings of the Lao Social

Indicator Survey (MoH & LSB, 2012) show that 76% of children aged 2–14 years experience some form of violent discipline method at home and 42% of adults believe that physical punishment is necessary to properly raise a child. Health and child welfare professionals increasingly agree on the need to support parents 'in learning nonviolent, effective approaches to discipline' (Durrant & Ensom, 2012). There is, however, a gap in the scholarly literature about social and cultural norms in regards to parenting as well as help-seeking behaviours in Laos. A better understanding of circumstances surrounding and resulting from the use of violence as well as how it is handled within families and communities across socio-cultural groups is needed to inform effective courses of action.

In contrast with other domains, representations of artistic expression, religious ceremonies, and customary practices did not generate any ambivalence among participants. Children unanimously assessed images of Buddhist monks, novices and the alms giving ceremonies (a practice particularly visible in Luang Prabang) as protective. Similarly, Baci and Soukhouan ceremonies are practiced throughout Laos in very diverse circumstances, from physical or psychological illness of a family member to major life transitions such as a marriage or birth of a new child. Most notably, Baci is believed to transmit best wishes for good health and recovery, as well as personal and professional prosperity. Ceremonies also offer an opportunity for people to get together and celebrate around food, dance, and music (Thammavongsa, 2014). Children's appreciation of social time in a dirt-free setting (as illustrated by the ambivalent reactions to an image of a cock, an animal that soils the yard) highlight the importance of creating and maintaining safe spaces for children to play, develop, and express themselves. Safe play spaces have shown to increase the time that children spend outdoors and being physically active in other settings (Farley et al., 2007). In so doing, children's views of what a 'safe space' entails (i.e. absence of animal droppings, far from the road, and open water sources) need to be taken into consideration by urban planners, teachers, community leaders, and those who manage playgrounds.

Findings from this study provide evidence of the usefulness of visual images in the manner hereby described as a diagnostic and an education tool. On the one hand, images serve to elicit young children's views of elements in their environment that facilitate or hinder well-being. Participants in our study visibly enjoyed the process and were able to articulate abstract concepts and to provide detailed descriptions by using images. Children were often drawn towards images that represented their own ethno-cultural group, thus underlining the need to contextualise images to facilitate young children's participation. On the other, considering the easiness of discussing the content of the images, this shows potential as a tool for public health education. For example, images can be used to explain the difference between minor bruises, such as those that may occur while playing, and major injuries resulting from a road accident. Although some searchable online image libraries exist to this end (e.g. http://www.cdc.gov/healthyplaces/images.htm), these are not always accessible, representative of all cultural groups and settings, or used in contextually appropriate educational applications. The flexibility of the method applied in this study to adapt to different social and cultural contexts is one of its strengths in global research. Rendering existing and future images accessible through free, open-access sites and supporting their integration into public health campaigns for specific contexts requires the attention of researchers and decision-makers. Researchers will first need to assess the appropriateness of using visual methods and also how to carry them out in a particular cultural environment, as there is evidence that not all societies are pictorial (Clark, 2011).

Involving young children in the selection of the initial set of images may enhance the efficacy of the method, increase the likelihood that a broader variety of images are selected by their peers, and enrich researchers' understanding of children's lived experiences and the environments in which they grow. Similarly, researchers may ponder whether to use cut-outs in map-making to enhance participation at the expense of surfacing more nuanced children's views. Ultimately, the purpose is to facilitate ways for young children to contribute to their own communities. There is evidence that 'programs working colla-boratively or achieving shared leadership with a community can lead to behaviour change and cost-effective sustained transformation to improve critical health behaviours and reduce poor health outcomes in low- and middle-income countries' (p. 68) yet children are more often than not considered as part of the desired target group or outcome rather than key actors in effective community mobilisation and participation (Farnsworth et al., 2014).

There are numerous benefits to involving young people and their insights in commu-nity development and planning processes (Driskell, 2002), including in the context of risk prevention and reduction interventions (Mitchell, Haynes, Wei, & Oven, 2008; Tanner, 2010). Incorporating children's perceptions of risk and safety can help develop effective strategies for the promotion of child physical and psychological development as well as risk and injury prevention, for example, in the context of pedestrian and traffic safety (Clancy, Rucklidge, & Owen, 2006). There is evidence that enhancing the neighbourhood social environment and traffic safety (e.g. through the construction of sidewalks and appropriate road signalling) may increase children's independent mobility, physical activity, and outdoor play, particularly for girls and of children with diverse ethno-cultural backgrounds (Aarts, de Vries, van Oers, & Schuit, 2012; Mitra, Faulkner, Buliung, & Stone, 2014). Caretakers also need to provide or make arrangements for close supervision of chil-dren around water at all times to prevent children from drowning (Balaban & Sleet, 2011; Rubio et al., 2015). While some children commented on teachers and other adults accom-panying them to swim in the river, they also admitted to sometimes going there with friends unsupervised. Broader initiatives to support working families (e.g. social policies facilitating access to public childcare) are thus needed as research in low- and middle-income countries has shown that children are more likely to end up unsupervised in families with poor working conditions, low income and education, and limited support networks (Ruiz-Casares & Heymann, 2009). Interventions focused on children's agency and capacity (e.g. to teach children safe water practices and peer protection strategies) are also recommended (Peterson, 1984; Petrass & Blitvich, 2014). Photo-elicitation has proven useful in uncovering children's family routines and distribution of tasks and responsibilities (McCloy, White, Lee Bunting, & Forwell, 2014), information needed for planning health promotion and prevention interventions to ensure adequate child supervision.

Children were not always consistent in the selection and interpretation of images that represent safety or risk. The contrast in the interpretation of the same or similar images not only among children in the same community but also by children in very different countries (Ruiz-Casares et al., 2013) highlights the flexibility of this method and its ability to be adapted to any given setting. This flexibility in turn facilitates the surfacing of context-specific knowledge and perceptions, including the relative importance of selected themes. For example, in contrast with the aforementioned study conducted in Liberia (Ruiz-Casares et al., 2013), no child in our sample selected any image of interpersonal violence as representing a protective factor, nor did any child in Laos interpret abundance of food as a risk factor. While others have highlighted the usefulness of using photos taken by children to challenge adults' prior assumptions (Samuels, 2004), our study showed that a diverse collection of visual prompts selected by the research team can also encourage adults to question their own assumptions.

Some limitations of this work should be noted. First, this study involved children aged 7–11 years old living in family-based and in residential care in Luang Prabang and Xayabury provinces only. Given its cross-sectional, qualitative design, the results of this study cannot be generalised to all children in Laos nor in the participating provinces. Implementation of selection criteria by local authorities in different communities may have resulted in divergent interpretations and, as result, potential exclusion of certain subgroups of children. Despite participation of boys and girls from different ethno-cultural groups, disaggregation of results is not possible to assess differences by group. It is, however, advisable that future studies carefully record and transcribe group discussions to allow for an uncovering of the latent meanings of images and the cultural and historical context from which participants operate. Similarly, the use of cut-outs instead of child-drawn map features may have prevented nuances about children's interpretations of safety and risk from emerging. Lastly, future studies could involve both children and adults in co-creating the images that later become the object of research (Banks, 2014). The use of project-generated images would likely enhance the dissemination of results.

Conclusion

This study presents results of consultation with young children in Northern Laos on elements in their communities that foster or hinder good health and well-being. It contributes to the very limited literature on public health, community development, and children's geographies in Laos, while advancing children's rights and particularly child participation. The use of visual prompts and community mapping can be adapted to the developmental, cultural, and other characteristics of participants and their environment in order to make the process engaging and meaningful for children while generating valid information. Ambivalent interpretations of images of food, living conditions, and physical activity challenge pre-conceived notions of dangerous and protective practices and call for further study to validate these interpretations with a larger group of children. Future studies would benefit from involving children in the initial selection of images and using open-access images to enhance the dissemination of research findings. By researching childhood-based risk perceptions this study put forth children as an information source to be trusted and engaged in child and community development initiatives. Researchers and decision-makers at different levels will benefit from adopting this method with young children and adapting it to their context in order to advance child well-being and promote children's participation.

Notes

1. Leapfrog is a game in which children successively jump over each other's stooped backs by straddling legs wide apart on each side. One image showed a group of children playing leap-frog outdoors.
2. In this context, cane wood is often used to make brooms.
3. The practice of almsgiving in Laos and other Theravada Buddhist contexts allows laypeople the opportunity to pay respects to Buddhist monks, nuns, and novices, and to make merit by providing them with food.
4. Children in orphanage attended the school situated on the same premises so children did not have to leave the fenced area on a daily bases.
5. In Laos, the traditional manner of eating is communal and by hand, with food served in a series of small plates from which all diners take directly with their hands (except liquids).

Acknowledgements

Thank you to all the children who generously contributed their time and ideas and to the research team from the National University of Laos and Save the Children (Laos) for their tireless contribution to data collection. Special gratitude to Chanphet Vongmathep, Soulivong Soukchandy, Souphunsa Xaphan, and Sisouphanh Phommahaxay for their skilful facilitation of group discussions. Thank you also to Cécile Rousseau and Tinka Markham Piper for her input during the preparation of this manuscript.

Disclosure statement

No potential conflict of interest was reported by the author.

Funding

This work was supported by Save the Children (Laos) and Start-Up Research Funds from the Centre de Santé et de Services Sociaux de la Montagne to the author.

References

Aarts, M. J., de Vries, S. I., van Oers, H. A. M., & Schuit, A. J. (2012). Outdoor play among children in relation to neighborhood characteristics: A cross-sectional neighborhood observation study. *The International Journal of Behavioral Nutrition and Physical Activity, 9,* 98–98. doi:10.1186/1479-5868-9-98

Aldiss, S., Horstman, M., O'Leary, C., Richardson, A., & Gibson, F. (2009). What is important to young children who have cancer while in hospital? *Children & Society, 23*(2), 85–98. doi:10.1111/j.1099-0860.2008.00162.x

Annim, S. K., & Imai, K. S. (2014). *Nutritional status of children, food consumption diversity and ethnicity in Lao PDR* (Economics Discussion Paper Series. EDP-1404). Manchester: School of Social Sciences, The University of Manchester.

Aubrey, C., & Dahl, S. (2006). Children's voices: The views of vulnerable children on their service providers and the relevance of services they receive. *British Journal of Social Work, 36*(1), 21–39. doi:10.1093/bjsw/bch249

Balaban, V., & Sleet, D. (2011). Injury prevention. In D. M. Kamat & P. R. Fischer (Eds.), *AAP textbook of global child health* (pp. 321–343). Elk Grove Village, IL: American Academy of Pediatrics.

Banks, M. (2014). Analysing images. In U. Flick (Ed.), *The SAGE handbook of qualitative data analysis* (pp. 394–408). Thousand Oaks, CA: Sage.

Cadag, J. R. D., & Gaillard, J. C. (2012). Integrating knowledge and actions in disaster risk reduction: The contribution of participatory mapping. *Area*, *44*(1), 100–109. doi:10.1111/j.1475-4762.2011.01065.x

Cavet, J., & Sloper, P. (2004). The participation of children and young people in decisions about UK service development. *Child: Care, Health and Development*, *30*(6), 613–621. doi:10.1111/j.1365-2214.2004.00470.x

Chongsuvivatwong, V., Phua, K. H., Yap, M. T., Pocock, N. S., Hashim, J. H., Chhem, R., … Lopez, A. D. (2011). Health and health-care systems in Southeast Asia: Diversity and transitions. *The Lancet*, *377*(9763), 429–437. doi:10.1016/S0140-6736(10)61507-3

Clancy, T. A., Rucklidge, J. J., & Owen, D. (2006). Road-crossing safety in virtual reality: A comparison of adolescents with and without ADHD. *Journal of Clinical Child & Adolescent Psychology*, *35*(2), 203–215. doi:10.1207/s15374424jccp3502_4

Clark, A. (2005). Listening to and involving young children: A review of research and practice. *Early Child Development and Care*, *175*(6), 489–505. doi:10.1080/03004430500131288

Clark, C. D. (1999). The autodriven interview: A photographic viewfinder into children's experience. *Visual Sociology*, *14*(1), 39–50. doi:10.1080/14725869908583801

Clark, C. D. (2011). *In a younger voice: Doing child-centered qualitative research*. New York, NY: Oxford University Press.

Clark-Ibáñez, M. (2004). Framing the social world with photo-elicitation interviews. *American Behavioral Scientist*, *47*(12), 1507–1527. doi:10.1177/0002764204266236

Clark, A., & P. Moss. (2001). *Listening to children: the mosaic approach*. London: National Children's Bureau.

Cousins, W., & Milner, S. (2006). Children's rights: A cross-border study of residential care. *Irish Journal of Psychology*, *37*(1–2), 88–96.

Davies, J., & Wright, J. (2008). Children's voices: A review of the literature pertinent to looked-after children's views of mental health services. *Child and Adolescent Mental Health*, *13*(1), 26–31. doi:10.1111/j.1475-3588.2007.00458.x

Desai, A., Sinclair, R. G. G., Rawson, D. S., & Gamboa, T. (2013). *Building sustainable water and sanitation infrastructure to improve health status of northern Laotians*. American Public Health Association 141st annual meeting and Expo, Boston, MA.

Dockett, S., & Perry, B. (2005). You need to know how to play safe': Children's experiences of starting school. *Contemporary Issues in Early Childhood*, *6*, 4–18. doi:10.2304/ciec.2005.6.1.7

Dommen, A., Lafont, P.-B., Osborne, M. E., Silverstein, J., & Zasloff, J. (2013). Laos. In *Encyclopaedia Britannica*. Retrieved from http://www.britannica.com/place/Laos

Driskell, D. (2002). *Creating better cities with children and youth: A manual for participation*. Paris: UNESCO; London: Earthscan.

Durham, J., & Hoy, D. (2013). Burden of injury from explosive remnants of conflict in Lao PDR and Cambodia. *Asia-Pacific Journal of Public Health*, *25*(2), 124–133. doi:10.1177/1010539513478149

Durrant, J., & Ensom, R. (2012). Physical punishment of children: Lessons from 20 years of research. *Canadian Medical Association Journal*, *184*(12), 1373–1377. doi:10.1503/cmaj.101314

Farley, T. A., Meriwether, R. A., Baker, E. T., Watkins, L. T., Johnson, C. C., & Webber, L. S. (2007). Safe play spaces to promote physical activity in inner-city children: Results from a pilot study of an environmental intervention. *Amercan Journal of Public Health*, *97*(9), 1625–1631. doi:10.2105/AJPH.2006.092692

Farnsworth, S. K., Böse, K., Fajobi, O., Souza, P. P., Peniston, A., Davidson, L. L., … Hodgins, S. (2014). Community engagement to enhance child survival and early development in low- and middle-income countries: An evidence review. *Journal of Health Communication*, *19*(suppl.1), 67–88. doi:10.1080/10810730.2014.941519

Global Road Safety Partnership. (2014). *Laos. Country summary*. Retrieved from http://grsp.drupalgardens.com/what-we-do/geography/asia/laos.

Haines, A., Bruce, N., Cairncross, S., Davies, M., Greenland, K., Hiscox, A., … Wilkinson, P. (2013). Promoting health and advancing development through improved housing in low-income settings. *Journal of Urban Health*, *90*(5), 810–831. doi:10.1007/s11524-012-9773-8

Harper, D. (2002). Talking about pictures: A case for photo elicitation. *Visual Studies, 17*(1), 13–26. doi:10.1080/14725860220137345

Harper, D. (2004). Wednesday-night bowling: Reflections on cultures of a rural working class. In C. Knowles & P. Sweetman (Eds.), *Picturing the social landscape: Visual methods and the sociological imagination* (pp. 93–114). London: Routledge.

Hart, R. A. (1997). *Children's participation. The theory and practice of involving young citizens in community development and environmental care.* New York: UNICEF & London: Earthscan.

Hunleth, J. (2011). Beyond on or with: Questioning power dynamics and knowledge production in 'child-oriented' research methodology. *Childhood, 18*(1), 81–93. doi:10.1177/0907568210371234

Ichikawa, M., Nakahara, S., Phommachanh, S., Mayxay, M., & Kimura, A. (2013). Roadside observation of secondary school students' commuting to school in Vientiane, Laos. *International Journal of Injury Control and Safety Promotion*, 1–5. doi:10.1080/17457300.2013.843570

Jacquez, F., Vaughn, L., & Wagner, E. (2013). Youth as partners, participants or passive recipients: A review of children and adolescents in community-based participatory research (CBPR). *American Journal of Community Psychology, 51*(1–2), 176–189. doi:10.1007/s10464-012-9533-7

Kamiya, Y. (2011). Socioeconomic determinants of nutritional status of children in Lao PDR: Effects of household and community factors. *Journal of Health, Population and Nutrition, 29* (4), 339–348.

Krueger, R., & Casey, M. (2009). *Focus groups: A practical guide for applied research* (4th ed.). Thousand Oaks, CA: Sage.

Lao Statistics Bureau. (2005). *National census – Lao Peoples Democratic Republic.* Vientiane: Lao Statistics Bureau.

McCloy, L., White, S., Lee Bunting, K., & Forwell, S. (2016). Photo-elicitation interviewing to capture Children's perspectives on family routines. *Journal of Occupational Science, 23*(1), 1–14. doi:10.1080/14427591.2014.986666

Miles, M. B., Huberman, A. M., & Saldaña, J. (2014). *Qualitative data analysis: A methods sourcebook* (3rd ed.). London: Sage.

Mitchell, T., Haynes, K., Wei, C., & Oven, K. (2008). The roles of children and youth in communicating disaster risk. *Children, Youth & Environments, 18*(1), 254–279.

Mitra, R., Faulkner, G. E., Buliung, R. N., & Stone, M. R. (2014). Do parental perceptions of the neighbourhood environment influence children's independent mobility? Evidence from Toronto, Canada. *Urban Studies, 51*(16), 3401–3419. doi:10.1177/0042098013519140

MoH, & LSB. (2012). *Lao social indicator survey (LSIS) 2011–12* (Final Report). Vientiane.

Ordoñez-Jasis, R., & Jasis, P. (2011). Mapping literacy, mapping lives: Teachers exploring the sociopolitical context of literacy and learning. *Multicultural Perspectives, 13*(4), 189–196. doi:10.1080/15210960.2011.616824

Ordoñez-Jasis, R., & Myck-Wayne, J. (2012). Community mapping in action: Uncovering resources and assets for young children and their families. *Young Exceptional Children, 15*(3), 31–45. doi:10.1177/1096250612451756

Peterson, L. (1984). Teaching home safety and survival skills to latch-key children: A comparison of two manuals and methods. *Journal of Applied Behavior Analysis, 17*(3), 279–293. doi:10.1901/jaba.1984.17-279

Petrass, L. A., & Blitvich, J. D. (2014). Preventing adolescent drowning: Understanding water safety knowledge, attitudes and swimming ability. The effect of a short water safety intervention. *Accident Analysis & Prevention, 70*(0), 188–194. doi:10.1016/j.aap.2014.04.006.

Pink, S. (2003). Interdisciplinary agendas in visual research: Re-situating visual anthropology. *Visual Studies, 18*(2), 179–192. doi:10.1080/14725860310001632029

Pink, S. (2013). *Doing visual ethnography* (3rd ed.). Thousand Oaks, CA: Sage.

Powell, M. A., & Smith, A. B. (2009). Children's participation rights in research. *Childhood, 16*(1), 124–142. doi:10.1177/0907568208101694

Pyle, A. (2013). Engaging young children in research through photo elicitation. *Early Child Development and Care, 183*(11), 1544–1558. doi:10.1080/03004430.2012.733944

Rampazzo, E., & Twahirwa, A. (2010). *Baseline study. Children's perceptions of child protection measures existing at community level in Rwanda* (Final report). Kigali, Rwanda. Retrieved from http://resourcecentre.savethechildren.se/node/4081

Rubio, B., Yagüe, F., Benítez, M. T., Esparza, M. J., González, J. C., Sánchez, F., ... Mintegi, S. (2015). Recommendations for the prevention of drowning. *Anales de Pediatría* (English Edition), *82*(1), 43.e1. doi:10.1016/j.anpede.2014.06.002.

Ruiz-Casares, M., & Heymann, J. (2009). Children home alone unsupervised: Modeling parental decisions and associated factors in Botswana, Mexico, and Vietnam. *Child Abuse and Neglect*, *33*(5), 312–323. doi:10.1016/j.chiabu.2008.09.010

Ruiz-Casares, M., Rousseau, C., Morlu, J., & Browne, C. (2013). Eliciting children's perspectives of risk and protection in Liberia: How to do it and why does it matter? *Child and Youth Care Forum*, *42*(5), 425–437. doi:10.1007/s10566-013-9208-z

Ruiz-Casares, M., & Thompson, J. (2014). Obtaining meaningful informed consent: Preliminary results of a study to develop visual informed consent forms with children. *Children's Geographies*, *14*(1), 35–45. doi:10.1080/14733285.2014.971713

Sa, J. D., Bouttasing, N., Sampson, L., Perks, C., Osrin, D., & Prost, A. (2013). Identifying priorities to improve maternal and child nutrition among the Khmu ethnic group, Laos: A formative study. *Maternal & Child Nutrition*, *9*(4), 452–466. doi:10.1111/j.1740-8709.2012.00406.x

Samuels, J. (2004). Breaking the ethnographer's frames: Reflections on the use of photo elicitation in understanding Sri Lankan monastic culture. *American Behavioral Scientist*, *47*(12), 1528–1550. doi:10.1177/0002764204266238

Save the Children. (2012). *Baseline survey on child protection in Luang Prabang and Sayaboury Provinces, Lao PDR*. Vientiane: Author.

Schreier, M. (2014). Qualitative content analysis. In U. Flick (Ed.), *The SAGE handbook of qualitative data analysis* (pp. 170–183). Thousand Oaks, CA: Sage.

Sharples, M., Davison, L., Thomas, G. V., & Rudman, P. D. (2003). Children as photographers: An analysis of children's photographic behaviour and intentions at three age levels. *Visual Communication*, *2*(3), 303–330. doi:10.1177/14703572030023004

Tanner, T. (2010). Shifting the narrative: Child-led responses to climate change and disasters in El Salvador and the Philippines. *Children & Society*, *24*(4), 339–351. doi:10.1111/j.1099-0860.2010.00316.x

Thammavongsa, P. (2014). Signification des cérémonies de baci et de soukhouane. *Le Rénovateur*, 779. Retrieved from http://www.ambafrance-laos.org/Signification-des-ceremonies-de

Tindle, K., Leconte, P., Buchanan, L., & Taymans, J. M. (2005). *Transition planning: Community mapping as a tool for teachers and students* (Research to Practice Brief, Vol. 4). National Center on Secondary Education and Transition (NCSE).

UN. (2014). *World statistics pocketbook*. Retrieved from http://data.un.org

UNDP. (2007). *Assessment of development results Lao P.D.R. Evaluation of UNDP's contribution*. New York, NY: Author.

UNDP. (2013). *The rise of the south: Human progress in a diverse world* (Human Development Report 2013). New York, NY: Author.

Vis, S. A., Strandbu, A., Holtan, A., & Thomas, N. (2011). Participation and health – A research review of child participation in planning and decision-making. *Child & Family Social Work*, *16*(3), 325–335. doi:10.1111/j.1365-2206.2010.00743.x

Whiting, L. (2009). Involving children in research. *Paediatric Nursing*, *21*, 32–36.

WHO. (2013). *Global status report on road safety 2013*. Retrieved from https://http://www.iru.org/cms-filesystem-action/policies/sustainable_development/road_safety/gsrrs_en.pdf

WHO. (2014). *Lao People's democratic Republic. Country cooperation strategy at a glance*. Geneva: Author.

Wiles, R., Prosser, J., Bagnoli, A., Clark, A., Davies, K., Holland, S., & Renold, E. (2008). *Visual ethics: Ethical issues in visual research*. Swindon: Economic & Social Research Council, National Centre for Research Methods.

Woolfson, R. C., Heffernan, E., Paul, M., & Brown, M. (2010). Young people's views of the child protection system in Scotland. *British Journal of Social Work*, *40*(7), 2069–2085. doi:10.1093/bjsw/bcp120

World Bank. (2014). *World development indicators: Laos 2012*. Washington, DC: Author.

Wridt, P. (2010). A qualitative GIS approach to mapping urban neighborhoods with children to promote physical activity and child-friendly community planning. *Environment and Planning B: Planning and Design*, *37*(1), 129–147. doi:10.1068/b35002

Zartler, U., & Richter, R. (2014). My family through the lens. Photo interviews with children and sensitive aspects of family life. *Children & Society*, *28*(1), 42–54. doi:10.1111/j.1099-0860.2012.00447.x

Participatory mapping in low-resource settings: Three novel methods used to engage Kenyan youth and other community members in community-based HIV prevention research

Eric P. Green[a], Virginia Rieck Warren[a], Sherryl Broverman[a,b,c], Benson Ogwang[b] and Eve S. Puffer[a,d]

[a]Duke Global Health Institute, Durham, NC, USA; [b]Women's Institute for Secondary Education and Research, Muhuru Bay, Kenya; [c]Department of Biology, Duke University, Durham, NC, USA; [d]Department of Psychology and Neuroscience, Duke University, Durham, NC, USA

ABSTRACT
Understanding the link between health and place can strengthen the design of health interventions, particularly in the context of HIV prevention. Individuals who might one day participate in such interventions – including youth – may further improve the design if engaged in a meaningful way in the formative research process. Increasingly, participatory mapping methods are being used to achieve both aims. We describe the development of three innovative mapping methods for engaging youth in formative community-based research: 'dot map' focus groups, geocaching games, and satellite imagery-assisted daily activity logs. We demonstrate that these methods are feasible and acceptable in a low-resource, rural African setting. The discussion outlines the merits of each method and considers possible limitations.

Introduction

Characteristics of the social and physical environment – the social ecology – can positively or negatively influence the health and well-being of adolescents, including their ability to avoid contracting HIV and other sexually transmitted diseases (Sumartojo, 2000). This environmental/structural view suggests that risk for HIV cannot be solely explained by characteristics of individuals, such as knowledge of HIV transmission or attitudes towards risky sexual behaviour (Blankenship, Friedman, Dworkin, & Mantell, 2006; Coates, Richter, & Caceres, 2008; Gupta, Parkhurst, Ogden, Aggleton, & Mahal, 2008; Latkin & Knowlton, 2005; O'Reilly & Piot, 1996; Sumartojo, 2000; Sumartojo, Doll, Holt-grave, Gayle, & Merson, 2000). The broader social ecology – from micro-level influences such as household resources, neighbourhood disorder (Latkin, Williams, Wang, & Curry, 2005), and social networks (Latkin, Hua, & Forman, 2003) to macro-level factors such as laws and policies (Rojanapithayakorn & Hanenberg, 1996) – can restrict or enhance individual agency to avoid risk (Blankenship et al., 2006). Thus in developing HIV prevention interventions, it is necessary to understand and address social–ecological factors that influence HIV transmission in a particular context.

Various frameworks have been offered to classify these extra-individual factors that influence HIV risk and also serve as points of intervention (Barnett & Whiteside, 2002; Sumartojo et al., 2000; Sweat & Denison, 1995), yet our knowledge of where and how to best intervene throughout the social ecology remains limited. In large part, prevention efforts have focused on the individual while research on the social determinants of risk has concentrated on the structural (or societal) level, such as poverty – the two extremes of the social ecology.

In the HIV prevention intervention literature, for instance, most interventions have attempted to change characteristics of individuals, not environments or social structures (DiClemente, Salazar, & Crosby, 2007). Though individual-level approaches have proven to be efficacious in the short term, effects typically diminish over time. There is some indication that multilevel interventions increase the likelihood of reducing risk behaviours (Coates et al., 2008), though there is limited empirical evidence on the effectiveness of 'structural' approaches to HIV prevention (Gupta et al., 2008).

On the other hand, and with a few notable exceptions (Campbell, 1997, 2003), research on the social determinants of HIV risk has too often been silent on the local mechanisms of disease transmission – finding, for instance, that poverty is an important risk factor for HIV without articulating *how* poverty increases risk in a particular setting. Thus the conclusion of this research is often limited to general prescriptions for change (Blankenship et al., 2006) rather than specific targets for intervention.

Concordant with the growing recognition of the role of social–ecological factors in disease transmission and the benefits of intervening at multiple levels, there is a specific need for knowledge of how the immediate physical and social environments increase behavioural risk factors for HIV and are amenable to sustainable change. Social settings represent important proximal targets for intervention that would complement individual- and structural-level approaches.

The systematic study of social settings, however, has been frustrated by measurement challenges (Blankenship et al., 2006; Gupta et al., 2008; Poundstone, Strathdee, & Celentano, 2004) and an emphasis on individuals as the unit of analysis (Tseng & Seidman, 2007). We lack critical information on setting development, functioning, and outcomes. This study directly addresses these limitations by developing and evaluating new methods for collaborating with local communities to understand social settings.

Frameworks for studying social settings

The social–ecological perspective (Bronfenbrenner, 1979; Moos, 1974; Moos & Bromet, 1986) offers a useful framework for conceptualising the transactional relationships between individuals and their environments that increase or decrease HIV risk. In Bronfenbrenner's concentric circle model, the individual is placed at the centre of an expanding system of inter-related environmental influences – from the immediate family to the neighbourhood to the broader context of culture, time, laws, and policies. Poundstone and colleagues presented a similar model specific to HIV transmission dynamics that diagrams individual, social, and structural factors (Poundstone et al., 2004). The current study draws upon two publications that advanced the study of social settings: (a) Tseng and Seidman's systems framework (Tseng & Seidman, 2007) for understanding youths' social settings; and (b) Latkin and Knowlton's (2005) application of Barker's concept of behaviour settings (Barker, 1963, 1978; Barker & Gump, 1964; Barker & Wright, 1954) to HIV prevention.

Social settings

Tseng and Seidman (2007) made a major contribution to the field by advancing a systems framework for understanding youths' social settings. Interested primarily in the end goal of setting-level interventions, the authors described social settings as consisting of several systems that are amenable to change, including resources (e.g. human, economic, physical, temporal), the organisation of resources, and proximal social processes – the interactions between people and their everyday environments. This conceptualisation of youths' social settings can inform our understanding of the context of HIV prevention and ultimately identify targets for intervention. How resources are physically organised in communities, and how does this organisation impact daily social processes? Where do youths spend their time? Are there certain geographic locations that are associated with risky behaviours like transactional sex? If so, what are the social norms and relationships that characterise these locations? How could resources (e.g. parental monitoring) be rearranged to alter these social processes? Broadly speaking, what is the immediate social ecology of the risky behaviours that could be targets for interventions?

Behaviour settings

Another useful conceptual framework for studying the role of social settings in HIV trans-mission is Barker's notion of behaviour settings that describes how particular settings are associated with defined patterns of behaviour (Barker, 1963, 1978; Barker & Gump, 1964; Barker & Wright, 1954). Applying this theory to HIV prevention, Latkin and Knowlton (2005) described a behaviour setting as ' … a venue in which individuals may be linked by various forms of social interaction and meaning-imbued physical space and attendant behav-iour norms' (p. S104). The authors cited research on drug users in American cities to explain how certain settings are governed by routine behaviours that are associated with increased risk – for example, sharing needles in shooting galleries. HIV risk is further elevated in these environments by the clustering of high-risk people who adhere to the norms of the setting.

Developing innovative methods for studying social settings

In designing this study, we set out to address the measurement challenges that limit progress in developing interventions and evaluating social settings. As part of a broader mixed-methods approach that included surveys, interviews, and focus groups with a broad range of community stakeholders (Puffer et al., 2011; Puffer, Watt, Sikkema, Ogwang-Odhiambo, & Broverman, 2012), we developed and tested several innovative participatory mapping methods for collecting data on social settings and involving youth in the process.

Participatory mapping

In the past decade, geospatial technologies – which include geographic information systems (GIS), remote sensing (e.g. satellite imagery) and global positioning systems

(GPS) – have emerged as useful tools for studying contextual and social–ecological aspects of communities across the social and behavioural sciences (Luke, 2005). This is particularly true in quantitative domain (Goodchild, Anselin, Appelbaum, & Harthorn, 2000), but there have also been interesting applications to qualitative research (Elwood, 2006; Knigge & Cope, 2006).

GIS technology itself dates back to the 1960s, but early work was limited to technical audiences. As GIS became more integrated in planning and policy over the years, a new approach called 'Public Participation GIS' (PPGIS) grew out of a concern that the non-technical public would be excluded from the policy-making process (Obermeyer, 1998). Different variations on this approach have since emerged, and PPGIS has been classified more generally as a subtype of 'Participatory GIS' (PGIS; Dunn, 2007). In general, PGIS models seek to incorporate local knowledge through public participation. In public health, community psychology, and other health-focused disciplines, the same concerns about integrating local knowledge and pursuing wider public participation have been addressed under the framework of community-based participatory research (CBPR; Israel et al., 2008; Jason, Keys, Suarez-Balcazar, Taylor, & Davis, 2004). Proponents of these participatory methods assume that the knowledge derived from CBPR, like PGIS, will be more representative, will gain access to data not available with standard methods, and will be more useful in addressing health concerns of research participants (Jason et al., 2004; Townley, Kloos, & Wright, 2009), including children and youth (Jacquez, Vaughn, & Wagner, 2013; Vaughn, Wagner, & Jacquez, 2013) and populations affected by HIV and AIDS (Puffer, Pian, Sikkema, Ogwang-Odhiambo, & Broverman, 2013).

The literature on participatory mapping approaches with young people is small but growing. Youth have been active participants in community mapping (Lundine, Kovacic, & Poggiali, 2012) and spatially informed public health evaluation (Amsden & VanWynsberghe, 2005), as well as key informants about community life and local context (Literat, 2013; Pearce et al., 2009; Robinson & Oreskovic, 2013). Innovative methods for exploring how youth interact with their environment have been developed, including Participatory Photo Mapping (Dennis, Gaulocher, Carpiano, & Brown, 2009), Ecological Interviews (Mason, Cheung, & Walker, 2004), and GPS tracking (Oreskovic et al., 2012). The current study adds to this literature by introducing methods suitable for low-resource settings: 'dot map' focus groups; geocaching games; and satellite imagery-assisted daily activity logs. Our focus in this article is the implementation of these methods, rather than the specific results of using the methods to study the ecological nature of HIV risk in this particular setting. We focus on the latter only to the extent necessary to explain how the information gathered could be useful to researchers and programme planners.

Methods

Setting and participants

This study took place in 2009 in Muhuru Bay, a small fishing town located in Kenya's (former) Nyanza Province and situated on the shores of Lake Victoria and the country's northernmost border with Tanzania. Two factors influenced the decision to work in Muhuru Bay: (i) this region of Kenya has the highest prevalence rate of HIV in the country – 14.9% at the time of the study; and (ii) our study was part of a larger HIV prevention intervention development effort based in this community (Puffer et al., 2013).

At the time of fieldwork, Kenya had five administrative levels: provinces (8), districts (46), divisions (262), locations (2427), and sub-locations (6612). Muhuru Bay Division had four locations and eight sub-locations. Following enactment of the new constitution that voters approved in 2010 and the elections in 2013, a system of devolved government took effect and counties and sub-counties became the new administrative levels, replacing the existing structure. Muhuru Bay is located in the newly formed Migori County (population 1,028,579).

As described below, activities involved youth ages 10–18, their parents, their teachers, community leaders, and health workers from local medical facilities. Recruitment strategies are described in Puffer et al. (2011) as this study was part of a larger effort.

Procedures

This study was conducted in four stages. In the first stage, the research team worked with the local community to develop a digital basemap, a basic map of the community depicting boundaries, main roads, and points of interest such as schools. The research team then conducted mapping activities and focus groups with youth, parents, and teachers and used the results to design a participatory mapping game for youth. In the final stage, youth participated in individual mapping interviews to document daily activities.

Community mapping

The goal of the first stage was to create the basemap of the community. A team of three young adults, including author BO, were recruited from the community and trained to use consumer grade, hand-held GPS devices to identify and locate community features that would be used to create the map. This step was necessary because the community did not have accurate paper or digital maps. The only paper map of the community that we found was a hand-drawn poster (not to scale) that was several years old and in poor condition. We were able to locate a shapefile – a common spatial data format for depicting points (e.g. villages), lines (e.g. roads), and polygons (e.g. administrative boundaries) – that outlined the division, and we used this as the extent of our basemap; the metadata for this file could not be located.

The mapping team created all of the other features by travelling throughout the division over the course of two weeks to capture waypoints (coordinates of latitude and longitude depicting specific locations) and routes (strings of coordinates depicting the path traversed). To complete this work, the team talked with dozens of residents they encountered and crosschecked information about location and sub-location boundaries with these informants. There were no paved roads in the division, so most of the work was done on foot or by motorbike. High-resolution satellite imagery (less than 0.5 m) captured a few months prior by the GeoEye-1 satellite was used to guide the team's efforts (Chen, 2008). With imagery of this resolution, it was possible to identify ground structures and distinguish between buildings and dwellings. We used the imagery to plan daily mapping activities and resolve discrepancies in field-mapped waypoints and routes. All spatial data were compiled into basemap layers using the free, open-source desktop GIS program QGIS (version 1.1; QGIS Development Team, n.d.).

Dot map focus groups

Once the basemap was finalised, 'dot map' focus groups followed to identify important places within the community with an emphasis on locations of positive and negative youth activity. Paper copies of the basemap were printed and presented to focus group participants (see Figure A1 in the Online Appendix). A total of 15 focus groups involving 82 individuals were conducted: 1 with health workers ($n = 5$); 1 with traditional male chiefs ($n = 7$); 1 with women leaders ($n = 4$); and 12 with parents ($n = 26$), teachers ($n = 16$), and youth ($n = 24$) across the 4 locations (segmented by school and parent/teacher/youth). Each participant was provided with one paper copy of the map and a sheet of coloured sticker dots (1/8 inch diameter). Two members of the research team (one American and one Kenyan) facilitated the group activities and discussion. The Kenyan team member translated English to Dholuo and vice versa for youth and parent focus groups (other groups preferred to conduct the session in English).

Following a brief orientation to the map, basic map reading knowledge was tested by asking the participants to use a sticker to indicate the location of four commonly known points of interest in the community (e.g. the health clinic, a particular beach, a cultural landmark). Participants were then asked a series of questions (e.g. What are places where youth can get into trouble?) and instructed to place certain coloured dots on the map that corresponded to that specific question (see Table A1 in the Online Appendix). Once participants completed the activity, the facilitators asked individuals to explain their maps to the group as a way of initiating discussion about associations between the locations' certain types of youth behaviour (e.g. alcohol use).

The resulting paper dot maps (see Figure A2 in the Online Appendix as an example) were scanned and saved in the portable document format (PDF). The PDF of each map was then imported into another desktop GIS program called *ArcGIS* (version 9.3) and georectified (ESRI, 2008). In this process, the digital scans of the paper maps were aligned with the original digital shapefiles. Once aligned, the centre of each colour sticker was converted into a map waypoint. Each waypoint was linked to the original participant's unique identifier.

Since the map was drawn at a scale of 1:50,000, it was only useful for discussions about the larger community and did not allow participants to pinpoint specific neighbourhood locations. Thus, following the paper map exercise, facilitators used a projector running on generator power (as focus group locations were not on the power grid) to show participants recently captured high-resolution satellite imagery of their local neighbourhoods. The activity began with volunteers locating their homes on the screen as a way of orienting participants to the imagery. Facilitators then continued the discussion from the previous exercise and focused on local community features. The facilitator operating the laptop created digital waypoints that corresponded to locations participants discussed. The activities and discussions lasted 45–75 minutes.

Geocaching games

Stage 3 then aimed to gather more detailed information from youths' perspectives about the locations identified during the focus groups as important to understanding positive youth development and risky behaviour. To do this, the research team designed four photo 'scavenger hunt' games for youth, one for each school participating in the focus group discussions. The games were inspired by the popular outdoor activity called geo-caching and the Participatory Photo Mapping method (Dennis et al., 2009). Geocaching is an activity in which participants hide small objects in public places and post the coor-dinates, or clues to the coordinates, on geocaching websites. Other geocachers then use GPS devices to navigate to the coordinates and find the hidden object. Anyone who locates a geocache may take the object in exchange for another object of similar value.

A different game was organised at each school, and two teams of four youth from the school participated ($n = 32$ overall). Teams were provided with hand-held GPS units (with built-in two-way radios) for navigation, and smartphones with a built-in camera and GPS to geotag locations of photos. They were given a list of five geocache coordinates to locate that required them to travel a 3–5-km route. As they travelled between geocaches along the route, they were instructed to find and photograph locations that fit a list of seven scaven-ger hunt categories related to youth behaviour, such as places 'where you have seen people having sex' or 'places to have fun'. The research team identified the coordinates and sca-venger hunt categories based on the focus group discussions. When teams completed the activities, the youth and the facilitators reviewed the photographs to label them with the appropriate categories and to discuss why the student teams captured the images and what could be learned about the community. The games and review sessions lasted about 90 minutes.

Satellite imagery-assisted activity logs

In the final activity, 325 youth ages 10–18 years taking part in a cross-sectional survey of psychosocial correlates of HIV risk behaviour (Puffer et al., 2011) were invited to partici-pate in individual interviews about their daily activities. This sample of youth was ran-domly selected from student rosters collected from 14 area schools (grade standards 5–8). Pairs of the research team (one American, one Kenyan) interviewed each youth in a private setting. One member of the team asked questions (see Table A2 in the Online Appendix) and operated a laptop that displayed the high-resolution satellite imagery while the other member of the team recorded the youth's answers on a paper form. Inter-views lasted about 20 minutes.

At the start of the interview, the participant described where she lives and the research team navigated to this location on the satellite image. When the participant and the team located the participant's home, the facilitators would mark a digital waypoint (latitude and longitude coordinates) in a shapefile created for the interviewee. The participant then recounted all of her activities on a specific day within the past week, starting with the time and place she woke up. As the participant described where she went throughout the day, the facilitators helped her to identify locations using the satellite imagery. The facilitators created waypoints for each location and recorded the ID numbers on a paper form. The result was a personalised log documenting times, spatial locations, and typical frequency of the participant's activities. As shown in Table A2, the facilitators also asked participants to identify other places where they go (and how often they go there) when they have free time.

Process surveys

Following each study activity, all participants were invited to complete a brief, anonymous survey about their experience. Survey items were translated from English to Dholuo and presented in writing. Kenyan facilitators were available to help any participants who struggled to read the items. Participants responded to each item on a 4-point scale: strongly disagree (1); disagree (2); agree (3); and strongly agree (4). Higher numbers represent greater satisfaction.

Analysis

Focus group transcripts were analysed by the research team to identify salient themes and community locations for follow-up investigation during the geocaching games. The georectified dot maps were aggregated in *QGIS* and heat maps were generated using the 'Heatmap' plugin. Heat maps plot the geographic clustering of spatial features, in this case the density of participants' sticker placements. For instance, in Figure 1, part A, darker red patches show locations most commonly identified as places where youth get into trouble. This analysis tool functions by applying kernel density estimation to a set of input points and interpolates a density raster. To create the heat maps shown in Figure 1, the search radius was set to 500 m and the 'triweight' kernel function was selected to give more weight to closer points. Photographs captured during the geocaching games were labelled by students and summarised. The standard deviational ellipse method of calculating activity spaces (Sherman, Spencer, Preisser, Gesler, & Arcury, 2005) was used to analyse daily activity logs, though those results are not reported here. Summary statistics of dot map placements and counts of photographs by domain were calculated in Stata 12MP (StataCorp, 2011).

Ethical review

The research protocol was reviewed and approved by ethical review boards at Duke University and the Kenya Medical Research Institute.

Results

A total of 316 youth participated in the spatial activity logs, and a subset played the geocaching games (*n* = 32) and took part in focus group discussions (*n* = 24). Participant demographics are listed in Table 1.

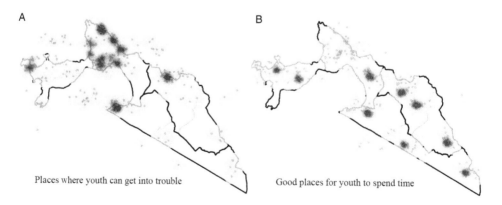

Figure 1. Hotspot analysis of 'bad' (a) and 'good' (b) places for youth to spend time, pooled analysis.

Table 1. Participant demographics.

Participants	n	Female (%)	Age		Education (years)		Married (%)
			Mean	SD	Mean	SD	
Focus groups							
Parents	26	38	40.5	16.6	8.2	3.4	96
Teachers	15	20	35.5	12.3	12.7	0.4	80
Youth	24	50	14.0	1.3	7.3	0.8	0
Chiefs	7	0	50.1	3.7	11.1	1.8	100
Women leaders	5	100	54.3	6.5	9.5	2.6	100
Health workers	4	40	34.2	12.5	12.2	1.3	60
Geocaching							
Youth	32	50					
Activity logs							
Youth	316	51	14.0	1.6	5.6	1.2	0

Note: Age, education, and marital status not documented for youth participants in geocaching game.

Community mapping

With significant community support, the research team mapped the majority of community features over the course of two weeks. Features included the locations of 72 villages, 65 churches, 32 businesses, 30 primary and secondary schools, 10 beaches, and 1 public medical facility. The team also traced numerous tertiary roads (all unpaved), major footpaths, and the boundaries for all four locations and eight sub-locations within Muhuru Bay Division. A paper map depicting the locations of schools and beaches is shown in Figure A1. A large version of the map was printed for the division's administrative offices and was their first formal map of the community.

Dot map focus groups

Across the 15 focus groups, 81 participants (1 missing) used a total of 1374 stickers to respond to facilitator questions. An example map from one youth participant is shown in Figure A2. Table 2 reports counts, means, and standard deviations of the number of sticker dots used by each type of participant to identify overall differences in patterns of responding. On average, the traditional chiefs identified 3.1 more 'bad' (red) places for young people to spend time compared to the youth participants. On average, parents and teachers also identified more 'bad' places than the youth.

Figure 1 displays the heat maps of 'bad' and 'good' places pooled across participants. There is no notable overlap in 'bad' and 'good' hotspots, suggesting that participants believe there are defined areas youth should avoid. Figure 2 shows the result of a hotspot analysis of 'bad' places according to adults and youth separately. Adults identified more beaches and a business district known as 'customs' compared to youth. Youth highlighted the dangers of fishing, a common income-generating activity for boys, by placing red stickers in Lake Victoria.

In describing the dangers of local beaches where fishermen disembark and sell their catch to female traders, a 50-year-old participant in the group of women's leaders explained:

> It is a bad place because the youth get spoiled in that place ... They are getting 'bhang' which they smoke. They get music and they dance, and they even watch videos. These things are bad, and they are spoiled by these things

Table 2. Count, mean, and standard deviation in the number of stickers used by sticker colour and participant type.

Group	n	Red			Blue			Green			Yellow		
		Count	Mean	SD	Count	Mean	SD	Count	Mean	SD	Count	Mean	SD
Parents	26	134	5.2	2.3	76	7.6	3.5	155	17.9	6.6	22	11.0	6.0
Teachers	15	90	6.0	1.9	97	12.9	3.0	89	19.1	4.9	5	20.0	0.0
Youth	24	111	4.6	1.6	105	8.8	2.9	96	12.0	5.8	72	12.0	3.9
Chiefs	7	54	7.7	0.5	54	15.4	1.5	56	24.0	0.0	0	0.0	0.0
Women leaders	5	15	3.8	1.0	32	16.0	0.0	28	21.0	4.2	15	15.0	2.0
Health workers	4	10	2.0	1.0	31	12.4	5.0	12	7.2	3.4	15	12.0	6.3

Notes: Chiefs were not asked the question about parental supervision, thus they used zero yellow stickers. See Table A1 for the link between sticker colour and focus group questions.

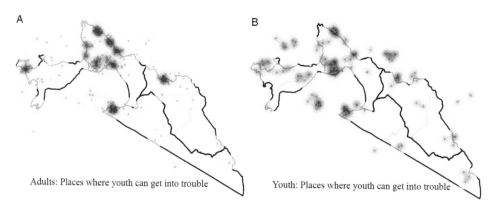

Figure 2. Hotspot analysis of 'bad' places for youth to spend time according to adults (a) and youth (b).

A 45-year-old mother of one of the youth participants added:

> At the beaches there are different people, especially women who are not having their husbands. They are staying at the beaches, so if the youths go there, these women attract them and engage in sex, so it is a bad place.

The adult participants – and the youth to a large extent – frequently endorsed these sentiments. Health workers made the link between sexual behaviour at beaches and the increased risk of contracting HIV.

Geocaching games

The 8 student teams captured a total of 263 geotagged photos during the geocaching activity (see Table 3). Students classified two-fifths of the photos as locations associated with 'risky' behaviours or behaviours that adults labelled detrimental to youth. A total of 40% of the photos were identified as places to have fun.

Process surveys

The results of the process surveys are presented in Table 4. Scores on every item show a high level of satisfaction with little variability. This could reflect excitement over new techniques and technologies that participants had not encountered previously.

Table 3. Photo descriptives.

Photo tags	Tagged photos	% of tags	% of photos (263)
Places where alcohol can be purchased	27	9.3	10.3
Places where you have seen people doing drugs	34	11.7	12.9
Places where you have seen people having sex	34	11.7	12.9
Places where you buy items for your family	57	19.7	21.7
Places to have fun	38	13.1	14.4
Places to watch videos	15	5.2	5.7
Important places	83	28.6	31.6
Other	2	0.7	0.8
Total	290	100.0	110.3

Note: Photos could be tagged with more than category, so the final column (percentage of photos) exceeds 100%.

Discussion

In this paper, we demonstrate three simple participatory mapping methods for engaging youth in research: focus group discussions with a dot map activity and review of high-resolution satellite imagery; geocaching 'games'; and daily activity geologs. Participants found each activity to be fun, easy, and informative. The 'hands-on' nature of the mapping exercises enabled information to flow both ways – from the community to the external members of the research team and from the research team to the community. Through the use of recent, high-resolution satellite imagery, participants gained a new perspective on their community – in a both literal and figurative sense. By anchoring this new perspective in engaging activities, participants and researchers were able to work together to create new knowledge about the community context.

Each method described here offers the researcher or programme planner something unique in terms of community engagement and information gathering. Community mapping is an established, but underused methodology. Community members can be involved in a number of ways, from leading the actual mapping to providing input and context. What we call 'dot map' focus groups is an easy way to get community input about broad issues that are linked to place. The activity is interactive and can be used to involve any community member regardless of educational background or literacy. The maps produced represent data about individuals' perceptions as well as focus group content for further discussion and debate. Geocaching games are particularly well-suited for engaging youth as the activity is designed to make data collection fun. Unlike the focus groups, these games have a hyper-local focus as teams have to walk (or run) a set course. For this reason, the games can be a good follow-up exercise to the broad and introductory focus group exercises. Finally, the satellite imagery-assisted activity logs can elicit individual-level data on youth (or adult) activity spaces without the need to physically visit the home of every participant. Geospatial data can also be linked to more traditional survey data to examine potential associations between place and behaviour.

An essential consideration in technology-based CBPR methods is whether methods match specific contexts. Results of this study suggest that these participatory mapping activities were particularly well-suited for a rural, low-resource environment. The youth who collaborated on this research come from a very poor community located in one of the poorest regions of a low-income country. At the time of the study, few residents had access to reliable electricity. Most adults have not completed secondary school.

Table 4. Process survey results.

Process questions	Youth (n = 24) m	Youth (n = 24) SD	Parents (n = 26) m	Parents (n = 26) SD	Teacher (n = 15) m	Teacher (n = 15) SD	Chiefs (n = 7) m	Chiefs (n = 7) SD	Women leaders (n = 5) m	Women leaders (n = 5) SD	Health workers (n = 5) m	Health workers (n = 5) SD	All (n = 82) m	All (n = 82) SD
Focus groups: Sticker dots and satellite imagery														
I liked putting stickers on the maps to share my views about Muhuru Bay.	4.0	0.0	3.9	0.3	3.6	0.8	4.0	0.0	4.0	0.0	3.6	0.6	3.9	0.4
I thought it was easy to use stickers to share my views about Muhuru Bay.	4.0	0.2	3.8	0.4	3.7	0.8	3.9	0.4	3.8	0.5	3.6	0.6	3.8	0.5
The sticker map I made helped me to explain things about life in Muhuru Bay.	3.8	0.4	3.9	0.4	3.9	0.4	4.0	0.0	3.6	0.6	3.6	0.6	3.8	0.4
I learned something new from discussing everyone's sticker maps.	3.8	0.4	3.9	0.3	3.7	0.5	3.9	0.4	4.0	0.0	3.8	0.5	3.8	0.4
I liked looking at the picture of Muhuru Bay.	3.8	0.5	3.9	0.3	4.0	0.0	3.9	0.4	3.8	0.5	3.4	0.9	3.9	0.4
I thought it was easy to recognise places on the picture of Muhuru Bay.	3.6	0.5	3.9	0.4	3.7	0.5	3.4	1.1	3.4	0.6	3.6	0.6	3.7	0.6
I learned something new from discussing the picture of Muhuru Bay.	3.9	0.3	3.9	0.3	3.8	0.4	4.0	0.0	4.0	0.0	3.8	0.5	3.9	0.3
Geocaching games: Youth only (n = 41)														
I liked using the GPS units.	4.0	0.2												
I liked using the camera phones.	4.0	0.0												
I thought it was easy to find places using the GPS units.	4.0	0.2												
I thought it was easy to use the camera phones.	4.0	0.2												
I thought the game was fun.	4.0	0.2												
I liked seeing my team's photos on the computer.	4.0	0.0												
Activity logs: Youth only (n = 323)														
I liked looking at the picture of Muhuru Bay.	3.9	0.3												
I thought it was easy to recognise places on the picture of Muhuru Bay.	3.8	0.5												
I could recognise my home and places around my home.	3.9	0.4												
I learned something new from discussing the picture of Muhuru Bay.	3.9	0.4												

Note: Participants were invited to complete anonymous surveys following each study activity. Response options: strongly disagree (1); disagree (2); agree (3); strongly agree (4). The number of youth completing process surveys for the activity log exercise exceeded the number of youth who actually completed the exercise by 7.

Food insecurity and health challenges like malaria and HIV steal time, money, and energy from just about every household. Yet none of these traditional 'barriers' limited the success of the study.

In fact, the rural backdrop of this work likely increased the probability of success. The community welcomed the research team, and local leaders found value in the ability to use modern technology to create a new community map. Residents guided the mapping team through fields and homesteads in search of a common understanding of boundaries. The absence of land conflict in this community meant that such an exercise did not run the risk of sparking or inflaming local disputes. Furthermore, without many vehicles on the road, it was safe to let youth race through the bush and over green hills, guided by GPS devices as they documented their journey. With relatively few huts dotting the landscape, it was also possible to sit with youth and pan through high-resolution satellite imagery to locate their homes, the places where they fetch water, the routes they travel to school, the areas they avoid, and the spots where they spend time with friends. Other initiatives like *MapKibera* have shown that such work is possible in Kenya's urban slums (Hagen, 2011), but the rural setting makes some aspects of the work easier to manage.

The feasibility of using technology-based participatory mapping tools in very low-resource settings is ever increasing. This makes it a promising approach for future studies in which understanding a community's geography and learning about specific locations can shed light on youths' behaviours and well-being. New tools and technologies are continuing to reduce the cost and difficulty of what was already a relatively inexpensive and easy endeavour in 2009. Smartphone prices are falling as the capability of the most basic models is expanding. When we conducted this work, we determined we needed two devices: a smartphone with a camera and a separate GPS unit for geocaching. If we had conducted the same study 3–5 years earlier, we would have needed to exchange the smartphone for a point-and-shoot camera. Today, a single smartphone device would suffice. Increasingly these devices can be found in the pockets of Africa's youth. Mobile subscriptions on the continent will hit 1 billion by 2015 on the way to 1.2 billion by 2018 (Informa, 2013). Smartphone ownership is projected to increase more than 5-fold in the next 4 years, from 79 million to 412 million.

In addition to advances in hardware, there are new software platforms that are lowering barriers to entry. Possibly the most impressive of them is the free, open-source mapping platform OpenStreetMap (Neis & Zipf, 2012; OpenStreetMap, n.d.). Since its founding in 2004, more than 1.5 million registered users have uploaded almost 4 billion GPS points and edited billions of nodes (OpenStreetMap, 2014b). Several browser-based editors make it easy for non-technical users to create free accounts and contribute to the world map (OpenStreetMap, 2014a). We have done this for Muhuru Bay; using the high-resolution satellite imagery provided through OpenStreetMap's license agreements with companies like Bing, we have traced all of the major roads and footpaths in the community (OpenStreetMap Contributors, 2014). If conducting the study today, we would be able to rely almost completely on this freely available resource and give youth the ability to contribute directly to OpenStreetMap via laptops and smartphone applications. There are also new 'low-tech' paper options like Walking Papers that enable citizens to contribute to OpenStreetMap without having access to a computer or smartphone (Migurski, n.d.).

There is still a need for separate analysis tools, but this space has grown substantially over the past few years as well. We used two propriety software programmes over the course of this study – *Stata* and *ArcGIS* – but neither is essential. *ArcGIS* remains the industry leader in GIS, but the free, open-source alternative *QGIS* is capable of most tasks. The R statistical programming package, also free, open-source, and cross-platform, is also capable of carrying out many spatial analyses once only available in *ArcGIS* (R Development Core Team, n.d.).

Especially given this increasing feasibility, these methods also have a secondary community service dimension. First, they include training local community members, including youth, to learn to use new technologies, building both technical and analytical skills. Beyond training in the use of the equipment, which can be valuable, participants and local research team members also learn about the integration of data from different sources (e.g. data from GPS units and satellite imagery) and are exposed to data visualisation techniques. As young adults are often the primary demographic serving as local staff for research in such settings, this type of exposure and experience can be motivating and valuable when seeking out future employment and education opportunities. In addition, as these technologies are becoming more accessible, the training equips community members to replicate the methods to answer new questions about their community in the future.

Despite these positives, there are challenges to implementing these methods and limitations to the approach. No amount of technology will ever replace the process of relationship-building with host communities. In this study, even strong endorsements from community leaders and an established presence in the community via a non-governmental organisation did not inoculate us to challenges of fieldwork. It is well-known that photo-documentary approaches can make bystanders uncomfortable if photographs are recorded without permission (Wang & Redwood-Jones, 2001). We experienced two occasions in which additional sensitisation of the community might have proved helpful. First, as students were racing to document their community during the geocaching games, a few shop owners expressed frustration to the facilitators that they were unaware of the nature of the activity and concerned about the implications. It was easy enough to address their concerns after the fact, but the experience taught us that we should have travelled the route first to introduce the activity to local residents. A similar situation occurred when a member of our research team was detained briefly by the local police for taking a photograph of the police station. The misunderstanding was also easily corrected, but better advance planning might have avoided the encounter altogether. Approval at the highest levels does not always flow quickly or completely to all segments of the community.

Nevertheless, with cheaper, more widely available hardware, easy to use platforms like *OpenStreetMap* with current high-resolution satellite imagery, and free and robust analysis tools like *QGIS* and *R*, it is possible for participants in low-income communities to participate in every aspect of this research. There will still be barriers to accessing computers and building computer literacy and technical skills for analysis, but barriers to this type of CBPR have never been lower.

Acknowledgements

The authors would like to thank Dyan Moses and Judith Andrew for their assistance carrying out the study, and the participants from Muhuru Bay for sharing their time and insights about the community.

Disclosure statement

No potential conflict of interest was reported by the authors.

References

Amsden, J., & VanWynsberghe, R. (2005). Community mapping as a research tool with youth. *Action Research, 3*, 357–381. doi:10.1177/1476750305058487

Barker, R. G. (1963). On the nature of the environment. *Journal of Social Issues, 19*(4), 17–38.

Barker, R. G. (1978). *Habitats, environments, and human behavior*. San Francisco, CA: Jossey-Bass.

Barker, R. G., & Gump, P. V. (1964). *Big school, small school: High school size and student behavior*. Stanford, CA: Stanford University Press.

Barker, R. G., & Wright, H. F. (1954). *Midwest and its children: The psychological ecology of an American town*. Hamden, CT: Archon Books.

Barnett, T., & Whiteside, A. (2002). *AIDS in the twenty-first century: Disease and globalization*. New York, NY: Palgrave Macmillan.

Blankenship, K. M., Friedman, S. R., Dworkin, S., & Mantell, J. E. (2006). Structural interventions: Concepts, challenges and opportunities for research. *Journal of Urban Health, 83*(1), 59–72. doi:10.1007/s11524-005-9007-4

Bronfenbrenner, U. (1979). *The ecology of human development: Experiments by nature and design*. Cambridge, MA: Harvard University Press.

Campbell, C. (1997). Migrancy, masculine identities and AIDS: The psychosocial context of HIV transmission on the South African gold mines. *Social Science & Medicine, 45*, 273–281. doi:10.1016/S0277-9536(96)00343-7

Campbell, C. (2003). *Letting them die: Why HIV/AIDS intervention programmes fail*. Oxford: James Currey.

Chen, B. X. (2008, October 8). Google's super satellite captures first image. *Wired.com*. Retrieved from http://www.wired.com/wiredscience/2008/10/geoeye-1-super/

Coates, T. J., Richter, L., & Caceres, C. (2008). Behavioural strategies to reduce HIV transmission: How to make them work better. *The Lancet, 372*, 669–684. doi:10.1016/S0140-6736(08)60886-7

Dennis Jr., S. F., Gaulocher, S., Carpiano, R. M., & Brown, D. (2009). Participatory photo mapping (PPM): Exploring an integrated method for health and place research with young people. *Health & Place, 15*, 466–473. doi:10.1016/j.healthplace.2008.08.004

DiClemente, R. J., Salazar, L. F., & Crosby, R. A. (2007). A review of STD/HIV preventive interventions for adolescents: Sustaining effects using an ecological approach. *Journal of Pediatric Psychology, 32*, 888–906. doi:10.1093/jpepsy/jsm056

Dunn, C. E. (2007). Participatory GIS—A people's GIS? *Progress in Human Geography, 31*, 616–637. doi:10.1177/0309132507081493

Elwood, S. (2006). Critical issues in participatory GIS: Deconstructions, reconstructions, and new research directions. *Transactions in GIS, 10*, 693–708. doi:10.1111/j.1467-9671.2006.01023.x

ESRI. (2008). *ArcGIS desktop: Release 9.3*. Redlands, CA: Environmental Systems Research Institute.

Goodchild, M. F., Anselin, L., Appelbaum, R. P., & Harthorn, B. H. (2000). Toward spatially integrated social science. *International Regional Science Review, 23*, 139–159. doi:10.1177/016001700761012701

Gupta, G. R., Parkhurst, J. O., Ogden, J. A., Aggleton, P., & Mahal, A. (2008). Structural approaches to HIV prevention. *The Lancet, 372*, 764–775. doi:10.1016/S0140-6736(08)60887-9

Hagen, E. (2011). Mapping change: Community information empowerment in Kibera (Innovations Case Narrative: Map Kibera). *Innovations: Technology, Governance, Globalization, 6*(1), 69–94. doi:10.1162/INOV_a_00059

Informa. (2013). Africa telecoms outlook. Informa telecoms & media. Retrieved from http://files.informatandm.com/uploads/2013/11/Africa_Telecoms_Outlook_Low_resolution.pdf

Israel, B. A., Schulz, A. J., Parker, E. A., Becker, A. B., Allen, A. J., & Guzman, J. R. (2008). Critical issues in developing and following community based participatory research principles. In M. Minkler, & N. Wallerstein (Eds.), *Community-based participatory research for health: from process to outcomes* (2nd ed., pp. 47–66). San Francisco, CA: Jossey-Bass.

Jacquez, F., Vaughn, L. M., & Wagner, E. (2013). Youth as partners, participants or passive recipients: A review of children and adolescents in community-based participatory research (CBPR). *American Journal of Community Psychology, 51*(1–2), 176–189. doi:10.1007/s10464-012-9533-7

Jason, L. A., Keys, C. B., Suarez-Balcazar, Y. E., Taylor, R. R., & Davis, M. I. (2004). *Participatory community research: Theories and methods in action*. Washington, DC: American Psychological Association. Retrieved from http://psycnet.apa.org/psycinfo/2003-88379-000/

Knigge, L., & Cope, M. (2006). Grounded visualization: Integrating the analysis of qualitative and quantitative data through grounded theory and visualization. *Environment and Planning A, 38*, 2021–2037. doi:10.1068/a37327

Latkin, C. A., Hua, W., & Forman, V. L. (2003). The relationship between social network charac-teristics and exchanging sex for drugs or money among drug users in Baltimore, MD, USA. *International Journal of STD & AIDS, 14*(11), 770–775.

Latkin, C. A., & Knowlton, A. R. (2005). Micro-social structural approaches to HIV prevention: A social ecological perspective. *AIDS Care, 17*, 102–113. doi:10.1080/09540120500121185

Latkin, C. A., Williams, C. T., Wang, J., & Curry, A. D. (2005). Neighborhood social disorder as a determinant of drug injection behaviors: A structural equation modeling approach. *Health Psychology, 24*(1), 96–100. doi:10.1037/0278-6133.24.1.96

Literat, I. (2013). Participatory mapping with urban youth: The visual elicitation of socio-spatial research data. *Learning, Media and Technology, 38*, 198–216. doi:10.1080/17439884.2013.782037

Luke, D. A. (2005). Getting the big picture in community science: Methods that capture context. *American Journal of Community Psychology, 35*(3–4), 185–200. doi:10.1007/s10464-005-3397-z

Lundine, J., Kovacic, P., & Poggiali, L. (2012). Youth and digital mapping in urban informal settle-ments: Lessons learned from participatory mapping processes in Mathare in Nairobi, Kenya. *Children Youth and Environments, 22*, 214–233. doi:10.7721/chilyoutenvi.22.2.0214

Mason, M., Cheung, I., & Walker, L. (2004). Substance use, social networks, and the geography of urban adolescents. *Substance Use & Misuse, 39*(10–12), 1751–1777. doi:10.1081/JA-200033222

Migurski, M., & Stamen Design. (n.d.). Walking papers. Retrieved from http://walking-papers.org/

Moos, R. H. (1974). *Evaluating treatment environments: A social ecological approach.* New York, NY: Wiley.

Moos, R. H., & Bromet, E. (1986). *The human context: Environmental determinants of behavior.* Malabar, FL: RE Krieger.

Neis, P., & Zipf, A. (2012). Analyzing the contributor activity of a volunteered geographic infor-mation project – The case of OpenStreetMap. *ISPRS International Journal of Geo-Information, 1*, 146–165. doi:10.3390/ijgi1020146

Obermeyer, N. J. (1998). The evolution of public participation GIS. *Cartography and Geographic Information Systems, 25*, 65–66.

OpenStreetMap. (2014a). Editing. Retrieved from http://wiki.openstreetmap.org/wiki/Editor

OpenStreetMap. (2014b). OpenStreetMap stats report. Retrieved from http://www.openstreetmap. org/stats/data_stats.html

OpenStreetMap. (n.d.). Retrieved from http://www.openstreetmap.org

OpenStreetMap Contributors. (2014). Muhuru Bay on OpenStreetMap. Retrieved from http:// www.openstreetmap.org/#map=13/-1.0283/34.1065

O'Reilly, K. R., & Piot, P. (1996). International perspectives on individual and community approaches to the prevention of sexually transmitted disease and human immunodeficiency virus infection. *Journal of Infect Diseases, 174*(2), S214–S222. doi:10.1093/infdis/174. Supplement_2.S214

Oreskovic, N. M., Blossom, J., Field, A. E., Chiang, S. R., Winickoff, J. P., & Kleinman, R. E. (2012). Combining global positioning system and accelerometer data to determine the locations of phys-ical activity in children. *Geospatial Health, 6*, 263–272. doi:10.4081/gh.2012.144

Pearce, A., Kirk, C., Cummins, S., Collins, M., Elliman, D., Connolly, A. M., & Law, C. (2009). Gaining children's perspectives: A multiple method approach to explore environmental influ-ences on healthy eating and physical activity. *Health & Place, 15*, 614–621. doi:10.1016/j. healthplace.2008.10.007

Poundstone, K. E., Strathdee, S. A., & Celentano, D. D. (2004). The social epidemiology of Human Immunodeficiency Virus/Acquired Immunodeficiency Syndrome. *Epidemiologic Reviews, 26*(1), 22–35. doi:10.1093/epirev/mxh005

Puffer, E. S., Meade, C. S., Drabkin, A. S., Broverman, S. A., Ogwang-Odhiambo, R. A., & Sikkema, K. J. (2011). Individual- and family-level psychosocial correlates of HIV risk behavior among youth in rural Kenya. *AIDS and Behavior, 15*, 1264–1274. doi:10.1007/s10461-010-9823-8

Puffer, E. S., Pian, J., Sikkema, K. J., Ogwang-Odhiambo, R. A., & Broverman, S. A. (2013). Developing a family-based HIV prevention intervention in Rural Kenya: Challenges in conducting community-based participatory research. *Journal of Empirical Research on Human Research Ethics: JERHRE, 8*, 119–128. doi:10.1525/jer.2013.8.2.119

Puffer, E. S., Watt, M. H., Sikkema, K. J., Ogwang-Odhiambo, R. A., & Broverman, S. A. (2012). The protective role of religious coping in adolescents' responses to poverty and sexual decision-making in rural Kenya. *Journal of Research on Adolescence, 22*(1), 1–7. doi:10.1111/j.1532-7795.2011.00760.x

QGIS Development Team. (n.d.). QGIS geographic information system. Open Source Geospatial Foundation Project. Retrieved from http://qgis.osgeo.org

R Development Core Team. (n.d.). R: A language and environment for statistical computing. Vienna, Austria: R Foundation for Statistical Computing. Retrieved from http://www.R-project.org

Robinson, A. I., & Oreskovic, N. M. (2013). Comparing self-identified and census-defined neighborhoods among adolescents using GPS and accelerometer. *International Journal of Health Geographics, 12*(1), 57. doi:10.1186/1476-072X-12-57

Rojanapithayakorn, W., & Hanenberg, R. (1996). The 100% condom program in Thailand. *AIDS, 10*(1), 1–8. doi:10.1097/00002030-199601000-00001

Sherman, J. E., Spencer, J., Preisser, J. S., Gesler, W. M., & Arcury, T. A. (2005). A suite of methods for representing activity space in a healthcare accessibility study. *International Journal of Health Geographics, 4*(1), 24. doi:10.1186/1476-072X-4-24

StataCorp. (2011). *Stata statistical software: Release 12*. College Station, TX: StataCorp LP.

Sumartojo, E. (2000). Structural factors in HIV prevention: Concepts, examples, and implications for research. *AIDS, 14*(11), S3–S10. doi:10.1097/00002030-200006001-00002

Sumartojo, E., Doll, L., Holtgrave, D., Gayle, H., & Merson, M. (2000). Enriching the mix: Incorporating structural factors into HIV prevention. *AIDS, 14*(11), S1–S2.

Sweat, M. D., & Denison, J. A. (1995). Reducing HIV incidence in developing countries with structural and environmental interventions. *AIDS, 9*, S251– S257.

Townley, G., Kloos, B., & Wright, P. A. (2009). Understanding the experience of place: Expanding methods to conceptualize and measure community integration of persons with serious mental illness. *Health & Place, 15*, 520–531. doi:10.1016/j.healthplace.2008.08.011

Tseng, V., & Seidman, E. (2007). A systems framework for understanding social settings. *American Journal of Community Psychology, 39*, 217–228. doi:10.1007/s10464-007-9101-8

Vaughn, L. M., Wagner, E., & Jacquez, F. (2013). A review of community-based participatory research in child health: MCN. *The American Journal of Maternal/Child Nursing, 38*(1), 48–53. doi:10.1097/NMC.0b013e31826591a3

Wang, C. C., & Redwood-Jones, Y. A. (2001). Photovoice ethics: Perspectives from flint photovoice. *Health Education & Behavior, 28*, 560–572. doi:10.1177/109019810102800504

Exploring social inclusion strategies for public health research and practice: The use of participatory visual methods to counter stigmas surrounding street-based substance abuse in Colombia

Amy E. Ritterbusch

School of Government, Universidad de los Andes, Bogotá, Colombia

ABSTRACT

This paper presents the participatory visual research design and findings from a qualitative assessment of the social impact of *bazuco* and inhalant/glue consumption among street youth in Bogotá, Colombia. The paper presents the visual methodologies our participatory action research (PAR) team employed in order to identify and overcome the stigmas and discrimination that street youth experience in society and within state-sponsored drug rehabilitation programmes. I call for critical reflection regarding the broad application of the terms 'participation' and 'participatory' in visual research and urge scholars and public health practitioners to consider the transformative potential of PAR for both the research and practice of global public health in general and rehabilitation programmes for street-based substance abuse in Colombia in particular. The paper concludes with recommendations as to how participatory visual methods can be used to promote social inclusion practices and to work against stigma and discrimination in health-related research and within health institutions.

Introduction

As illustrated in Figure 1, drawn by participants of the 'Beyond Glue and Bazuco' project in Bogotá, Colombia, street-connected adolescents do not want to be seen or labelled as drug addicts or drug-dependent. They want to be considered and treated as human beings. As part of this special issue's call for the use of participatory visual methods in public health research and practice in multiple contexts, this paper draws from a long-term, ongoing participatory action research (PAR) initiative with street-connected communities in Colombia.

This PAR initiative involves collective work with the community to assess and construct pathways to action surrounding their most immediate problems and concerns, many of which are health-related. Within the context of the 'Beyond Glue and Bazuco' project, participatory visual methods were used to achieve the social change objectives of the project aiming to counter stigmas surrounding street-connected adolescents and

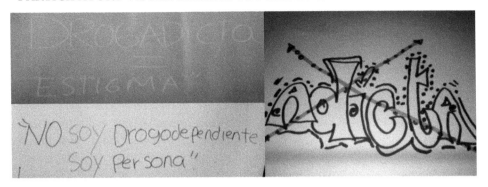

Figure 1. 'Drug addict = stigma', 'I am not drug-dependent … I'm a person', '[Don't call me an] addict'. Source: Focus group.

inhalant/glue and *bazuco*[1] addiction in Colombia. The project focused specifically on institutional stigma and visual strategies to transform the practices of health professionals who work directly with street-connected adolescents in a rehabilitation programme in Bogotá.

Based on these research experiences, I argue that it is essential to include participants and target populations in the design and implementation of both public health research and practice that aim to achieve a particular health-related social change objective. The incorporation of a participatory focus into research and practice enables scholars to contribute to a public health evidence base that better reflects participants' health-related needs and to design public health interventions that are more adequately equipped to promote positive change in the lives of target populations. Furthermore, I argue that the principles and critical praxis of PAR can be used to inform the design of more inclusive public health research.

In order to support this argument, this paper reviews relevant literature and previous studies that have engaged visual methods in health-related research and discusses three key principles and practices (reflexivity, critical dissemination practices, and sustainability). These key principles and practices guide participatory initiatives and should be considered by the research team for the project planning, implementation, and long-term social impact of the project. The paper then describes the research design and methodology underpinning the long-term PAR initiative as well as the specific design of the 'Beyond Glue and Bazuco' subproject. Finally, in the results section, the paper describes how reflexivity, critical dissemination practices, and sustainability were employed in each phase of the 'Beyond Glue and Bazuco' project to catalyse social change.

Through life histories, photographs, and a video visualising participants' experiences of stigmatisation and a description of the PAR process, the paper provides an example of a participatory visual methods project that has inspired critical hope in the lives and work of street-connected communities, university-based researchers, activists, and health workers.

Visual methods in health-related research

Visual methods have been employed in the global North and South to explore health-related issues such as homelessness and extreme poverty in the lives of street children (Joanou, 2009) and family dynamics surrounding autism and alternative therapeutic approaches for people with learning disabilities (Aldridge, 2007; Hwang, 2013). Studies have also focused on the evaluation of early childhood development programmes using the Mosaic approach (Clark, 2011), behavioural studies including sexuality research in secondary schools (Allen, 2008, 2009), and adults' active leisure participation (Annear et al., 2013).

In order to research health-related social problems, visual methods have also been used to contextualise participant perceptions of the factors impacting physical activity in Hispanic women (Balbale, Schwingel, Chodzko-Zajko, & Huhman, 2014) and the lived experiences of individuals with severe mental illness (Fullana, Pallisera, & Vilà, 2013). Previous studies have also researched food practices in the household and children's diets and nutrition (O'Connell, 2013), primary care for depression (Palmer, Dowrick, & Gunn, 2014), and love and sexuality in the disability community (Sitter, 2012).

While several of the previously mentioned studies present the research design within a participatory framework, the transformative objective of the projects are not clear and participation is framed in terms of the data collection techniques applied with participants rather than in terms of social transformation catalysed within the community. Although these projects employ creative visual techniques that involve participants in data collection and interpretation, the methods are used mainly to represent participants' understanding of their world and the particular health-related dilemmas studied by the research team.

As critical PAR scholars have argued, '[w]hen participation is presented as a set of techniques, rather than as a commitment to working with communities, it may result in the reproduction, rather than the challenging, of unequal power relations' (Cahill, Quijada, & Bradley, 2010, p. 408; Arieli, Friedman, & Agbaria, 2009; Cahill, 2007a; Cooke & Kothari, 2001; Mohan, 2001; Pain, Kesby, & Askins, 2011; Skelton, 2008). It is important to make this distinction when exploring the use and relevance of participatory visual methods for health research in order to avoid the broad application of the term 'participation' in the methodological framing of projects, which ' … may mask tokenism and provide an illusion of consultation' (Cahill et al., 2010, p. 408).

The transformative potential of participatory visual methods in public health research is therefore demonstrated through projects that engage communities *throughout* the research process and use the visual products collectively constructed by participants to catalyse social change in society. For example, a study in South Africa was designed as part of the 'Hope and Healing Campaign' and employed participatory visual methods to challenge HIV and AIDS-related stigma. Through this project, students became involved in activist initiatives and created dialogue about their loved ones living with HIV/AIDS as a means of breaking the silence generated by stigma and discrimination (Francis & Hemson, 2006).

The core principles of participatory visual methods for catalysing social change in public health research and practice

In order to ensure that participatory visual projects leave more than a set of photographs or videos with the community, our initiatives should facilitate a research context in which participants ' … present and represent their message in a contextualized way and in a visual and visible form that has the potential to educate and sensitize others about agency and social change' (De Lange & Mitchell, 2012, p. 323). For the purpose of shedding light on the transformative potential of participatory visual methods for public health research and practice, I focus on three principles and practices that are discussed in the visual methods and PAR literature in the context of social change: reflexivity, critical dissemination practices, and sustainability.

Reflexivity

Literature on PAR across multiple disciplines emphasises the importance of both collective and individual processes of reflection as fundamental praxis underpinning the social change objectives and outcomes of PAR projects (Cahill, 2004, 2007b; Pain, 2004; Pain et al., 2011). Additionally, PAR has been framed as a feminist praxis inspiring 'critical hope' in the lives of participants and as a means of achieving the research community's collectively established social justice goals (Cahill et al., 2010 ; Torre et al., 2001). Within the context of visual research, scholars have reflected on what the visual methods process provokes in the lives of participants and how this contributes to social justice and/or health-related goals. For example, a project with Ugandan women about sexual health used story making and performance in the production of a video that enabled participants 'to create individualized and powerful scenes to express their life-worlds and to explore embedded power relations' (Waite & Conn, 2012, p. 95). This project in Uganda provided practical pathways for the community-based exploration of difficult-to-address health-related issues and enabled participants to reflect individually and collectively about how to improve public health programmes that target their most pressing issues and needs. Furthermore, as discussed by Yang (2012), participatory visual initiatives should promote participant-centred reflexivity practice, provoking critical reflections on authorship, the relationship between filmmakers, film subjects and audiences, and constant communication between all those touched by the visual method process (see also Mitchell & De Lange, 2011).

Critical dissemination practices

As observed in the field of public health, dissemination provides a means of bridging the gap between public health policy and practice and is ' ... not an end in itself; its intended benefits depend on integration and implementation by the end users, who will also determine the relevance and usability of whatever is disseminated' (Green, Ottoson, García, & Hiatt, 2009, p. 178). Frequently used as the concluding phase of a participatory visual project, a public event or screening provides a platform for the team to share the project results with a broad audience and to devise steps for collective action. Mitchell urges scholars to ' ... be haunted by images and work with communities in ways that ensure that others are similarly haunted' (Mitchell, 2011, p. 200). How, then, can we employ critical dissemination practices to haunt others, particularly public health policy-makers and others who have the power and resources to catalyse change? In each research context, the appropriate strategies will differ depending on the actors and sectors involved.

In terms of the purpose of dissemination activities and the potential to catalyse change, public screenings can also be employed as a platform for exposing ' ... the issues about which people are silent – those issues which are "hidden" and around which community action is required' (Mitchell & De Lange, 2011, p. 179). Previous work has also demonstrated that successful dissemination strategies are not necessarily measured based on the quantity and span of the audience reached but rather strategically planning 'who sees it and what they do with it', particularly if the communicative purpose targets policy-makers (Miller & Smith, 2012, p. 345; Mitchell, 2011; Wheeler, 2012).

Sustainability

While ethical dilemmas and power dynamics implicit in visual projects have been explored in previous work (Bleiker & Kay, 2007; Joanou, 2009; Prins, 2010), the subsequent use of the images and footage captured by participatory photography and video projects is rarely discussed in detail. De Lange and Mitchell's (2012) work makes an important contribution to this gap in the literature through their call for reflection about 'what happens when we're gone' (p. 318) and what contributes to the sustainability and 'afterlife' of participatory video projects (De Lange & Mitchell, 2012, p. 319). This call beckons us to question what *can* and what *do* communities do with visual materials upon project completion.

In relation to participatory visual methods, social change has been conceptualised in terms of action within the research community and the academic community that is catalysed 'over time and [is] not some sort of "in and out" type of activity' (Mitchell & De Lange, 2011, p. 183). Additionally, Plush (2012) argues that,

> participatory video holds the potential to educate, persuade, and advocate in ways that bring positive change. To do so, participatory video projects designed explicitly for social change need to go beyond a process of community members telling their stories through video mainly for an external audience. (p. 68)

In order to push the use of visual methods beyond storytelling and to integrate participatory ideals within the process, Plush (2012) discusses the importance of incorporating mechanisms that strengthen the agency of participants and argues that the 'use of the final videos must be embedded into larger development projects and programs that incorporate empowering initiatives for community-led advocacy' (p. 81). Drawing from the field of visual anthropology, scholars also emphasise the importance of articulating the participatory visual research process with advocacy networks as a means of engaging the activist community in the dissemination of the participatory photographs and videos produced in the project (Mitchell & De Lange, 2011, p. 183).

The following section describes the research design and methodology guiding the ongoing PAR initiative as well as the specific design of the 'Beyond Glue and Bazuco' subproject. In the subsequent results section, I return to the three principles and practices discussed in this section and contextualise their importance for attaining the social justice objectives of the project.

PAR design and methodology

The qualitative and visual information presented in this paper draws from multiple phases and subprojects of a long-term PAR initiative with street-connected communities in Bogotá, Colombia. The long-term PAR initiative started in 2008 with a group of 10 street-connected female and transgender adolescents. They became community action research leaders throughout the process and were formally trained in qualitative, geo-ethnographic, and participatory methodologies. The PAR process has involved 63 street-connected adolescents and youth in formal research activities using different combinations of the above-mentioned methodologies and organised into the following subprojects: (1) the socio-spatial exclusion and violence against street-connected youth in Bogotá; (2) trafficking of minors and sexual exploitation; (3) gender-based violence in experiences of forced displacement; and (4) inhalant/glue and *bazuco* addiction ('Beyond Glue and Bazuco' project).

The 'Beyond Glue and Bazuco' project is a follow-up initiative catalysed by one of the community action research leaders of the long-term PAR initiative. The 'Beyond Glue and Bazuco' project used interview data from the first two subprojects to define the initial project objectives targeting substance abuse, which the team identified as an important challenge in the lives of street-connected adolescents. Additionally, this paper draws from qualitative data from the first subproject in order to contextualise the life histories of street-connected adolescents and youth. The first subproject on the socio-spatial exclusion of street-connected adolescents and youth was completed with a total research population of 33 participants, each of whom participated in 3 semi-structured interviews (exploratory, auto-photographic, and cognitive and activity mapping interviews). In addition to the 99 interviews conducted, 5 roving focus groups were also conducted in order to capture additional socio-spatial variables of exclusion that were not captured in other research phases. The roving focus groups were used to further stimulate conversation in a group setting referred to as 'talking whilst walking' through a particular zone of the study site (Anderson, 2004).

The research design of the 'Beyond Glue and Bazuco' subproject included ten semi-structured life history interviews and four cartographic focus groups with street-connected adolescents who have consumed glue and/or *bazuco* since early childhood. In this research context, the cartographic focus groups were used to catalyse a group conversation guided by a social mapping exercise aiming to destabilise dominant representations of urban space through the voices and vision of participants (Kwan, 2002).

After completing these data collection phases, we held several group analysis sessions. The sessions included university researchers and street-connected adolescents in order to collectively identify areas for action and advocacy. Based on the analysis session conclusions, the team then collectively designed the participatory visual research component as a means of working towards the social change objectives of the project. The participatory visual component of the 'Beyond Glue and Bazuco' subproject was completed with the 10 street-connected adolescents who participated in the previous phases and included their participation in each of the 5 phases detailed in Table 1.

Through each of the phases, the ethical framework underpinning this project seeks to move beyond the consideration of research ethics as limited to institutional ethics and informed consent procedures and towards a more comprehensive care ethics practice that prioritises empathy, mutual understanding, and respect in the development of relationships with participants and the broader research community (Ritterbusch, 2012).

Drawing from the various subprojects of the long-term PAR initiative and from the qualitative and participatory visual methods components of the 'Beyond Glue and Bazuco' project, the following section presents the project's results and social change activities designed and implemented by the PAR team.

Table 1. Details of the participatory visual methods process.

Visual component phases	Description
(1) Immersion activities and generation of trust between university and street-connected team members	These activities included a sleep over and bonfire with storytelling at the rehabilitation centre where university team members stayed the night, various self-empowerment workshops led by university team members and artistic activities including the decoration of coffee mugs and jewellery in order to cultivate the creativity of each team member and to collectively create an artistic product as a team
(2) Identification of transformative objectives of the project	During group analysis sessions, the street- and university-connected team members analysed the life history and cartography content from the previous phases in order to identify the principle problems to be addressed in the action component of the PAR project. The problems that the team decided to focus on for this project were stigma and discrimination
(3) Participatory photography design and implementation	This process included the naming of each phase/category of the photo shoot – see 'Participatory photography' section of 'Results' for more detail
(4) Participatory video process	See 'Participatory video' section of 'Results' for more detail
(5) Participatory forum	Including planning, rehearsal and de-brief – see 'Participatory forum' section of 'Results' for more detail

Results

The results section follows the conceptual logic presented in the literature review sections above, including a discussion of how the core principles of reflexivity, dissemination, and sustainability were incorporated within the project design and how they contributed to the achievement of the social change outcomes surrounding institutional stigma. The first three sections describe different ways in which reflexivity and group reflection were stimulated by the use of life histories, participatory photography, and participatory video, the fourth section describes the critical dissemination strategies used to catalyse social change and to mobilise different sectors of society towards action and the fifth section describes the 'afterlife' and sustainability of the project through the consolidation of the non-profit organisation PARCES.

Placing street-based substance abuse and institutional stigma in context: the use of life histories in the participatory visual methods process

Through the employment of life history methods during the initial phases of the project, our PAR team dedicated a great deal of time to the creation of safe spaces for mapping the common ground that unite the project-based goals and dreams of both university-based and street-based participatory researchers. As part of the process of generating consciousness about a particular health-related issue and preparing the terrain for critical social change praxis employed in the participatory visual methods process, the use of life history techniques can provide a productive space for reflexivity and group reflection surrounding the health-related problems being explored.

An emergent theme in the life history data collected during the initial phases of the 'Beyond Glue and Bazuco' study was participants' desire to be seen not as addicts but rather as human beings with particular histories and experiences that led them to seek refuge in drugs and in the streets. As stated by one of the participants, ' … my name is not "bazuco" … my name is Viviana … ' (Viviana, Exploratory Interview, 22 February 2013). This quote contextualises street-connected adolescents' frustrations with the manner in which their families, the media, health workers, and other public health professionals reduce their identities to the substances they consume in the streets.

Hunger, poverty, pain, abandonment, neglect, violent memories, and rage are some of the common feelings and realities that lead marginalised youth to inhalant/glue and *bazuco* abuse. A rough home life and childhood of domestic violence, rape, and the conditions of extreme impoverishment push children and adolescents to the streets of Bogotá in pursuit of opportunities and a better life.

In Camila's life history, she explains why she was forced to leave her home in Cali and fend for herself in the streets of Bogotá:

> … I got pregnant at an early age … mmm … my Mommy turned her back on me and I don't know my father's family … my Aunt beat me a lot and my uncle, well my Aunt's husband, raped me, and my Aunt's son also raped me … and I didn't have a relationship with anyone … not with my cousins or anyone … I was always alone … And my Dad is an alcoholic and lives in Medellin, he is a drug addict … My Mommy had me when she was 14 years old. And she left me with my grandmother … I told my mother about the rapes and she didn't believe me. She told me no, that I was a liar, that she knew my Aunt very well and what class of person she was, that how could I say such a thing … well the child welfare agency [ICBF] helped me make a legal case [against my Uncle] … but nothing ever came of it … And well my Mommy left me with ICBF declaring abandonment because of my pregnancy … and she left and since then I know nothing else of her … (Camila, Exploratory Interview, 11 February 2010)

The life history of Camila echoes the content of dozens of other interviews our team has conducted over the last six years and contextualises why youth seek refuge in the streets and in drugs in the absence of safety within the family unit.

While multiple child protection institutions exist at both the district and national scale in Colombia, many children and adolescents prefer to fend for themselves in the streets rather than face discrimination, abuse, and lack of emotional care and empathy in state institutions. Rehabilitation programmes rarely incorporate the training of public health professionals in order to provide them with non-judgemental and empathetic strategies for dealing with the complexities of street-connected adolescents' trauma-driven behaviours.

As revealed by Isabela, sexual and other forms of abuse and harassment often occur in child protection institutions:

> … when I was pregnant I was institutionalized and a nun sexually abused me … the room assignments placed two girls together and she never assigned me a roommate and she would come to my room at 10 at night to visit me and hug me … (Isabela, Exploratory Interview, 4 May 2010)

Several participants also mention experiences of verbal abuse and discrimination in different child protection and rehabilitation institutions:

> … there are professors that confront you about nothing and they tell you 'that you are a bitch' and you don't know why. (Paola, Exploratory Interview, 15 June 2010)

In addition to the abuse and discrimination experienced in early childhood both at home and in child protection institutions, street-connected adolescents also describe receiving mistreatment, mistrust, and judgement from public health professionals in reha-bilitation programmes:

> I have felt boxed in, for example in the moment when you go to talk with them [health workers] ... the psychologists always box you in ... They always do that ... they have the idea ... that the drug addict is a manipulator. That the drug addict is a liar ... that you can't believe everything a drug addict says ... for example ... something is hurting me and I express that something is hurting me and right away she [the psychologist] assumes that it is anxiety to consume [withdrawal]. No ... they can't believe that maybe something is really hurting ... this also affects me ... (Stella, Focus Group, 23 May 2013)

Stella's intervention in the focus group inspired extensive reflection among all partici-pants about the general lack of respect, empathy, and mutual understanding in their mul-tiple daily encounters with health workers and other institutional actors in the rehabilitation programme. Within state child protection and drug rehabilitation pro-grammes for children and adolescents, there is little or no emphasis on the importance of creating safe, caring, and empathetic spaces for productive interactions between health workers and programme participants. Rather than designing ways to establish trust and create the sensation of family, closeness and care, children and adolescents are kept at a distance and made to feel as less-than and different from health workers and other institutional actors.

Humanising 'addicts' through participatory visual methods: mobilising our voices and vision against stigma

Based on group analysis of participants' experiences of discrimination and violence, the team designed the participatory photography and video component of the project detailed in the following sections. Through the subversion of the traditional use of the camera in research, team members worked towards the social change objectives of the project by re-presenting young, street-connected 'addicts' to society in the way that they want to be seen thus presenting a new set of visually based meanings and working against institutional stigma through participatory photography and video.

Participatory photography: my photos, my fight against stigma

Based on the multiple institutional stigmas identified during the interview and focus group phases of the 'Beyond Glue and Bazuco' project, the participatory photography activities were organised into three categories representing participants' experiences of stigma and discrimination: (1) 'Gomelas[2]: How Society Wants Me to Be', (2) 'How Society Sees Me', and (3) 'How I Am'. During the focus group phase, multiple decisions were made about the photo shoot process including conversations in which all research actors decided how they wanted to be photographed, with what backdrop, with what clothing and make-up, and what props to use (including the creation of fake drug pipes, glue bags, cell phones, shoes, etc.). We used the participatory photography exercises as a space for both individual and collective reflection surrounding the ways participants wanted the photographs to be used, for what purpose and in what contexts (Figure 2).

Through this process of critical reflection that took place both while taking the photo-graphs and while reviewing how they turned out, project participants were able to com-municate their frustrations of being misunderstood and mistreated on a daily basis and

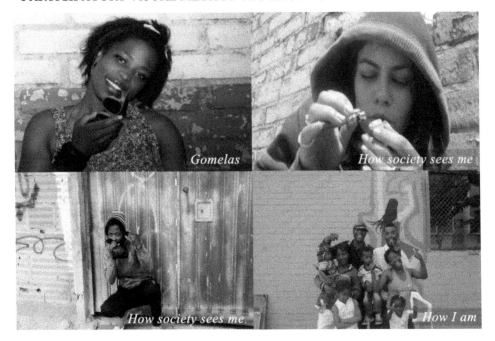

Figure 2. '*Gomelas*: How society wants me to be', 'How society sees me', 'How I am'.

were able to channel their message about how they want to be seen and treated: as human beings, smiling, as mothers, as sisters, as daughters, as friends, as lovers, and as citizens that deserve respect and care like everyone else.

Participatory video: 'Behind the veil'[3]

The participatory video process also included multiple conversations and reflections with project participants about how they wanted to re-present themselves to society, how they wanted to be filmed and what they wanted to be doing and wearing. The video includes the following scenes: project participant's jumping, walking, dancing, rapping, doing arts activities and painting, doing their make-up, laughing together, and smiling. These particular moments in the video humanise project participants, moving beyond traditional representations of glue and *bazuco* users and showing that they are just like any other group of adolescent girls in Colombia, capable of smiling, feeling, laughing, and entitled to the fundamental human rights that are often violated, even within institutions that ostensibly exist to provide care.

The video's song was written by one of the PAR team members and was inspired by his interaction with project participants during the focus group and reflection sessions. The principle message communicated through these lyrics is the desire to be seen as a human being and the desire for society to see the positive aspects of participants' personalities and life histories. In the use of participatory visual methods, the most important factor to consider when evaluating the quality and relevance of the visual product for the research community is whether participants feel represented by the images and videos being displayed. As discussed in postcolonial feminist literature, there are problems and ethical dilemmas implicit in the representation of marginalised communities through text or images (Spivak, 1988; Tuhiwai Smith, 1999). As presented by Tuhiwai Smith (1999), the problem arises when ' … we do see ourselves but can barely recognize ourselves through the representation' (p. 35). In the context of participatory visual projects, an important ethical protocol involves participant feedback on the final products in order to ensure that they feel identified with the images representing their daily lives and struggles. As was the case in our project, one way to achieve participant identification with visual products is their involvement in every stage of project design and the production of images and footage.

The participatory video making process included a profound process of reflection surrounding stigmas experienced by adolescent glue and *bazuco* users and reflections about the discrimination they experience on a daily basis because of their physical appearance. During the video planning phase and artistic interventions, participants reflected about the consequences of the stigmatising labels imposed on them by different actors in society and in the rehabilitation programme. Through these critical discussions, participants collectively constructed the content of their message to society in general and health workers in particular through the design of the posters used in the video to complete the phrase in the song 'behind the veil' with the following words: 'I'm the same as you', '[I have] The freedom and right to exercise my sexuality', 'I'm a mother', '[You must] Respect my rights', 'I'm brave' and 'I'm a warrior' (respectively, according to Figure 3). The poster phrases communicate multiple messages to a broad audience,

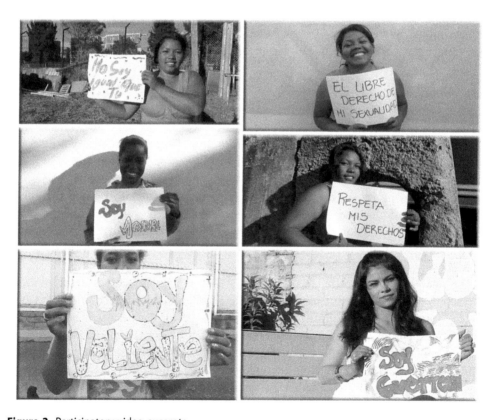

Figure 3. Participatory video excerpts.

including the stigmas public health and rehabilitation programmes should work to counter through programme activities and through the training of health workers to recognise street-connected adolescents as more than 'addicts' and most importantly as human beings. These phrases written by participants answer the following question posed by the research team: How do you want to be seen by the world? What is the veil (of stigma) hiding?.

Participatory forum against glue and 'bazuco' stigmas: exploring critical dissemination methods for social change

The participatory forum against glue and *bazuco*-related stigma was planned as the culmination of the participatory visual research process and for a diverse audience including public health, rehabilitation and drug policy-makers, toxicology specialists, academics across different health-related disciplines, students and activist organisations (Figure 4).

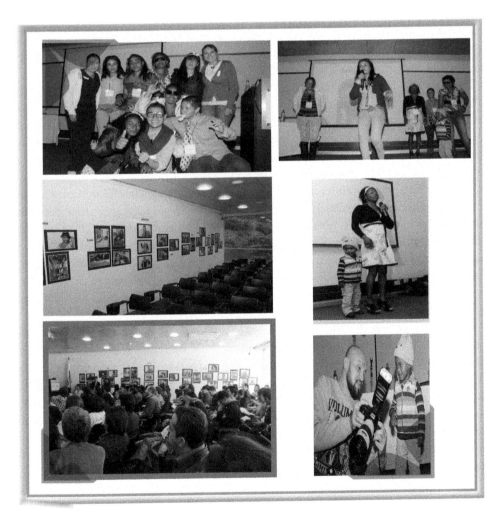

Figure 4. Participatory forum.

We planned the forum with the participants of the 'Beyond Glue and Bazuco' project as a place in which multiple actors could engage in an albeit uncomfortable yet productive conversation about the life histories leading to glue and *bazuco* addiction, the physiological consequences of consumption, the efficacy of rehabilitation programmes and the agencies designing state-driven outreach efforts with street-connected populations. The participatory forum sought to inspire reflection and debate between all attendees including the expert panels, a presentation of the participatory video, a presentation of life histories led by street-connected adolescents and a collective viewing of participant's photographs in a gallery posted on the wall of the auditorium.

Panel topics ranged from public health approaches to inhalant and *bazuco* addiction to street-connected adolescents' lived experiences of the effects of glue and *bazuco* in their daily lives. Panellists included academic, public sector and street-based experts including the director of the district's largest street-based substance abuse rehabilitation programme, a toxicology specialist, an analyst on drug policy from the national government, academics from different disciplines and street-connected adolescents who contributed their experiences in rehabilitation programmes and street life to the panel discussions.

At the end of every 'expert'-led discussion, street-connected adolescents posed questions to the panellists and opened the space for audience participation. Beyond just moderating and posing difficult questions, street-connected adolescents were also the principle panellists of the first featured panel on the lived experiences of addiction.

The diversity of perspectives and approaches to understanding the dynamics of glue, *bazuco,* and life in the streets was overwhelming for various panellists, including street-connected adolescents, and for the audience. The conversation was uncomfortable and at times aggressive, and the participatory methodology was disconcerting for academic panellists and government officials accustomed to being the experts within a context of order and authority in traditional academic conference settings.

In this forum, Bogotá's street-connected adolescents and 'addicts' also occupied a space of authority and were regarded as experts in the addictions and substance abuse they have faced throughout their lives. As a means of empowerment and in order to destabilise traditional hierarchies in academic research and conferences, these street-based experts were the hosts of the event and were the moderators of each panel including the diverse groups of experts mentioned previously. The street-connected adolescents were in charge of time keeping for each panel, commentary, and presentation of guiding questions following each panel presentation and the identification of questions from the audience.

Having control over the microphone and the moderation of the overall event was also a symbolic act of prioritising participants' voices in the dissemination process and placing them in direct dialogue with those who traditionally have decision-making power in rehabilitation programmes. One of the comments made by project participants during the public health panel included the following statement: ' ... just because I supposedly have a lower IQ than those individuals who didn't do glue when they were young doesn't mean that I can't study and achieve my dreams'. Through this participatory approach to the dissemination of research findings, participants felt more powerful than those who constantly reduce them to the substances they consume.

Although uncomfortable for all parties, our team made an effort to construct a safe space within the forum auditorium for reflection, debate and empathy between the diverse panellists and audiences, allowing participants to be themselves and re-present their image and life histories to society the way they want to be seen. Project participants stood up in front of more than 120 individuals and demanded to be treated with respect and care in both rehabilitation programmes and public spaces in Bogotá. It is important to create this safe space at the beginning of the event by stating that all perspectives and experiences can be freely expressed and by requesting that all forum participants act and intervene in a respectful, empathetic manner. A safe space for reflection and expression is the context in which solutions to public health problems can be collectively designed.

PARCES and the potential of 'critical hope' for sustainability

As questioned by participatory visual methods scholars in previous work, what happens after the forum? What is done with this knowledge that haunts policy-makers as they return to their offices the next day? What do community leaders and activists do with this knowledge after being inspired to action through a critical dissemination activity (see Cahill et al., 2010; De Lange & Mitchell, 2012)? In the case of the 'Beyond Glue and Bazuco' project, the beginnings of the afterlife of the participatory visual initiative were inspired by the development of a sense of community between university and street-connected activists and rehabilitation programme workers. Through the project, this diverse group of individuals identified the common goal of improving the quality of life and the protection of street-connected adolescents' human rights.

Two months after the forum, the non-profit organisation PARCES[4] (the Spanish acronym for Peers in Action-Reaction Against Social Exclusion), was founded by members of the 'Beyond Glue and Bazuco' project. This grassroots organisation continues to work towards the social justice objectives of the 'Beyond Glue and Bazuco' project through a formal alliance with the government in the implementation of the 'Youth for Peace' programme, a youth empowerment initiative within the state institution that houses the rehabilitation programme discussed in this article. Programme participants are trained in the principles of PAR and must complete an internship with a social organisation as the exit project of the internship. PARCES sponsors a group of interns from this programme each year and the current group of interns are working on the design of the 'Safe Spaces' programme to be implemented in the state institution. This training programme provides a means of working alongside street-connected adolescents in order to inform interventions that make a difference in their lives and those of their peers. Drawing from critical PAR scholars, the work of PARCES in the fight against inequality in Colombia echoes the definition of critical hope as a feminist practice 'where what could be is sought; where what has been, is critiqued; and where what is, is troubled' (Torre et al., 2001, p. 150; cited in Cahill et al., 2010, p. 407).

In a society fraught with civil strife and armed conflict and divided along the lines of geographic, racial, class, and gendered difference, it is not often that a diverse group of activists, university students and street-connected adolescents come together to challenge the invisible barbed wires that traditionally keep these groups at an 'acceptable' distance from one another in the city. The PAR initiatives of PARCES include the annual 'Sex Worker's Forum' in Bogotá fighting for youth sex worker's health rights and against police abuse, a human rights project with street-connected and LGBTQ populations in prison and a participatory photography project with street-connected youth involved in prostitution. PARCES has also designed and launched the 'Safe Spaces' programme for LGBTQ youth implemented in both government and educational institutions and a participatory photography project with transgender, street-connected youth who are victims of forced displacement. Through the collective planning and implementation of these PAR initiatives, long-lasting relationships are cultivated with community members involved in each project. What lives on after project completion are precisely these relationships and the bonds formed during the fight for a common purpose. These projects are sustained by the energy of the youth driving the PARCES movement and continue to create spaces for critical interventions that catalyse social transformations in the lives of street-connected adolescents in Colombia.

Conclusion

Aligned with the objective of mainstreaming the use of humanising praxis within public health research and practice at the global scale, this paper urges scholars to use participatory visual methods to contextualise and visualise the answers to health-related research questions and to capture information that is not easily or efficiently communicated verbally, textually, or quantitatively. This paper also illustrates the transformative potential of participatory visual dissemination methods for working against processes of stigmatisation in rehabilitation programmes and for destabilising the power relations implicit in traditional research methodologies. Finally, I argue that public health professionals can use participatory visual methodologies to counter stigmas surrounding multiple health-related issues and to generate empathetic, reciprocal, and caring relations between health workers and historically marginalised populations.

Notes

1. *Bazuco* is often equated to crack; however, chemically, *bazuco* is the 'intermediate product in the production of cocaine' and in some contexts is referred to as 'PBC' (*pasta básica de cocaina*) or cocaine paste (Joanou, 2009, p. 216).
2. A label used in Colombian society referring to dainty, rich girls and women (in this case, for gender).
3. See http://youtu.be/w1EoO2avtwU to view the participatory video (YouTube version).
4. In the Colombian context, the word *parce* in Spanish means friend, peer or companion in a relationship of trust and solidarity. See www.parces.org for more information about the organisation.

Acknowledgments

I would like to express my gratitude and appreciation of all research actors involved in and touched by the PAR process in the distinct projects mentioned in this article. I also thank my colleagues of PARCES who tirelessly fight for the human rights of sex workers, LGBTQ + communities, homeless and other street-connected populations in Colombia and who played an essential role in the development of this care ethics-grounded participatory visual methods project. Finally, I would like to express my gratitude directly to the youth from the rehabilitation institution, Laura Martínez Apráez (team leader of the participatory photography exercise), Rafael Bojaca (film-maker in charge of the participatory video exercise), María Inés Cubides Kovacsics (team leader in charge of action research and fieldwork coordination), Julian(a) Salamanca and Alejandro Lanz Sánchez (team leaders in charge of action-oriented activities, trust building and community–university relations), and Argenis Navarro Diaz (team leader in charge of street-based outreach and relationships within the rehabilitation institution).

Disclosure statement

No potential conflict of interest was reported by the authors.

Funding

This research was funded by the Center for the Study of Security and Drugs (CESED) and also draws from research funded by the National Science Foundation [grant number BCS-0903025].

References

Aldridge, J. (2007). Picture this: The use of participatory photographic research methods with people with learning disabilities. *Disability & Society, 22*(1), 1–17. doi:10.1080/09687590601056006

Allen, L. (2008). Young people's 'agency' in sexuality research using visual methods. *Journal of Youth Studies, 11*(6), 565–577. doi:10.1080/13676260802225744

Allen, L. (2009). 'Snapped': Researching the sexual cultures of schools using visual methods. *International Journal of Qualitative Studies in Education, 22*(5), 549–561. doi:10.1080/09518390903051523

Anderson, J. (2004). Talking whilst walking: A geographical archaeology of knowledge. *Area, 36*(3), 254–261. doi:10.1111/j.0004-0894.2004.00222.x

Annear, M., Cushman, G., Gidlow, B., Keeling, S., Wilkinson, T., & Hopkins, H. (2013). A place for visual research methods in the field of leisure studies? Evidence from two studies of older adults' active leisure. *Leisure Studies, 33*(6), 618–643. doi:10.1080/02614367.2013.841743

Arieli, D., Friedman, V. J., & Agbaria, K. (2009). The paradox of participation in action research. *Action Research, 7*(3), 263–290. doi:10.1177/1476750309336718

Balbale, S., Schwingel, A., Chodzko-Zajko, W., & Huhman, M. (2014). Visual and participatory research methods for the development of health messages for underserved populations. *Health Communication, 29*(7), 728–740. doi:10.1080/10410236.2013.800442

Bleiker, R., & Kay, A. (2007). Representing HIV/AIDS in Africa: Pluralist photography and local empowerment. *International Studies Quarterly, 51*(1), 139–163. doi:10.1111/j.1468-2478.2007.00443

Cahill, C. (2004). Defying gravity? Raising consciousness through collective research. *Children's Geographies, 2*(2), 273–286. doi:10.1080/14733280410001720557

Cahill, C. (2007a). Doing research with young people: Participatory research and the rituals of collective work. *Children's Geographies, 5*(3), 297–312. doi:10.1080/14733280701445895

Cahill, C. (2007b). Repositioning ethical commitments: Participatory action research as a relational praxis of social change. *ACME: An International E-Journal for Critical Geographies, 6*(3), 360–373. Retrieved from http://www.acme-journal.org/vol6/CC.pdf

Cahill, C., Quijada D. A., & Bradley, M. (2010). 'Dreaming of … ': Reflections on participatory action research as a feminist praxis of critical hope. *Affilia, 25*(4), 406–416. doi:10.1177/0886109910384576

Clark, A. (2011). Breaking methodological boundaries? Exploring visual, participatory methods with adults and young children. *European Early Childhood Education Research Journal, 19*(3), 321–330. doi:10.1080/1350293X.2011.597964

Cooke, B., & Kothari, U. (Eds.). (2001). *Participation: The new tyranny?* London: Zed Books.

De Lange, N., & Mitchell, C. (2012). Building sustainability into work with participatory video. In E.-J. Milne, C. Mitchell, & N. De Lange (Eds.), *Handbook of participatory video* (pp. 318–330). Plymouth: AltaMira Press.

Francis, D., & Hemson, C. (2006). 'See the Hope' – Using participatory visual arts methods to challenge HIV related stigma. *Education as Change, 10*(2), 53–65. doi:10.1080/168232006094 87139

Fullana, J., Pallisera, M., & Vilà, M. (2013). Advancing towards inclusive social research: Visual methods as opportunities for people with severe mental illness to participate in research. *International Journal of Social Research Methodology, 17*(6), 723–738. doi:10.1080/13645579. 2013.832049

Green, L. W., Ottoson, J. M., García, C., & Hiatt, R. A. (2009). Diffusion theory and knowledge dissemination, utilization, and integration in public health. *Annual Review of Public Health, 30*(1), 151–174. doi:10.1146/annurev.publhealth.031308.100049

Hwang, S. K. (2013). Home movies in participatory research: Children as movie-makers. *International Journal of Social Research Methodology, 16*(5), 445–456. doi:10.1080/13645579. 2012.729796

Joanou, J. P. (2009). The bad and the ugly: Ethical concerns in participatory photographic methods with children living and working on the streets of Lima, Peru. *Visual Studies, 24*(3), 214–223. doi:10.1080/14725860903309120

Kwan, M. P. (2002). Feminist visualization: Re-envisioning GIS as a method in feminist geographic research. *Annals of the Association of American Geographers, 92*(4), 645–661. doi:10.1111/1467-8306.00309

Miller, E., & Smith, M. (2012). Dissemination and ownership of knowledge. In E-J. Milne, C. Mitchell, & N. De Lange (Eds.), *Handbook of participatory video* (pp. 331–348). Plymouth: AltaMira Press.

Mitchell, C. (2011). *Doing visual research.* London: Sage.

Mitchell, C., & De Lange, N. (2011). Community-based participatory video and social action in rural South Africa. In E. Margolis & L. Pauwels (Eds.), *The Sage handbook of visual research methods* (pp. 171–185). London: Sage.

Mohan, G. (2001). Beyond participation: Strategies for deeper empowerment. In B. Cooke & U. Kothari (Eds.), *Participation the new tyranny?* (pp. 153–167). London: Zed Books.

O'Connell, R. (2013). The use of visual methods with children in a mixed methods study of family food practices. *International Journal of Social Research Methodology, 16*(1), 31–46. doi:10.1080/13645579.2011.647517

Pain, R. (2004) Social geography: Participatory research. *Progress in Human Geography, 28*(5), 652–663. doi:10.1191/0309132504ph511

Pain, R., Kesby, M., & Askins, K. (2011). Geographies of impact: Power, participation and potential. *Area, 43*(2), 183–188. doi:10.1111/j.1475-4762.2010.00978.x

Palmer, V. J., Dowrick, C. & Gunn, J. M. (2014). Mandalas as a visual research method for understanding primary care for depression. *International Journal of Social Research Methodology, 17*(5), 527–541. doi:10.1080/13645579.2013.796764

Plush, T. (2012). Fostering social change through participatory video: A conceptual framework. In E-J. Milne, C. Mitchell, & N. De Lange (Eds.), *Handbook of participatory video* (pp. 67–84). Plymouth: AltaMira Press.

Prins, E. (2010). Participatory photography: A tool for empowerment or surveillance? *Action Research, 8*(4), 426–443. doi:10.1177/1476750310374502

Ritterbusch, A. (2012). Bridging guidelines and practice: Toward a grounded care ethics in youth participatory action research. *The Professional Geographer, 64*(1), 16–24. doi:10.1080/00330124.2011.596783

Sitter, K. C. (2012). Participatory video: Toward a method, advocacy and voice (MAV) framework. *Intercultural Education, 23*(6), 541–554. doi:10.1080/14675986.2012.746842

Skelton, T. (2008). Research with children and young people: Exploring the tensions between ethics, competence and participation. *Children's Geographies, 6*(1), 21–36. doi:10.1080/1473328070 1791876

Spivak, G. C. (1988). Can the subaltern speak? In C. Nelson & L. Grossberg (Eds.), *Marxism and the interpretation of culture* (pp. 271–313). Basingstoke: Macmillan Education.

Torre, M. E., Fine, M., Boudin, K., Bowen, I., Clark, J., Hylton, D., & Upegui, D. (2001). A space for co-constructing counter stories under surveillance. *International Journal of Critical Psychology, 4,* 149–166.

Tuhiwai Smith, L. (1999). *Decolonizing methodologies: Research and indigenous peoples.* New York, NY: Zed Books.

Waite, L., & Conn, C. (2012). Participatory video: A feminist way of seeing? In E-J. Milne, C. Mitchell, & N. De Lange (Eds.), *Handbook of participatory video* (pp. 85–99). Plymouth: AltaMira Press.

Wheeler, J. (2012). Using participatory video to engage in policy processes: Representation, power, and knowledge in public screenings. In E-J. Milne, C. Mitchell, & N. De Lange (Eds.), *Handbook of participatory video* (pp. 365–379). Plymouth: AltaMira Press.

Yang, K. (2012). Reflexivity, participation and video. In E-J. Milne, C. Mitchell, & N. De Lange (Eds.), *Handbook of participatory video* (pp. 100–114). Plymouth: AltaMira Press.

Bodies as evidence: Mapping new terrain for teen pregnancy and parenting

Aline C. Gubrium[a,], Alice Fiddian-Green[a], Kasey Jernigan[b] and Elizabeth L. Krause[b]

[a]School of Public Health and Health Sciences, University of Massachusetts Amherst, Amherst, MA, USA;
[b]Department of Anthropology, University of Massachusetts Amherst, Amherst, MA, USA

ABSTRACT

Predominant approaches to teen pregnancy focus on decreasing numbers of teen mothers, babies born to them, and state dollars spent to support their families. This overshadows the structural violence interwoven into daily existence for these young parents. This paper argues for the increased use of participatory visual methods to compliment traditional research methods in shifting notions of what counts as evidence in response to teen pregnancy and parenting. We present the methods and results from a body mapping workshop as part of 'Hear Our Stories: Diasporic Youth for Sexual Rights and Justice', a project that examines structural barriers faced by young parenting Latinas and seeks to develop relevant messaging and programming to support and engage youth. Body mapping, as an engaging, innovative participatory visual methodology, involves young parenting women and other marginalised populations in drawing out a deeper understanding of sexual health inequities. Our findings highlight the ways body mapping elicits *bodies as evidence* to understand young motherhood and wellbeing.

Introduction

Teen pregnancy and birth are considered a major public health and social problem. Although birth rates among women aged 15–19 years are at a record low (31.3 per 1000) in the United States (Hamilton, Martin, & Ventura, 2012), teen pregnancy remains a national public health priority requiring targeted interventions (Shaw & Lawlor, 2007). It is considered simultaneously a medical, social, and economic problem for both the young mother and her child, as well as for society at large (Bonell, 2004; Hoffman, 2008; Kearney & Levine, 2012; Scally, 2010). According to the 2010 *Annual Review of Public Health*, teen pregnancy is associated with low educational attainment; increased unemployment, poverty, and welfare dependency; rapid repeat pregnancy; single motherhood and divorce. Furthermore, infants of teenage mothers are more likely to be premature, experience infant mortality, and, as children, do less well on health and social wellbeing indicators than children of older mothers (Santelli & Melnikas, 2010).

Our approach is at odds with what are often depicted as glaring truths. We shift notions of what counts as evidence in the construction of and response to teen parenting and youth sexuality through body mapping – a participatory visual methodology that engages young parenting women as artists incarnate. Body mapping is an arts-based research method in which participants are asked to draw, write, paint, or use other artistic means to respond to prompts, which correspond to different parts of the body, so as to explore their lives. The body mapping process stands out as an innovative approach for acknowledging and incorporating the multifaceted nature of people's lives, and recognises the limitations of traditional research methods and approaches to assessing and addressing health inequities. In this paper, we highlight the ways the technique, both empirically and critically, elicits bodies *as evidence otherwise not captured*, to map new terrain for understanding youth sexuality, motherhood, and wellbeing.

Existing approaches to teen pregnancy emphasise narrow, band-aid solutions myopically focused on individual-level behaviours and specifically aimed at the poor. They fail to use the relevant local knowledge of those targeted (i.e. youth deemed 'at risk' for teen pregnancy) and rarely take into account the marginalised existence of many young people who are systematically neglected by the state and whose communities have experienced histories of material dispossession. Thus, issues related to structural violence that become embodied – including housing and food insecurity, interpersonal and state-based violence, marginalisation in the public education system, and insecurity as a result of dispossession from the state system – are either ignored or, worse, used as 'rhetoric of blame' (Quesada, Hart, & Bourgois, 2011) to legitimise oft-cited negative outcomes of teen pregnancy and parenting.

We argue that negative outcomes that are presented as inherent to, or caused by, teen pregnancy (Santelli & Melnikas, 2010) are better attributed to the effects of social inequality, poverty, and racism (Geronimus, 2003; Geronimus & Korenman, 1993; Sisson, 2012). As such, the construction of teen pregnancy and young motherhood as a social and public health problem cannot be understood separately from the historical, political, moral, and economic fabric of individual communities (Holgate, Evans, & Yuen, 2006) and is always subject to shifting historical moments and social policies (Luker, 1996; Mulongo, 2006; Nathanson, 1991).

Bodies of evidence on teen pregnancy and parenting

Bodies of evidence surrounding teen pregnancy and the teen birth 'epidemic' are socially maneuvered to biopolitically manage and control the lives of young Latinas, positioning individuals who act outside of the expected 'norm' as errant, irresponsible, and a drain on public resources. Predicated on lowered rates and reduced statistics as evidence of effectiveness (i.e. *decreased* numbers of teen pregnancies, babies born to teen mothers, and state dollars spent to support their families), bodies of evidence inform a 'teen pregnancy industrial complex' (Chris Barcelos, 2014, personal communication), rather than supporting human dignity through meaningful engagement. Dominant notions of biocitizenship are hence constituted through a moral economy in which 'to be deemed a worthy, responsible American, each of us must become a virtuous biocitizen' (Greenhalgh & Carney, 2014). In the context of youth sexuality, a good biocitizen will graduate from high school, attend a college or university, earn a good wage and benefits, get married, and *then* have a child or children. Valuations on the body politic also inform the evidence. Chavez (2004) argues,

> Latina biological reproduction combines with its social reproduction to produce fears about the population growth of Latinos in American society, which in turn positions them as a possible threat to the 'nation', that is, the 'people' as conceived in demographic and racial terms. (p. 175)

Teen motherhood – itself a product of specific historical, cultural, and social processes that work to provide 'calibrations of ideal motherhood' (Smart, 1996, p. 46) – is conceptualized in terms of outcomes insofar as teen mothers are framed as psychologically immature and incapable of being good parents (Mulongo, 2006; Smart, 1996). A focus on the medical, psychological, and physical aspects of teenage pregnancy invokes an authoritative voice that at once decontextualizes young mothers' sexuality while ignoring the structural factors that influence how teen mothers experience their sexuality, motherhood, and selfhood (Mulongo, 2006). Our aim is to glean more nuanced bodies of evidence on teen pregnancy and parenting.

Bodies as evidence through body mapping

The current research paradigm in public health does little to consider evidence as it is contextualized and embodied. New approaches are needed to better get at context as it inflects public health and intervention (Edwards & diRuggiero, 2011). The exclusion of contextual considerations is a significant omission, particularly for people who have been directly and historically impacted by historical injustices; these histories cannot be erased, and they also should not be ignored in the context of health inequity (Edwards & diRuggiero, 2011).

Active participation in the creation of a visual artefact such as a body map is a process that can be both positive and enjoyable. The process 'has the potential to shift attention from a negative focus, in which the fixing of ill-health becomes codified as "health" and citizens continue to be seen as in need of reform or repair' (Putland, 2008, p. 273). Increased use of arts-based methods, including body mapping, for health promotion can create opportunities to re-evaluate the questions 'what is good health research' and 'what counts as evidence', to support this shift in research paradigms so that visual methodologies, biomedical science, and social science 'collide, coalesce, and restructure to become something' new (Finley, 2005, p. 684). Our study, conducted in the United States, intersects with and speaks in many ways to arts-based studies with teenage mothers that have been carried out in other countries (Levy & Weber, 2010, 2011), as well as domestically (Luttrell, 2003).

We intentionally focus on bodies *as* evidence to challenge the hegemony of expert knowledge around teen pregnancy and parenting, which is created through the production of statistics that surfaces a discourse of blame and shame. Body mapping has been used to explore other stigmatised topics, such as HIV and AIDS, undocumented migrant worker health, occupational health, and sexual health education (Chenhall, Davison, Fitz, Pearse, & Senior, 2013; Gastaldo, Magalhaes, Carrasco, & Davy, 2012; Gubrium & Shafer, 2014; Soloman, 2006). Data collected through body mapping mirror the dynamic nature of explanatory models of health and wellbeing (Guillemin, 2004).

Participants are encouraged to determine for themselves what should be added to their maps – what is important, what is valued, what problems exist (or not), and where any issues or challenges lie. This is an essential component of body mapping as it allows participants to determine which histories or experiences are given 'voice', and the trail of cultural, material, and physical evidence that has resulted from particular social and structural constraints.

In the following sections, we present the context and method behind the Hear Our Stories: Diasporic Youth for Sexual Rights and Justice project, review key findings from its body mapping workshop, and reflect on directions for shaping new bodies of evidence around teen pregnancy and parenting.

The Hear Our Stories project

In focusing on diasporic youth, we intentionally prioritise uprooted young parenting Latinas, whose material conditions and cultural worlds have placed them in tenuous positions, which are both socially constructed and experientially embodied. The ultimate aim of Hear Our Stories is to shift the often stigmatising and shaming discourse on teen parenting to shape a new, more supportive policy dialogue for young mothers and their families. It is situated in a reproductive justice framework as we broaden the focus from individual behaviours and choices to one that includes an analysis of economic, cultural, and structural constraints on praxis.

Project research questions centre on the ways young parenting women link social memories, structural violence, and lived experiences with sexual practices in their personal narratives, and how these linkages, and the way participants negotiate dominating discourses about 'fit' parenting, shape sexual practice dialogues between them and their children. We further examine if and how participatory visual methodologies, including body mapping, have the capacity to transform youth subjectivities and public conversations and policies surrounding sexuality, health, rights, and justice.

For the research design, we conceptualised the use of participatory visual methods as mechanisms for the collection of potentially transformative ethnographic data, to see how such a setting might provide a framework that not only 'reflect[s] ... multi-sensorial sense-making' (Sharf, Harter, Yamasaki, & Haidet, 2011, p. 45), but also creates a context that could trigger participants' sense of having come into sexuality, motherhood, and emerging adulthood. As 'sense-making' objects, we explore if/how body maps can serve as transformative evidence, pushing the production of evidence making – and just what counts as evidence – in new directions to inform the field, as well as policies (Krause & De Zordo, 2012).

Study location

The project research site is an alternative education (GED prep) programme for pregnant and parenting teens that we call 'The Centre'. The Centre serves young women between the ages of 16 and 21 and their children. Over the past five years, Centre students have reported a household income at or below 50% of the poverty level, and nearly two-thirds have been pushed out of high school by the tenth grade, the majority before becoming pregnant. Histories of dispossession underlie these inequities. The Centre is located in a postindustrial US city in western Massachusetts, here called 'The City', a former mill town that experienced considerable economic depression with the decline of manufacturing in the early- to mid-twentieth century. Throughout the 19th and 20th centuries, the town experienced several waves of im/migration; today nearly half of the population in the city is Latino/a, the majority of whom are Puerto Rican and speak Spanish as their first language.

Historically and currently, many citizens in The City face inequity: nearly a third of the population lives below the federal poverty level, unemployment is almost two times higher than the rest of the state (U.S. Census Bureau, 2012), and the high-school graduation rate is 53% (Massachusetts Department of Elementary and Secondary Education, 2013). More-over, The City has the third highest age-adjusted mortality rate in the state, influenced by a disproportionate burden of diabetes, heart disease, cancer, and HIV/AIDS (Massachusetts Department of Public Health, 2011); and the highest teen birth rate in the state (83.6 per 1000 in 2010). In the United States, Latina teen birth rates (32.6 per 1000) are above the national average and almost three times higher than white teen birth rates (11.3 per 1000) (Hamilton, Marin, & Ventura, 2012).

As a prominent body of evidence, leading health indicators often overshadow consider-ations of inequity as policymakers highlight the need for teen pregnancy prevention sol-utions. The standard evidence elides deeper dimensions of lives or the ways that those targeted make sense of and respond to their experiences, which may be used to create more meaningful ways to promote wellbeing. The data that figure as evidence for this paper are drawn from field notes written during Hear Our Stories project body mapping sessions, as well as from an analysis of the participant-produced body maps.

Study sample

Beginning in May 2013 until the present, we have organised a group of students from The Centre to develop their capacity as sexual and reproductive rights activists. Calling them-selves Women Organizing Across Ages (WOAA), the women have engaged in project-sponsored trainings, workshops, meetings, and conferences. In February 2014, five WOAA members took part in a body mapping workshop, with three participants com-pleting all three sessions of the workshop by that April.

The body mapping workshop

Body mapping involves tracing the shape of one's own or a partner's body on life-sized pieces of paper and responding to specific prompts that ask participants to think about and artistically express their lives on the body tracing. After completing a series of activi-ties and discussions, participants create a body map and a body-map key (a guide to key elements of their body map) (Figure 1).

Our body mapping workshop was entitled 'Body Mapping: Telling Your Life Story Through Art' and was facilitated by a 'Young Parent Policy Fellowship' specialist from the Massachusetts Alliance on Teen Pregnancy, a collaborating partner on the Hear

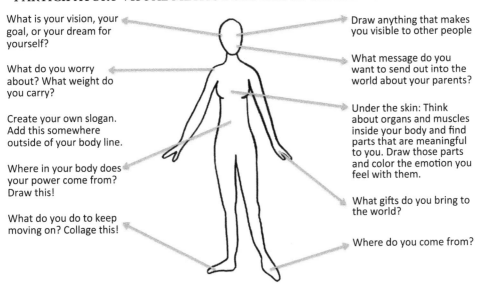

What is your vision, your goal, or your dream for yourself?

What do you worry about? What weight do you carry?

Create your own slogan. Add this somewhere outside of your body line.

Where in your body does your power come from? Draw this!

What do you do to keep moving on? Collage this!

Draw anything that makes you visible to other people

What message do you want to send out into the world about your parents?

Under the skin: Think about organs and muscles inside your body and find parts that are meaningful to you. Draw those parts and color the emotion you feel with them.

What gifts do you bring to the world?

Where do you come from?

Figure 1. Body map key.

Our Stories project. Each of the three sessions took place during two–and-a-half-hour meetings, held once per month over the course of three months.

Session one: body tracing and expression of identity

During the first session, mapping prompts were organised to consider multiplicity in embodiment – addressing micro- to macro-considerations, as well as moving beyond Cartesian binaries. We began the first session by pairing participants, asking them to trace each other's bodies on large sheets of newsprint and then to respond symbolically to various prompts intended to elicit expressions of identity. Prompts included questions pertaining to teen parenting, such as 'When you hear the words "teen parent", what are some of the images that you think people see?' and 'What are the images or words you think of when you think about your own teen parent story?'.

Next, we asked participants to consider their current social location and what they envision for their futures. Prompts included 'Where do you come from?' to encourage representation of the various places they have lived, their communities, and cultures. We also asked participants to represent their life trajectories, their 'visions, goals, or dreams' for themselves and their children, and to consider what they were moving toward. They then linked where they come from with where they are going by skilfully connecting one point to the other across the map.

Final prompts in the first session focused on physical and emotional markers and sources of strength and support. We asked participants to draw visible marks (tattoos, scars, things on their skin others see) and, if they felt comfortable, to write the story of how those marks got on their bodies. Next, we focused on 'under our skin', asking participants to draw important internal organs and colour the emotions they felt with them. Then we shifted to support systems; we asked participants to write down names of those who have supported them in getting where they are today. Throughout the process, participants discussed their depictions with each other.

Session two: meaning-making, embodiment, and resilience

In the second session, we focused on life trajectories and embodiment. We began by asking each participant to think of a question that they identify as relevant and important to answer in their lives. Throughout the rest of the session, each participant asked her question, with other participants artfully responding to the question on their body maps. The activity encouraged active engagement among participants in determining the direction and shape of the resulting body maps.

Next, we took a sensory orientation to encourage participants to think about 'home' temporally and spatially. Participants depicted the places they had lived and who had lived with them, using colour to symbolise how they felt in each of these places, until they reached the place where they currently lived. We also asked participants to think more metaphorically about their bodies, encouraging them to reflect on how their lived experience is internally embodied. On their shoulders, they were asked to represent what they worry about; on their eyes, to focus on how they see the world their child/ren is being born into; on their hands to elicit what gifts they know they bring to the world; and finally on their skin: 'going deeper than the tattoos on our bodies', to focus on embodiment.

Participants were then asked to think about how they felt when they first found out they were pregnant and to use a symbolic colour to represent these feelings. Participants drew a symbol to represent this emotion in the location of the body where it was felt, as well as to add the date of this time and the date of their child or children's births to their maps. Finally, participants used colours, shapes, and symbols to depict where they 'feel or have felt pain and strength in [their bodies] and why?'

Shifting to focus on participant self-care and resilience, we asked the young women what they do to 'keep moving on' in their lives. Participants were encouraged to collage with magazine cutouts and glue to depict these things on their body maps. At the end of the second session participants created their 'own slogan', which could be the words of a song, something a close friend says to them, or just something they say to themselves when the 'going gets tough'. They added these expressions to their body maps.

Session three: message to the world

On the third and final session, we asked participants to consider messaging around their body maps. First, they responded to the prompt: 'What message do you want to send out to the world about teen parents?' Messages were written anywhere outside of the body tracings on their maps. The rest of the session was spent on group reflection and picture taking, with each participant standing next to her body map for an 'artist's photo'. Body maps were posted on the wall around the room, and participants presented their body maps to each other. Participants also worked on creating captions, which would eventually be posted next to their body maps to highlight key elements when they were mounted for exhibition at a community forum held in The City later that month.

With regard to these 'artist's photos' (see Figure 2), we recognise the significant ethical implications involved in using a mosaic effect on the body map artist's face in their presentation here, specifically the inherent tension of divorcing the artist from her claim to knowledge production by making her face unrecognisable. We do so here because we

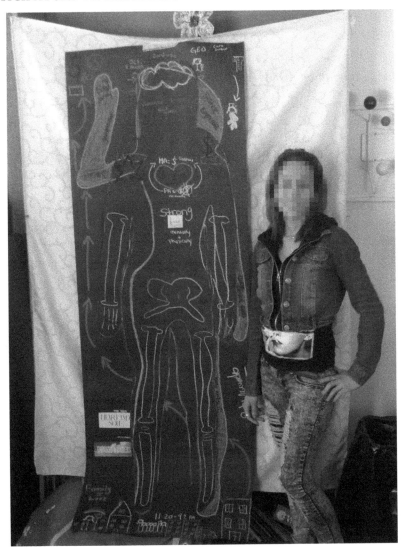

Figure 2. Body map example from Hear Our Stories project.

are presenting the body map work as part of a research project that is governed by our institutional human subjects review board, which expects that we protect potentially vulnerable participants through their anonymity. While the erasure of the subject is one issue, so are our institutional requirements to protect subjects, especially those defined as vulnerable, even as engagement and arts shift into our research endeavours. We appreciate these different ethical standpoints and that different contexts require different treatments of visual material.

Results

Three participants (Reyna, Fabiola, and Eva)[1] completed the body mapping workshop, with five participants (including Annalisse and Rose) completing at least two of the sessions. Two key contrasting themes arose through the process of drawing and discussion: (1) positive valuations and support systems and (2) embodied trauma.

Do not judge a book by its cover: positive valuations and support systems

We used body mapping to explore identity construction and meaning-making around teen motherhood. The first session focused on the process of unpacking identity. When asked to name an image or images associated with the label 'teen parent', participants called out: 'young' and 'irresponsible'. Taking a different tack, another student responded, 'being more into the GED',[2] that is, more into education as a result of being a teen parent. Relatedly, when asked to depict and discuss 'where they were headed', participants' faces lit up. They became jovial, with many depictions focused on future careers. Annalisse drew the symbol for nursing (the Caduceus) on the top of her body map, spending a lot of time to 'get it right'. Other participants said that they wanted to be nurses or medical assistants. Explaining that she wanted to be a parole officer so that she could 'help people, especially those in trouble with the law', Eva drew a badge with the initials PO and identification numbers listed in the centre of it.

Continuing in a positive vein, Reyna said that 'teen parents are the best parents', opening up discussion beyond discursive binaries. Seemingly reinforcing the notion of teen parents as good (responsible and focused) parents, Eva noted, 'when you have your children when you're young, then when you're older (middle aged) you can enjoy life'. Fabiola also agreed: 'You're less outgoing when you have children as a teen', and then clarified that teen parents go out less, with their priorities now on their child or children. The students discussed the TV show *16 and Pregnant*, and one participant said, 'life is edited out of the show'. Ironically, the day-to-day realities of young mothers featured on this reality television show did not capture the participant's sense of the experience.

In the third session, when participants were asked to write their 'message to the world' they drew symbols and wrote slogans about being strong, good parents. In the middle of her map, Reyna wrote the word 'strong', with a collaged magazine cutout of a woman pumping her arm in the air to connote strength, placed below. Underneath the cutout she wrote 'mentally and physically'. When asked to discuss her drawing, Reyna stated vehemently: 'Wherever you go, people will criticize teen parents. But we're powerful, we can withstand a lot'. The statement spoke volumes, foreshadowing depictions of challenging lives that would be drawn and discussed throughout the workshop. At the end of the workshop participants were asked to write captions, which would be displayed alongside their body maps at a city community forum. Fabiola wrote: 'Don't judge a book by its cover', explaining that she liked participating in the body mapping workshop because it gave her a chance to 'show and explain a little about myself – so people who have judged me, or are going to judge me, can see where I am coming from and how as a teen parent I can still have a future'.

Affirmative representations were highlighted as participants 'filled in the gaps' between their own body tracings and those of their partners on their body maps, with written names and drawings used to signify people who served as supportive figures in their lives. Notably, family and friends were not the only figures referenced. Social service providers were deemed as especially supportive; The Centre was depicted as particularly so. Reyna noted that, along with helping to prepare her to take the GED test, The Centre also helped her to manage her appointments. Drawings of the building, with its telltale pink clapboard Victorian structure, were prominently displayed on several body maps.

Participants also noted the supportive role of other social service providers in their lives. Fabiola and Annalisse both wrote the name of their 'parent support advocate', whom they both shared in common. Annalisse noted that the advocate helped her with transportation issues and in her interactions with the Department of Children and Families (DCF); this woman was working *for* Annalisse by treating her with respect. Along with family members, she also added the name of her DCF caseworker. Fabiola also listed the names of social service providers, listing the names of staff at the shelter where she lived that helped her and her family to find housing. Eva also highlighted the support she received from a social service provider, writing 'DCF' and saying that 'they help my kids financially, with education and day care. They help with my house, buying a refrigerator'. Finally, as Reyna elaborated on sources of support in her life, she mentioned her therapist as a being a source of support. Other participants agreed by nodding their heads, apparently having forgotten to list their therapists.

Embodied trauma

More often than not, participants focused on embodied trauma, the ways that bodies experience, feel, and internalise trauma; this includes violence that occurs at any level. Typical examples included discussions of family abuse, neglect and rejection, depression and mental health issues, housing and food insecurity, disinvestment from the public education system, and intimate partner violence. Depictions and discussions in this light could be connected to interpersonal and/or structural violence in participant's lives (i.e. intimate partner violence leading to interactions with flawed social service systems).

Embodied traumas were mapped by participants: beginning at the feet to signify where they had 'come from', traced through intergenerational histories of violence and dispossession, and quite often led to worries about the future as noted in the upper body. Challenges faced by participants were depicted as occurring inside the body whereas affirmative aspects of everyday lives were represented outside of the body, often up in the air above the head, as if out of reach. The centre of the body was a hot spot for conveying stress, anxiety, and heartache.

Home/place and insecurity

In visualising where they had lived, in the past and in the present, and where they saw themselves in the future, participants discussed 'homeplace' (Hooks, 1990). We define homeplace here as different senses, such as smells, sights, tastes, sounds, tactile or felt sensations, that remind participants of home, and are often connected to memories. A common theme that surfaced was the tension between home and community/place. Fabiola began, saying that she was 'trying to stay positive among all the negative' around her. She spoke of growing up in a town neighbouring The City and drew a glowing peace symbol near one foot of her body tracing. Around the symbol she drew what she termed a 'ring of fire', explaining that she came 'from a place of peace', but that it was situated in a 'living hell'. Collectively, we talked about what participants might use to signify or symbolise The City. Describing The City as a 'world of violence',

Reyna brainstormed with the group about the pictures she might use to depict everyday experiences in her community: 'it could be burning buildings, gangs'. On one foot on her body map, Reyna depicted where she was coming from by drawing an image of an apartment on fire and a figure of a person who had been stabbed standing outside the building. Blood was spewing out of the person's throat. On her other foot, Reyna drew a rainbow in reference to the sizable LGBT contingent in the city. Yet Reyna quickly changed course, proceeding to talk about life in The City and expressing worries for her young son who she was raising there.

Eva and Rose, whom each have two young sons, chimed in as well, agreeing that The City was not a good place to raise their boys. Eva elaborated: her son was now in the first grade and was starting to follow what his friends did and 'hang out with the older boys'. 'He's up to no good', she said, and worried about this a lot. A potentially common conversation in any household, Reyna and Eva discussed the ways they restricted their children's video game use. Not as common, they commiserated that while outsiders might see them as raising their children 'all ghetto', that they were 'old school', trying to teach their sons right from wrong.

Reyna continued, telling a story about her own young son. Her son is often at her grandmother's place in The City 'ghetto', as she helps to take care of him. Reyna described the ghetto as having a 'lot of loud conversation and swearing going on'. The ghetto was sensed and described by participants through its sonic qualities – loud swearing, crude language, and gunshots. 'Toxic noise', said one participant. Eva jumped in with where she had left off, saying that she had recently been out with her older son and he said to her, 'Mommy, I'm a gangster'. She was taken aback. All together, the participants talked about boys in The City emulating gangsters and traced this to the city's violence, as well as a general sense of insecurity and lack of control over what may come of young men in their community.

Annalisse, who lived in another neighbouring city, said that she had grown up 'in a house with a whole family' and drew a house with its own door and mailbox to indicate that her house was inhabited by only one family, thus distancing herself from the norm of multi-family housing (i.e. multiplexes) for disadvantaged citizens living in The City and surrounding areas. In contrast, when asked to talk about her present community and supports offered, she curled up her face and said, 'I live in the ghetto' – meaning that it was no place to live.

During the session that focused on participants' housing journeys, each focused on where they were born and places they had lived; all spoke about difficulties they faced to obtain or keep their housing. Participants referred to living in 'the slum', 'the hood', and about everyday acts of violence pervading these areas. Some spoke of not being able to 'get into' housing, and living in shelters instead. Highlighting the sense of insecurity ever-present in participants' lives, and ways this is seasonally circumscribed, participants talked about being 'not sure what to do' about housing in the wintertime, with this winter's weather being particularly brutal.

Frequent movement was depicted on the bottom of body maps, near tracings of participants' feet. Reyna's body map was especially illustrative. She spoke of living in 'the projects' in both The City and in Pennsylvania, where she lived for a brief time. She had recently moved to a house. Like Annalisse, she clarified that the place was not 'an apartment or a place in another place', but her 'own home', with only her boyfriend and child living there with her. Her body map vividly displayed her trail of movement from one place to another over the course of her still young life: sparse buildings with blank windows and rows of stick figure people lined up out front. Reyna wrote dates and locations above each building to mark the time and place of each move, ultimately conveying a sense of rootlessness.

The educational system: power and deprivation

The educational system was similarly a prominent source of trauma depicted in participants' body maps. When participants were asked to draw a symbol that represents 'the power within you', most often they noted the importance of obtaining an education. Eva drew a brain – and talked about going to college as 'money' – with dollar signs framing it. On the chest of her body tracing she drew a picture of a female figure holding a certificate. Describing this drawing she said: 'once I have my major (in college) I can give my all'. Fabiola drew a set of stairs on her chest to symbolise 'moving up' in the world by getting her GED, and concluded that she 'hasn't given up on life. People give up, kill themselves, I keep going'.

However, much of the talk and many of the depictions around education were less glowing. Reyna talked about dropping out of school, initially taking on a discourse of blame and shame: it was '[her] fault' that she dropped out of school: she was smoking, wanting to hang out, party – she had hated school. She elaborated: 'I couldn't go there to learn' – she always had to 'watch [her] back' instead. Over the course of discussion, participants increasingly began to resituate 'individual decision-making' to take into account structural circumstances that informed their experiences with schooling. Eva talked about making it to the ninth grade – but then giving birth to her son – she was not supported by the system to continue in school.

When prompted to depict and discuss what they worried about, participants talked about experiencing depression and anxiety, often related to experiences with the educational system. Eva talked about the 'biggest weight' in her life being the worry that she 'never gets an education' and does not 'progress in life'. Reyna drew a picture of a heart on her body map, with a line drawn through it to convey a 'broken heart'. She wrote 'GED' right outside the heart to signify a breaking point. 'The GED is the biggest weight', she said.

Participants spoke of the link between frequent moves and school credits being lost, and feelings of humiliation and exasperation at having to repeat a grade due to systemic errors. Encircling the outside of her head, Rose wrote in blue about her path of dispossession through the educational system. She described this trajectory: having her first baby when she was in the ninth grade; that she was a 'drop out'. Upon returning to school Rose was told that she was missing credits and could not progress to the tenth grade. After meeting her husband she had a second baby. 'Problems at school' and 'went away' were written on her body map to convey her sense of alienation from the educational system.

Interpersonal violence

Interpersonal violence was another significant subtheme of embodied trauma. Responding to the prompt of what on their body made them visible to others, Fabiola drew bright skeletal bones inside her body tracing, instead of drawing tattoos and piercings, as had other participants. The bones were meant to reflect 'all of the hell I've been through'. Fabiola's body map caption, which was written at the end of the workshop and displayed alongside her the map, read:

> The part of my body that bothers me sometimes is my tininess. I used to look very healthy but I don't anymore because of some health issues. When you look at my body map, you can see my bones. That shows how thin I am. But to be honest, it doesn't bother me much, because I know the reasons why I am like this.

Rose's depictions and descriptions were especially evocative of embodied trauma from interpersonal violence. Over the course of her participation in the Hear Our Stories project Rose changed markedly in how she presented herself. By the end of her stay at The Centre she looked better on the outside: her hair had grown out, she had dyed it a striking shade of red, and she had a happy glow about her. Her voice, though, still had the same quake of worry and tinge of anxiety that it held when we met her a few months back. In another project activity, held earlier, Rose had produced a digital story focused on the physical abuse she experienced from her husband, as well as intergenerational histories of trauma inflicted on women in her family. She had shared photos on her cell phone of bruises and lacerations as evidence of this violence. Now returned to The Centre, she told how she had left The Centre abruptly, right after completing her digital story. She reshaped her story to be more about her mother-in-law kicking her out and less about the brutal violence she had experienced at the hands of her husband.

A theme of escape seemed to pervade Rose's life, in her digital story and now in the body mapping process. Rose talked about her relocation to a nearby city (about 50 miles away, resulting from a policy meant to protect 'victims of abuse' from their perpetrators) to live in a shelter with her two boys. She knew no one, was not going to school, and mostly felt trapped because she 'kept inside' at the shelter with nothing to do, nowhere to go. Rose returned to The City, got back together with her husband, and was living with him and her two sons in a family shelter close to The Centre. They had just received word that they got their 'own place' through the housing authority. Over the course of the body mapping workshop, Rose paced back and forth, whispering on her phone, talking with her husband, checking in. By the last body mapping session Rose was already gone. She had left town with her two sons.

Discussion

The topic of teen pregnancy commonly positions young parents as either redeemable good mothers or irresponsible, bad biocitizens (Greenhalgh & Carney, 2014), without considering whole lives and lived experiences (Barcelos & Gubrium, 2014). The value of a participatory methodology such as body mapping is that rather than being an object to be analysed and mined for data, the research participant becomes a co-creator of knowledge and information. As co-creator, their knowledge, meaning-making, and lived experiences are valued as assets. All too often value (or lack thereof) is assigned to individuals based on assumptions that lack validity.

Here, body mapping was used as an additional source of data collection, deepening and strengthening initial findings from other project research-based activities, in which participants shared their experiences as young parents. Having established a basic relationship with participants through the other activities, body mapping allowed us to further explore their lived experiences. A critical step in the process was to ensure that both researcher and participant had a role in the evaluation of the final body map artefact. Body maps are co-created; as such, co-analysis is essential. In this way, both researcher and participant are valued for the contribution of their specific expertise: the participant in generating and interpreting their map, and the researcher in identifying themes, conducting analysis, summarizing theory, and drawing conclusions (Guillemin & Drew, 2010).

Through this process of body mapping with young parenting Latinas, critical issues surfaced that are often missing from teen pregnancy and parenting discourses: physical violence, insecurity of place, structural barriers within the educational system, and the resultant embodiment of stress. Because students at The Centre experience high rates of displacement, the impact of rootlessness is a critical component to integrate into future efforts to support Latino/a youth. Rootlessness and disruption of links to family, friends, and locations are a common thread among individuals who have relocated. This experience of 'community dispossession threaten[s] ties between individuals and their social-support networks and also undermine[s] claims to the spaces that serve as geographic anchors for these social ties' (Keene, Padilla, & Geronimus, 2010, p. 276). The simultaneous experience of rootlessness and lack of social support can compound feelings of isolation, perceived stigmatisation, and stress.

Contrary to the widely held perception that girls drop out of school as a result of a pregnancy, many young women of colour are in fact 'pushed out' of school prior to their first pregnancy. A range of policies, 'including fiscal inequality, unequal distribution of certified educators, high-stakes testing, and a retreat from bilingual education and affirmative action, have colluded to produce a grossly uneven landscape of public education' that has the greatest impact on students of colour, immigrants, and low-income individuals (Fine & McClelland, 2006, p. 302). In considering teen pregnancy, it is important to remember that it serves as a barometer 'for the interrelationship between, housing, environmental, economic, and other social stressors' (Mullings & Wali, 2001, p. 162). Lived experiences such as intimate partner violence, insecure housing, economic and food insecurity, and lack of social support are compounded during pregnancy, adding to the experience of stress for young parents.

A significant advantage to body mapping is that, in contrast to participatory visual methods such as photovoice and digital storytelling that require access to and funding for technology, and facilitators trained in those technologies, the process requires only basic supplies that are relatively low cost: butcher block paper, drawing supplies, magazines, glue sticks, scissors, pen, and paper. Body mapping can be used as a point of departure for discussions that revolve around varied topics pertaining to health and wellness. As such, it can be adapted in multiple contexts, increasing its utility.

Programmes that remain strictly focused on bodies of evidence such as lowered rates of teen pregnancy and sexually transmitted infections and increased rates of access to and use of contraceptives will continue to be limited in their approach, in particular for marginalised communities. Participatory visual methods such as body mapping present the opportunity for participants and researchers to identify significant challenges faced by populations that are integral to the development of relevant, context-specific, and ultimately more sustainable health promotion efforts.

Limitations

Our initial findings are based on a small sample size that self-selected into the body mapping workshop. Of the 31 Hear Our Stories participants, five enrolled in the workshop. Of those five, two completed all three sessions and two completed two sessions. Findings from this project are strictly exploratory and are therefore not generalisable right now.

Conclusion

As ethnographers, we are particularly interested in meaning-making around youth sexuality – even when direct reference to sexual practice is silent. Participants voiced a sense of stigma and shame. The stories and discussions in and around the body maps illuminated linkages between social memories, structural violence, lived experience, and sexual practices, especially the ways participants negotiate dominating discourses about 'fit' parenting and describe instances of dehumanization in the system and a felt sense of isolation and insecurity.

The process illuminated how structural violence impacts dominant cultural understandings and hierarchies that circulate about young parenting Latinas (Ginsburg & Rapp, 1995). It made not only visible but also *visceral* the often invisible reverberations of structural violence – in the form of intergenerational poverty and its effect on families and intimate partner relationships, and systematic dispossession from state supports in the form of education and housing. Participants face an 'unending cyclone of requirements' (Elizabeth Silver, personal communication, December 2013) to negotiate support for themselves and their families in everyday life. Indignities mount.

It is important to consider how the lives of pregnant and parenting young women are shaped by larger bodies of evidence around youth sexuality and parenthood and equally so how young mothers (and other marginalised social groups) may reclaim the evidence, dialogically and strategically shaping it using their own embodied understandings as a basis. Body mapping is a critical tool that can elicit questions and issues researchers may never know to ask, which, by remaining silenced, perpetuate the health inequities that persist across all health indicators. Integration of participatory visual methods such as body mapping can upend traditional evidence-based methods. The approach creates space for the expression of multiple health beliefs in varied forms that can reveal 'personal, recent, and embodied history[ies] that [are] rooted in national and international historical movements that shape people's' lives' (Gastaldo et al., 2012, p. 11). Not only can body mapping deepen our understandings of health and wellbeing, but it can also serve to redress the power dynamics inherent in traditional approaches by valuing and prioritizing the voices of the communities they intend to promote.

Notes

1. Pseudonyms are used for all participants.

2. GED stands for the 'General Educational Development' test, which was used in the US until the end of 2013 to indicate that a student possessed high-school-level academic skills. The High School Equivalency Exam (HiSET) replaced this exam in 2014.

Acknowledgments

We are particularly grateful to the young women from The Centre for participating in body mapping and other project-related workshops and activities. We also wish to acknowledge support from our project partner, the Massachusetts Alliance on Teen Pregnancy, and particularly the work of Katherine Bright, who facilitated the body mapping workshops; and acknowledge our wonderful team of research assistants: Chris Barcelos, Iesha Ramos, and Miriam Shafer.

Disclosure statement

No potential conflict of interest was reported by the authors.

Funding

A research grant from a Ford Foundation initiative 'Sexuality, Health and Rights Among Youth in the United States: Transforming Public Policy and Public Understanding Through Social Science Research' supported the project 'Hear Our Stories: Diasporic Youth for Sexual and Reproductive Health'.

References

Barcelos, C., & Gubrium, A. (2014). Reproducing stories: Strategic narratives of teen pregnancy and motherhood. *Social Problems, 61*(3), 466–481. doi:10.1525/sp.2014.12241

Bonell, C. (2004). Why is teenage pregnancy conceptualized as a social problem? A review of quantitative research from the USA and UK. *Culture, Health & Sexuality, 6*(3), 255–272. doi:10.1080/13691050310001643025

Chavez, L. R. (2004). A glass half empty: Latina reproduction and public discourse. *Human Organization, 63*, 173–188. doi:10.17730/humo.63.2.hmk4m0mfey10n51k

Chenhall, R., Davison, B., Fitz, J., Pearse, T., & Senior, K. (2013). Engaging youth in sexual health research: Refining a "youth friendly" method in the northern territory, Australia. *Visual Anthropology Review, 29*(2), 123–132. doi:10.1111/var.12009

Edwards, N., & diRuggiero, E. (2011). Exploring which context matters in the study of health inequities and their mitigation. *Scandinavian Journal of Public Health, 39*(6), 43–49. doi:10.1177/1403494810393558.

Fine, M., & McClelland, S. (2006). Sexuality education and desire: Still missing after all these years. *Harvard Educational Review, 76*(3), 297–338. doi:10.17763/haer.76.3.w5042g23122n6703

Finley, S. (2005). Arts-based inquiry: Performing revolutionary pedagogy. In N. Denzin & Y. Lincoln (Eds.), *The Sage handbook of qualitative research* (3rd ed., pp. 681–694). London: Sage Publications.

Gastaldo, D., Magalhaes, L., Carrasco, C., & Davy, C. (2012). *Body-map storytelling as research: Methodological considerations for telling the stories of undocumented workers through body mapping.* Retrieved from http://www.migrationhealth.ca/undocumented-workers-ontario/body-mapping

Geronimus, A. (2003). Damned if you do: Culture, identity, privilege, and teenage childbearing in the United States. *Social Science & Medicine, 57*(5), 881–893.

Geronimus, A., & Korenman, S. (1993). Maternal youth or family background? On the health disadvantages of infants with teenage mothers. *American Journal of Epidemiology, 137*(2), 213–225. doi:10.1016/S0277-9536(02)00456-2

Ginsburg, F., & Rapp, R. (Eds.). (1995). *Conceiving the new world order: The global politics of repro-duction*. Berkeley: University of California Press.

Greenhalgh, S., & Carney, M. A. (2014). Bad biocitizens? Latinos and the US 'obesity epidemic'. *Human Organization, 73*(3), 267–276. doi:10.17730/humo.73.3.w53hh1t413038240

Gubrium, A., & Shafer, M. (2014). Sensual sexuality education with young parenting women. *Health Education Research, 29*(4), 649–661. doi:10.1093/her/cyu001

Guillemin, M. (2004). Understanding illness: Using drawings as a research method. *Qualitative Health Research, 14*(2), 272–289. doi:10.1177/1049732303260445

Guillemin, M., & Drew, S. (2010). Questions of process in participant-generated visual method-ologies. *Visual Studies, 25*(2), 175–188. doi:10.1080/1472586X.2010.502676

Hamilton, B. E., Marin, J. A., & Ventura, S. J. (2012). *Births: Preliminary data for 2011* (National Vital Statistics Reports No. 61(5)). Hyattsville, MD: National Center for Health Statistics.

Hoffman, S. D. (2008). *Kids having kids: Economic costs and social consequences of teen pregnancy*. Washington, D.C.: Urban Institute.

Holgate, H., Evans, R., & Yuen, F. K. O. (2006). *Teenage pregnancy and parenthood: Global perspec-tives, issues and interventions*. New York: Routledge.

Hooks, B. (1990). *Yearning: Race, gender, and cultural politics*. Boston, MA: South End Press.

Kearney, M. S., & Levine, P. B. (2012). Why is the teen birth rate in the United States so high and why does it matter? *The Journal of Economic Perspectives, 26*(2), 141–166. doi:10.1257/jep.26.2.141

Keene, D., Padilla, M., & Geronimus, A. (2010). Leaving Chicago for Iowa's 'fields of opportunity': Community dispossession, rootlessness, and the quest for somewhere to 'be OK'. *Human Organization, 69*(3), 275–284.

Krause, E. L., & De Zordo, S. (2012). Introduction. Ethnography and biopolitics: Tracing 'rational-ities' of reproduction across the north-south divide. *Anthropology & Medicine, 19*(2), 137–151. doi:10.1080/13648470.2012.675050

Levy, L., & Weber, S. (2010). 'Yes I am a mother and I am still a teenager': Teen moms use digital photography to share their views. *Girlhood Studies, 3*(20), 129–139. doi:10.3167/ghs.2010.030208

Levy, L., & Weber, S. (2011). Teenmom.ca: A community arts-based new media empowerment project for teenage mothers. *Studies in Art Education, 52*(4), 292–309.

Luker, K. (1996). *Dubious conceptions: The politics of teenage pregnancy*. Cambridge, MA: Harvard University Press.

Luttrell, W. (2003). *Pregnant minds, fertile bodies: Gender, race, and the schooling of pregnant teens*. New York, NY: Routledge.

Massachusetts Department of Public Health. (2011). *Massachusetts community health information profile: Health status indicators report for Holyoke*. Retrieved from http://www.mass.gov/eohhs/researcher/community-health/masschip/topics/health-status-indicators

Massachusetts Department of Elementary and Secondary Education. (2013). *Graduation rates*. Retrieved from http://www.doe.mass.edu/infoservices/reports/gradrate

Mullings, L., & Wali, A. (2001). *Stress and resilience: The social context of reproduction in central Harlem*. New York: Springer.

Mulongo, E. (2006). *Young single motherhood: Contested notions of motherhood and sexuality in policy discourses/program interventions*. ISS Working Paper Series/General Series. Retrieved from http://repub.eur.nl/res/pub/19183/wp423.pdf

Nathanson, C. (1991). *Dangerous passages: The social control of sexuality in women's adolescence*. Philadelphia: Temple University Press.

Putland, C. (2008). Lost in translation: The question of evidence linking community-based arts and health promotion. *Journal of Health Psychology, 13*(2), 265–276. doi:10.1177/1359105307086706

Quesada, J., Hart, L. K., & Bourgois, P. (2011). Structural vulnerability and health: Latino migrant laborers in the United States. *Medical Anthropology, 30*(4), 339–362. doi:10.1080/01459740.2011.576725

Santelli, J.S., & Melnikas, A.J. (2010). Teen fertility in transition: Recent and historic trends in the United States. *Annual Review of Public Health, 31*(1), 371–383. doi:10.1146/annurev.publhealth.29.020907.090830

Scally, G. (2010). Too much too young? Teenage pregnancy is a public health, not a clinical, problem. *International Journal of Epidemiology, 31*(3), 554–555. doi:10.1093/ije/31.3.554

Sharf, B. F., Harter, L. M., Yamasaki, J., & Haidet, P. (2011). Narrative turns epic: Continuous developments in health narrative scholarship. In T. L. Thompson, R. Parrott, & J. F. Nussbaum (Eds.), *The Routledge handbook of health communication* (pp. 36–51). New York: Routledge.

Shaw, M. E., & Lawlor, D. A. (2007). Why we measure teenage pregnancy but do not count teenage mothers? *Critical Public Health, 17*(4), 311–316. doi:10.1080/09581590701302281

Sisson, G. (2012). Finding a way to offer something more: Reframing teen pregnancy prevention. *Sexuality Research and Social Policy, 9*(1), 57–69.

Smart, C. (1996). Deconstructing motherhood. In E. B. Silva (Ed.), *Good enough mothering? Feminist perspectives on lone motherhood* (pp. 37–57). New York, NY: Routledge.

Soloman, J. (2006). *Living with X: A body mapping journey in the time of HIV and AIDS. Facilitator's guide.* Johannesburg: REPSSI.

US Census Bureau. (2012). *2007–2011 American community survey.* Retrieved from http://quickfacts.census.gov/qfd/index.html

From informed consent to dissemination: Using participatory visual methods with young people with long-term conditions at different stages of research

Cecilia Vindrola-Padros[a], Ana Martins[b], Imelda Coyne[c], Gemma Bryan[b] and Faith Gibson[b,d]

[a]Department of Applied Health Research, University College London, London, UK; [b]Department of Children's Nursing, London South Bank University, London, UK; [c]School of Nursing & Midwifery, Trinity College Dublin, Dublin, Ireland; [d]Great Ormond Street Hospital NHS Foundation Trust, London, UK

ABSTRACT

Research with young people suffering from a long-term illness has more recently incorporated the use of visual methods to foster engagement of research participants from a wide age range, capture the longitudinal and complex factors involved in young people's experiences of care, and allow young people to express their views in multiple ways. Despite its contributions, these methods are not always easy to implement and there is a possibility that they might not generate the results or engagement initially anticipated by researchers. We hope to expand on the emerging discussion on the use of participatory visual methods by presenting the practical issues we have faced while using this methodology during different stages of research: informed assent/consent, data collection, and the dissemination of findings. We propose a combination of techniques to make sure that the research design is flexible enough to allow research participants to shape the research process according to their needs and interests.

Introduction

Research with young people increasingly involves the use of one or multiple types of visual methods. Visual methods, and in particular those involving creative or arts-based approaches, have gained popularity in the field of research with young people because they make participating in research an enjoyable experience, facilitate communication by allowing the young person to express their ideas in non-verbal ways, and allow the researcher to gain a new insight into the everyday lives of young people (Carter & Ford, 2013; Johnson, Pfister, & Vindrola-Padros, 2012; Pfister, Vindrola-Padros, & Johnson, 2014). Furthermore, researchers commonly argue that visual methods are participatory as they alter age, status, and research-based hierarchies and allow the young person to shape the research process (Close, 2007; Drew, Duncan, & Sawyer, 2010). Research designs using visual methods with young people are inherently flexible as they involve a wide range of approaches for young people to choose from and use open-ended instructions or guidelines where participants have the opportunity to create their own outputs (Weller, 2012). Flexible designs suit a range of development-related capacities; an important issue to consider when study participants span a broad age group (Drew et al., 2010).

We hope to expand on the emerging discussion on the use of participatory visual methods by presenting the practical issues we have faced while using this methodology during different stages of research: informed assent/consent, data collection, and the dissemination of findings. Each stage, method, and research setting created particular, often unanticipated, challenges that led our team to make decisions around the degree of participation, the impact of our research, and the factors we should take into consideration while designing future studies. We share here the lessons we have learned and strategies we have used along the way in order to make a contribution to the further development of participatory visual methods both in young and older populations.

Young people with long-term illness

Visual methods have been rapidly incorporated into health research with young people, particularly in research exploring experiences of long-term illness (Sartain, Clarke, & Heyman, 2000). These methods have been used successfully in the exploration of young people's perceptions of health and disease and how their feelings and ideas change throughout medical treatment (Rollins, 2005). As Sartain et al. (2000) have argued, young people living with long-term conditions have continuous contact with health care services and their daily lives unfold in close connection with their disease. There is a particular longitudinal quality to their experiences that is difficult to grasp in research (as most research only captures a snapshot of the child's life), but visual methods have proven effective in documenting the biographical changes and disruptions faced by young people with chronic conditions, as well as the wide diversity of individual illness experiences (Sartain et al., 2000).

Participatory visual methods in practice

Despite the many advantages, these methods are not always easy to implement and there is a possibility that they might not generate the results or engagement initially anticipated by researchers. Some methods can be time consuming, require prior training, and create a burden for participants (Drew et al., 2010; Pain, 2012). Not all methods are suitable for all groups of young people or for all research contexts (Carter & Ford, 2013; Coyne, Hayes, & Gallagher, 2009; Johnson et al., 2012). Some young people might actually prefer verbal communication and feel visual methods are not the best way to convey their experience to the researcher. Furthermore, the inclusion of visual methods in the research design does not automatically make it 'participatory' as young people's voices might not be considered as important as the voice of the researcher or other adults or they might not have avenues or the 'tools' for shaping the research process (Barker & Smith, 2012; Lomax, 2012).

Most of the evidence we currently have on the use of visual methods focuses on data collection, while other phases of research are often overlooked (Weller, 2012). The details of methods used to analyse visual data are often missing from publications (Pfister et al., 2014) and few studies have incorporated visual methods during the informed assent/consent process or when disseminating the findings of a study (Ford, Sankey, & Crisp, 2007; Lambert & Glacken, 2011; Weller, 2012). The use of visual methods during these phases is important because as Dockett, Perry, and Kearney (2013) have argued, 'the format of the information provided can influence children's understandings of the research itself and what is involved in participation' (p. 805). The use of visual methods in multiple phases of studies represents an attempt to create more active ways of fully involving young people in research (Brannen, 2002; Weller, 2012).

The following sections of the article present examples where the authors have used participatory visual methods in three stages of research: informed assent/consent, data collection, and the dissemination of findings. In each example, the authors describe the study, present the rationale for including visual methods in the research design, identify the methods' contributions and limitations, and discuss the lessons they learned from use of these methods in practice. All three examples are based on research with young people. We define young people as a study population including children, teenagers, and young adults: aged 4–24.

Informed assent/consent in the 'Talking with children study'

The 'Talking with children study' was an ethnographic study with families of children newly diagnosed with leukaemia. Data collection took place on the oncology units of a children's hospital in the U.K. between May 2011 and May 2012. The aim of this study was to explore children's knowledge of their disease to inform good practice in communication within childhood cancer. Families of children newly diagnosed with leukaemia aged between 4 and 11 years old were invited to take part. Seven children (average age 7.4 years old) and their families were recruited to take part in the study. Three of the children were female. A child-centred approach to negotiating informed assent and consent was taken (Dell Clark, 2010). This approach respected a child's capacity to be involved in informed decision-making while simultaneously recognising the parents' responsibility as protective gatekeepers (Lambert & Glacken, 2011). Prior to gaining ethical approval, members of our study advisory group (a parent and two children aged between 4 and 11) sent comments on the participatory visual methods.

Description of participatory visual methods

Informed consent and assent was negotiated in four stages. A member of ward staff first approached the family to ask if they would be willing to speak to the researcher. If the answer was yes, the researcher then met the family and explained the study to the parents and gave them the parent information sheet, which detailed the purpose, possible benefits and disadvantages of the family taking part in the research, privacy, confidentiality and child protection issues, and the contact information for the research team and local research office. In the third stage, 24 hours later, the researcher returned to ask for permission to speak with the child about the study. If permission was granted, the researchers then introduced themselves and briefly explained the study. The child was then shown two types of patient information sheets: one in a comic book style aimed at children between 4

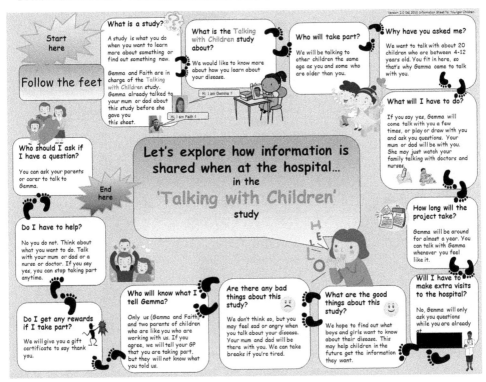

Figure 1. Information sheet for younger children used in the 'Talking with children' study.

and 7 years old (Figure 1) and one with more text aimed at 3- to 11-year olds (Figure 2), and asked to select the one they preferred. No reference was made to an age range on the documents to avoid any potential for influencing children's choice. Both documents used child-friendly words and images and included photographs of members of the research team. The younger child's comic book also utilised 'footprints' to move the reader through the comic and indicate which box they should look at next.

The researcher and the child read through the chosen information sheet together. After answering any questions, the child was asked to choose between two assent activities to explore the purpose of the research and what their participation would involve: a storyboard with symbols replacing missing words aimed at younger children (Figure 3), and a word search aimed at older children (Figure 4), in which key words such as 'observe' and 'participate' were scrambled. Each time the word was found in the word search or replaced in the storyboard, the child was asked to explain what the word meant in their own context and then again in a research context. These methods were used to determine whether the child understood the key issues of what being involved in the study would require them to do, including that participation was voluntary, that they could withdraw at any time, and the possible risks and benefits of taking part.

The child was then asked if they would like to take part in the study. Older children who gave assent were subsequently asked to complete and sign the assent form (Figure 5), which was countersigned by a parent and the researcher. For practical reasons, younger children who gave assent but were yet to start, or who had just started school, did not

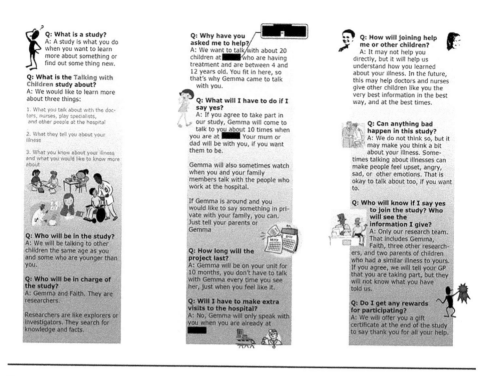

Figure 2. First page of the information sheet for the 'Talking with children' study aimed at older children.

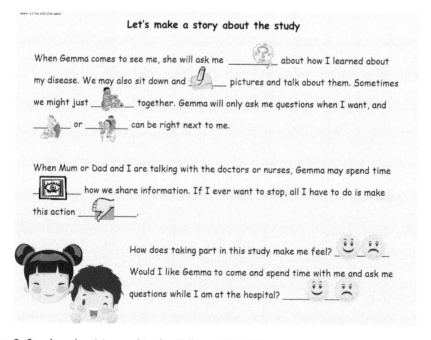

Figure 3. Storyboard activity used in the 'Talking with children' study.

The Talking with Children Study

WORD SEARCH

All of the words written below are hidden in the grid. Can you find them?

P	A	R	T	I	C	I	P	A	T	E	P
F	G	H	R	L	G	E	F	D	P	B	M
R	R	A	L	K	S	B	I	V	N	L	S
P	E	O	M	X	A	F	L	N	X	R	T
T	E	B	N	Z	F	K	H	O	D	E	I
H	V	S	E	I	R	E	T	B	L	D	G
D	I	F	C	G	C	A	Y	E	G	R	Y
A	Q	U	O	S	I	D	L	V	F	O	R
J	L	G	P	M	U	B	P	G	A	C	M
T	N	R	C	T	F	X	R	C	F	E	P
V	O	B	S	E	R	V	E	I	B	R	J
S	C	Z	A	P	E	L	O	N	Y	A	S

We are doing a **STUDY** to understand how information about your illness is shared among children, their parents and health professionals. We would like you to **PARTICIPATE**. If you **AGREE**, we will ask you to speak in an interview, or draw a picture and describe it. Sometimes we may just **OBSERVE** what is happening when you are at the hospital. This could happen many times, or just a few over almost a year. We will use a voice **RECORDER** to record our discussions. It won't be **DIFFICULT** for you, but you can **SAY NO**.

Figure 4. Word search activity used in the 'Talking with children' study.

complete this form and instead circled the smiley faces on the storyboard activity to indicate assent. Parents were asked to provide parental consent for themselves and their child to take part only when the child had provided assent. During this process, the researcher was mindful of obvious and subtle signs of child, or parental, refusal such as a child's body language (Lambert & Glacken, 2011). The child's assent to participate in the study was not viewed as a one-off event and was constantly re-negotiated verbally. In order to enhance the children's ability to take a break or withdraw from the research (Lambert & Glacken, 2011), children who joined the study were taught a sign (a thumbs down signal) to demonstrate that they would like the researcher to leave. A picture of this signal was also included in the children's information sheets. The signal was practiced in three hypothetical situations (a mock interview question, during play, and during interactions with clinicians) to coach the child to be confident in using the sign (Kumpunen, Shipway, Taylor, Aldiss, & Gibson, 2012).

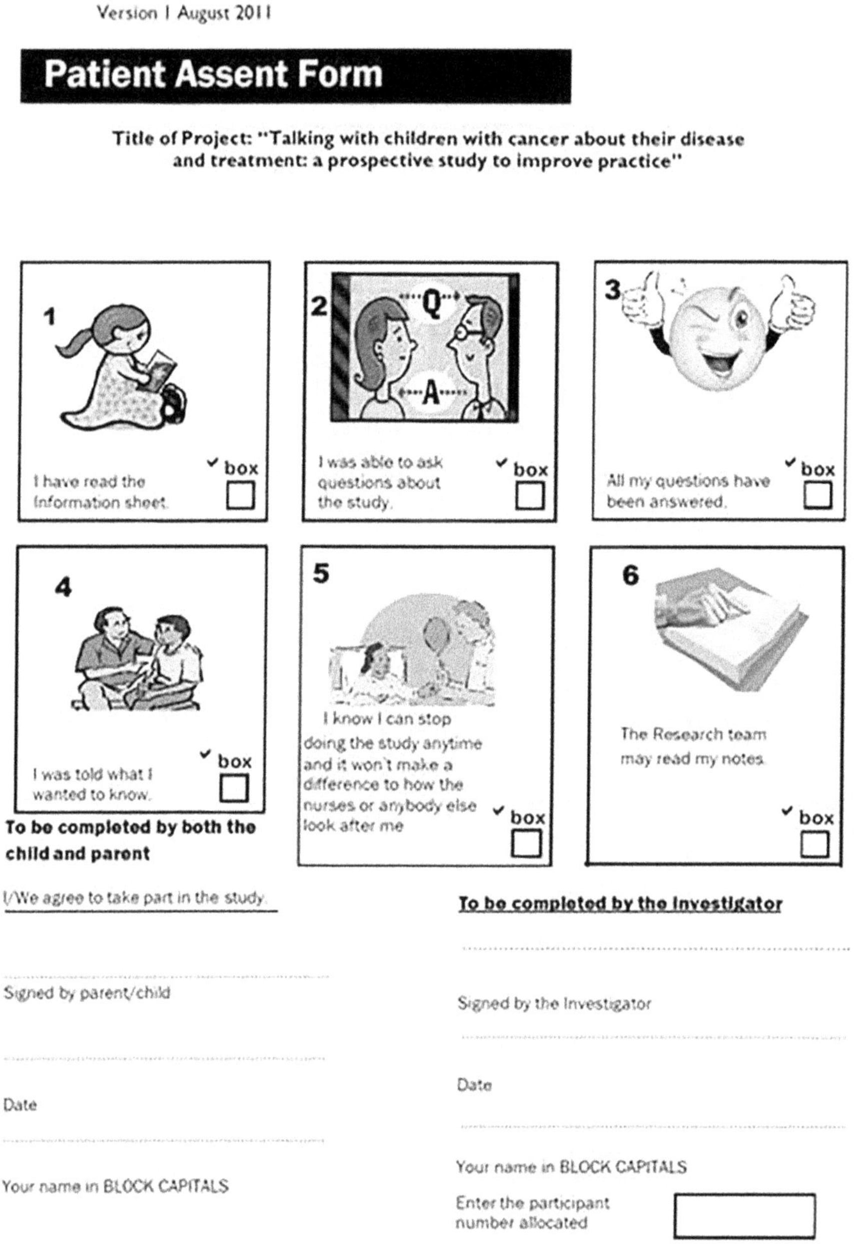

Version 1 August 2011

Patient Assent Form

Title of Project: "Talking with children with cancer about their disease and treatment: a prospective study to improve practice"

1 I have read the information sheet. ✔ box ☐

2 I was able to ask questions about the study. ✔ box ☐

3 All my questions have been answered. ✔ box ☐

4 I was told what I wanted to know. ✔ box ☐

5 I know I can stop doing the study anytime and it won't make a difference to how the nurses or anybody else look after me ✔ box ☐

6 The Research team may read my notes ✔ box ☐

To be completed by both the child and parent

I/We agree to take part in the study.

Signed by parent/child

Date

Your name in BLOCK CAPITALS

To be completed by the Investigator

Signed by the Investigator

Date

Your name in BLOCK CAPITALS

Enter the participant number allocated

Figure 5. Assent form for older children used in the 'Talking with children' study.

Lessons learned

The research team has a long history of using visual methods in the assent/consent process (Kumpunen et al., 2012). Visual methods convey information about the study to families in a clear and accessible format. The visual nature of the information sheets was engaging and helped the researcher to quickly build rapport and establish a dialogue with children.

The use of visual methods in informed assent/consent is not however without its challenges. Recruitment took place on a busy ward, where space was at a premium. This meant that recruitment had to take place at the bedside. The assent process took some time and was subject to constant interruption from members of the clinical team. There were two different information sheets to choose from, and one older boy recruited into the study was scornful of the 'babyish' nature of the younger child's information sheet. However, other children of similar age did not voice this opinion. In fact, the younger children's information sheet proved to be the more popular of the two.

Although careful consideration was given to all the images included in the documents and comments were received on the assent documents from children in our advisory group, issues were identified with the storyboard assent activity during recruitment. This document used a symbol of an eye to represent the missing word 'observe', which some of the children misidentified as the symbol for the television show Big Brother despite an apparent lack of similarity between the images from the researcher's perspective. Likewise, the picture representing the missing word 'mother' also included a cake and was consequently frequently misidentified as 'birthday cake'. So although review of information sheets in advance by children was helpful, the individual nature of understanding 'what we see' means that explanation might still be required.

We relied on Microsoft Word Clipart for the pictures for the information sheets and assent activities used in this study. In the future, we would consider purchasing pictures from a stock photograph and diagram resource to obtain a greater range of images. Although the majority of children selected the younger child's information sheet, this was viewed as too 'babyish' by one child. The use of two different styles of information sheet in future studies to respond to individual preferences is therefore warranted. The inclusion of visual methods in children's information sheets is a worthwhile, albeit time consuming, process that requires further evaluation by children.

Data collection in the 'Mapping study'

The Mapping Teenage and Young Adult Cancer Services in England study sought to provide an overview of the way care is organised across the main centres where young people (13–24 years of age) with cancer receive care. The researcher spent from 1 to 3 days in 11 centres and interviewed 34 staff members, 21 young people, and 15 family members, carried out observations on the units, and used photography and drawing techniques (adapted from the Mosaic Approach described by Clark & Moss, 2011) with young people to create maps of their care.

The Mosaic approach integrates visual and verbal techniques such as photographs, tours, maps, conversations with the researcher, and observations (Clark & Moss, 2011). It was selected as the main approach for this study because it relies on the combination of multiple methods; it focuses on the lived experience of the research participants and their interaction with the daily environment; and it is participatory and reflexive (viewing participants as co-constructors of knowledge) (Clark & Moss, 2011).

Description of participatory visual methods

Our initial idea in the Mapping study was to bring together a group of young people (who were on the ward at the time when the researcher was carrying out observations) to develop a map of their care. We originally envisioned young people using the cameras we provided to move around the ward individually or in groups and photograph areas they considered important parts of their care. They would then come together and discuss which photographs they thought should be a part of their map. They would draw the map together on a large piece of paper and paste the photographs in the relevant areas. This process would be documented by the researcher, and the map would be used as an elicitation device, to enable young people to talk about their experiences of care.

In practice, however, we encountered unanticipated situations that led us to change our original plans. The researcher was only able to visit the wards for a few days due to time constraints for study completion (produced by delays in the local Research and Development [R&D] approval process). This meant that sometimes there were only a few young people available on the ward and the group activity could not be arranged. When we could find larger groups of young people on the ward, they often did not want to participate in a group activity and preferred to create the map on their own. This was an issue frequently discussed with the youth coordinators on the wards who indicated that integrating young people of this age into group activities was challenging and many preferred the privacy of their own rooms.

Many of the young people on the wards were in delicate health condition, often dealing with side effects of treatment such as fatigue and nausea, and did not feel well enough to get out of bed. Regardless of this, some young people still wanted to take part in the study, so we adapted the methodology to allow them to carry out the activity from their bed. For instance, one young person asked her mother to take pictures of specific areas of the ward while another participant only included pictures of areas she could capture lying down. A case that surprised us was that of a young woman who had been very ill all week and had refused to get out of bed. When asked if she wanted to participate in the photography and drawing activity, however, she immediately agreed and asked the researcher to walk with her around the ward to make sure she did not fall while she took the photographs.

Another situation we encountered was the high number of young people who said that they preferred to talk about their experiences instead of taking photographs and drawing the map. Some participants indicated that they were not good with that 'stuff' and preferred to have a conversation with the researcher in their rooms.

Lessons learned

The Mapping study allowed us to see that participatory visual methods need to be adapted to suit the needs of the participants and the research context. Many times we assume that young people will prefer these types of method over interviews or focus groups because they are fun and creative, but as the Mapping study showed, these preferences will depend on the mood, personality, and health condition of the young person. When working with ill participants our research design needs to be flexible enough to adapt to the way they are feeling on the day of the interview. By offering research participants different alternatives for taking part in our studies, we are empowering them to shape the research process according to their needs and encouraging them to engage with the methods they feel most comfortable with at that particular time. The more choices we include, the more participatory our design will be.

Dissemination of findings from the 'Children's participation in decision-making study'

This study used a qualitative approach to explore parents, doctors, nurses and allied healthcare professionals' perspectives on triadic decision-making in a children's hospital in Ireland. Interviews and participatory methods (photo voice, sorting cards, stick a star quiz, and diamond ranking exercises) were used to elicit the views and experiences of participation in decision-making from 23 children and young people (aged 8–16 years with chronic and acute illnesses). These participatory 'tools' complemented the information gathered through the interviews and enhanced the quality of interactions and data obtained. On completion of the study, the team was anxious to find a means of disseminating the research findings beyond academic formats. Research reports and short summaries are typically tailored for a more adult audience. To reach an audience such as children and young people in hospital, it was important to utilise both visual and verbal techniques and to involve children and young people in the co-development of an information-leaflet on decision-making.

Description of participatory visual methods

The aim was to distil the key findings from the study into an information-leaflet that would be accessible to children aged approximately 7–16 years old (Figure 6). The leaflet had to be visually appealing and the information had to be concise but informative. Thus, visual methods were used with focus group discussions to enable dialogue about aspects of decision-making and to co-produce the leaflet. We set up a co-design group consisting of children with long-term conditions (7–14 years) and a group of healthy children (11–13 years) and used images (of children) and sorting cards (key statements on decision-making). Our participatory approach was guided by four key principles: consultation and cooperation with relevant stakeholders, experimentation with alternative designs, contextualisation (testing with users and providers), and iterative development (modification in response to evaluation) (Waller, Franklin, Pagliari, & Greene, 2006). This was an iterative process as we (researchers, children, and graphic design person) experimented with different wording and designs in three participatory workshops.

The diamond ranking exercise (O'Kane, 2000) was used to elicit children's views about what was important to include in the leaflet about decision-making in hospital. The data were summarised in key statements placed on cards and children worked within the focus group (or individually) to rank them according to order of importance in a diamond shape so that the most and least important statements were placed from the tip to the base of the diamond. At the end of the diamond ranking process, children were asked to provide feedback and offer a rationale for their choice of placement of the most/least points. Although this exercise helped to reduce the findings to a key list of most important points, the wording had to be re-worked several times to meet with children's approval. For example, when the draft content was reviewed in the third focus group, the wording underwent significant revision as children thought the information needed to be phrased simply and the content needed to convey information as empowering rather than negatively.

This exercise complemented the information gathered through the photo voice exercise where different photos of children in hospital settings were shown. The children disliked

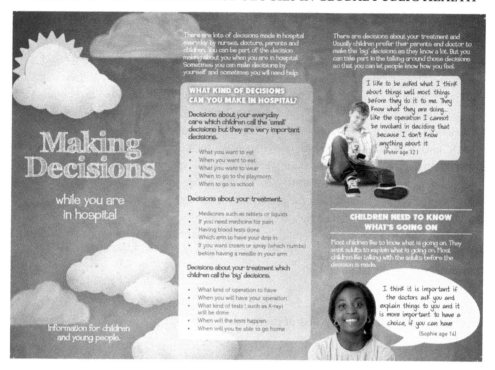

Figure 6. Information leaflet produced in the 'Children's participation in decision-making' study.

the images selected by the graphic design person and instead chose images of happy children of different ages and ethnic origin. They asked for children's quotes to be placed in a 'voice bubble' beside the image to make the content more visually appealing. The content and format were tested and modified in response to evaluations by children primarily and latterly by other stakeholders (parent, children's nurse, children's lecturer, and member of the Children in Hospital Ireland (CHI)).

Lessons learned

The participatory workshops worked well and the children found the process stimulating and easy to do. Since the group of healthy children had never been hospitalised, before they could contribute, the researcher had to provide fuller explanations using pictorial representation of decisions to explain the different types of decisions that children might be involved in hospital settings. Using pictures helped children to understand and discuss decisions and then to select the key points for inclusion in the leaflet. The visual methods helped make the focus groups enjoyable and enabled children of different ages with varied literacy skills to participate. Involving children in each step of the co-design process greatly assisted in the refinement and phrasing of content, layout, colour, formatting, and style. The sorting of the pictures and data (on cards) by the children led to a personal investment in those tasks and facilitated the discussion. Although the rationale for the diamond ranking exercise was explained, some children had some initial difficulty sorting the cards as they felt that all the data were important.

Improving our use of participatory visual methods

The three studies described here have pointed to common issues faced while using participatory visual methods with young people receiving long-term medical treatment. These experiences point to the fact that guaranteeing the participation of young people in research is not a simple and linear process. While reflecting on the use of participatory methods with children, Kefyalew (1996) has argued, 'participatory techniques were only effective when false expectations were not raised, when resources were properly used and stereotypical views (of both methodologies and children) were set aside' (p. 210). To these thoughts, we would add the following strategies to assist researchers in promoting the active engagement of research participants:

(1) Individualisation of approaches
(2) Contextualisation of approaches
(3) Taking the time required to design and apply participatory visual methods

Active engagement is facilitated by the long-term presence of the researcher in research settings, and fostering of relationships with young people. This immersion in the research context can help researchers consider different approaches for engaging young people. Flexible research designs include a wide range of methods young people can choose from to take part in the study depending on their individual preferences or how they feel on the day. Flexible designs allow for the need to make changes in the research instruments based on feedback from young people or problems encountered while piloting the method (as mentioned before in the example of the interpretation of images in the child information sheets). The aim of flexible research designs providing ample methodological choices is to give children the opportunity to participate on their own terms (James, Jenks, & Prout, 1998).

O'Kane (2000) has indicated that the effective use of participatory methods with children relies on 'creating a space which enables children to speak up and be heard' (p. 126). The creation of this space entails reflecting on the conditions under which the method will be used, so that proper measures can be taken to ensure active engagement when the method is applied. In the case of the studies presented here, this process could have entailed recognising the fact that most young people were hospitalised and ill, thus maybe not feeling energetic enough to carry out demanding tasks and not having plenty of room at their bedside for using large visual materials. For instance, in the Mapping study, we tried to adapt the Mosaic approach, which was originally developed in a school setting with well children (Clark & Moss, 2011), to the work we wanted to carry out in a hospital setting with inpatients. We now realise that we should have carried out further work to make sure our research method was suitable for the setting and characteristics of our research participants. Having said that it was a method that seemed to energise at least one participant, reinforcing the complexity of accommodating the 'individual' in any research design.

Lack of privacy is another issue encountered in clinical settings and should be factored into the considerations made by the researchers during the research design. By thinking carefully about the context where the research will be carried out and the characteristics of the young people who will be asked to take part, researchers can anticipate some of the common problems we discussed in the previous sections. Similarly, greater use of and evaluation of such methods will ensure that they are embedded into many clinical studies, resulting in increased patience of clinical staff/reduction in interruptions through recognition of the value and difference such techniques might add, particularly to the assent/ consent process.

In our experience, the design and implementation of visual methods requires a great deal of time and effort (see also O'Kane, 2000; Pretty, Guijt, Thompson, & Scoones, 1995). When visual material is used to elicit children's participation, as in the 'Talking with Children' study, attention needs to be paid to the details of the images, format, colour, font, etc. The researchers also need to be open to making iterative reformulations of the research methods to suit the needs and preferences of the children involved. Nieuwenhuys (1996) has spoken in favour of establishing a 'continuous dialogue' with children throughout the research process to ensure that research methods are effective. This ongoing dialogue might be difficult to arrange and certainly increases the researchers' workload, but in the end it gives research participants the direct opportunity to shape the research process. This capacity to shape the research provides researchers with several advantages such as: to ensure that participants' consent to participate is informed and voluntary, deliver study findings that better reflect the views and experiences of those involved in the study, and provide mechanisms for disseminating research findings that will guarantee they are assimilated to a greater extent by the groups involved in the research (hopefully producing greater impact).

Conclusions

Participatory visual methods are excellent 'tools' for engaging young people in health research, but participation needs to be envisioned from initial stages of research design and throughout subsequent stages of a study. The use of visual methods in itself does not guarantee a participatory research process; participation in the form of active engagement has to be fostered by the researcher to allow young people to fully express their views and mould the study according to their preferences and interests. To do this successfully, the researcher will need to be competent and confident in the use of such methods, be sensitive and responsive to the needs of the research participants, and be prepared to be flexible in all situations.

In our experience, active engagement is achieved through the long-term presence of the researcher in the research setting, through flexible research designs, and the consideration of the particular conditions where, when, and with whom the study is carried out. We hope that the examples presented here have illustrated how visual methods can be useful 'tools' for obtaining informed consent/assent, collecting data, and dissemination of findings, and have pointed to ways in which we can continue to improve our use of these methods in health-care settings with populations across the age range.

We hope that future studies can continue to explore the advantages and disadvantages of using participatory visual methods in different settings and at different stages of research. We certainly need more evidence on the use of participatory visual methods to obtain informed consent and disseminate study findings. An important avenue of future study concerns the role the research site, population, and study aims play in the shaping of both the research methods and the process of participation of research participants, thus leading to more context-sensitive research approaches. We must continue to be brave in our endeavours, to continue to refine our approaches based on reflections of use in practice, as well as feedback from young people. We must continue to share what works well and less well, and in what context, so that as a research community we build evidence that is available to others.

Disclosure statement

No potential conflict of interest was reported by the authors.

Funding

The work of Prof Imelda Coyne was supported by Health Research Board, Ireland. The work of Dr Gemma Bryan was supported by the Olivia Hodson Cancer Fund. The work of Dr Cecilia Vindrola-Padros was supported by London South Bank University.

References

Barker, J., & Smith, F. (2012). What's in focus? A critical discussion of photography, children and young people. *International Journal of Social Research Methodology, 15*, 91–103. doi:10.1080/13645579.2012.649406

Brannen, J. (2002). The use of video in research dissemination: Children as experts on their own family lives. *International Journal of Social Research Methodology, 5*, 173–180. doi:10.1080/13645570110118700

Carter, B., & Ford, K. (2013). Researching children's health experiences: The place for participatory, child-centered, arts-based approaches. *Research in Nursing and Health, 36*, 95–107. doi:10.1002/nur.21517

Clark, A., & Moss, P. (2011). *Listening to young children: The Mosaic approach* (2nd ed.). London: National Children's Bureau.

Close, H. (2007). The use of photography as a qualitative research tool. *Nurse Research, 15*, 27–36.

Coyne, I., Hayes, E., & Gallagher, P. (2009). Research with hospitalized children: Ethical, methodological and organizational challenges. *Childhood, 16*, 413–429. doi:10.1177/0907568209335319

Dell Clark, C. (2010). *In a younger voice: Doing child-centered qualitative research*. Berkshire: Open University Press.

Dockett, S., Perry, B., & Kearney, E. (2013). Promoting children's informed assent in research participation. *International Journal of Qualitative Studies in Education, 26*, 802–828. doi:10.1080/09518398.2012.666289

Drew, S. E., Duncan, R. E., & Sawyer, S. M. (2010). Visual storytelling: A beneficial but challenging method for health research with young people. *Qualitative Health Research, 20*, 1677–1688. doi:10.1177/1049732310377455

Ford, K., Sankey, J., & Crisp, J. (2007). Development of children's assent documents using a child-centred approach. *Journal of Child Health Care, 11*, 19–28. doi:10.1177/1367493507073058

James, A., Jenks, C., & Prout, A. (1998). *Theorizing childhood*. Cambridge: Polity.

Johnson, G. A., Pfister, A. E., & Vindrola-Padros, C. (2012). Drawings, photos, and performances: Using visual methods with children. *Visual Anthropology Review, 28*, 164–178. doi:10.1111/j.1548-7458.2012.01122.x

Kefyalew, F. (1996). The reality of child participation in research: Experience from a capacity-building programme. *Childhood, 3*, 203–213. doi:10.1177/0907568296003002007

Kumpunen, S. Shipway, L., Taylor, R. M. Aldiss, S., & Gibson, F. (2012). Practical approaches to seeking assent from children. *Nurse Researcher, 19*, 23 27.

Lambert, V. & Glacken, M. (2011). Engaging with children in research: Theoretical and practical implications of negotiating informed consent/assent. *Nursing Ethics, 18*, 781–801. doi:10.1177/0969733011401122

Lomax, H. (2012). Contested voices? Methodological tensions in creative visual research with children. *International Journal of Social Research Methodology, 15*, 105–117. doi:10.1080/13645579.2012.649408

Nieuwenhuys, O. (1996). Action research with street children: A role for street educators. *PLA Notes, 25*, 52–55.

O'Kane, C. (2000). The development of participatory techniques: Facilitating children's views about decisions which affect them. In P. Christensen & A. James (Eds.), *Research with children: Perspectives and practices* (pp. 125–155). London: Falmer Press.

Pain, H. (2012). A literature review to evaluate the choice and use of visual methods. *International Journal of Qualitative Methods, 11*, 303–319.

Pfister, A., Vindrola-Padros, C., & Johnson, G. (2014). Together, we can show you: Using participant-generated visual data in collaborative research. *Collaborative Anthropologies, 7*, 26–49. doi:10.1353/cla.2014.0005

Pretty, J. N., Guijt, I., Thompson, J., & Scoones, I. (1995). *Participatory learning and action: A trainers guide*. London: IIED Participatory Methodology Series.

Rollins, J. A. (2005). Tell me about it: Drawing as a communication tool for children with cancer. *Journal of Pediatric Oncology Nursing, 22*, 203–221. doi:10.1177/1043454205277103

Sartain, S. A., Clarke, C. L., & Heyman, R. (2000). Hearing the voices of children with chronic illness. *Journal of Advanced Nursing, 32*, 913–921. doi:10.1046/j.1365-2648.2000.01556.x

Waller, A., Franklin, V., Pagliari, C., & Greene, S. (2006). Participatory design of a text message scheduling system to support young people with diabetes. *Health Informatics Journal, 12*, 304–318. doi:10.1177/1460458206070023

Weller, S. (2012). Evolving creativity in qualitative longitudinal research with children and teenagers. *International Journal of Social Research Methodology, 15*, 119–133. doi:10.1080/13645579.2012.649412

Beyond engagement in working with children in eight Nairobi slums to address safety, security, and housing: Digital tools for policy and community dialogue

Claudia Mitchell[a], Fatuma Chege[b], Lucy Maina[c] and Margot Rothman[d]

[a]Department of Integrated Studies in Education, McGill University, Montréal, Canada; [b]Department of Educational Foundations, Kenyatta University, Nairobi, Kenya; [c]Department of Sociology, Kenyatta University, Nairobi, Kenya; [d]Groupe-conseil INTERALIA, Montréal, Canada

ABSTRACT
This article studies the ways in which researchers working in the area of health and social research and using participatory visual methods might extend the reach of participant-generated creations such as photos and drawings to engage community leaders and policymakers. Framed as going 'beyond engagement', the article explores the idea of the production of researcher-led digital dialogue tools, focusing on one example, based on a series of visual arts-based workshops with children from eight slums in Nairobi addressing issues of safety, security, and well-being in relation to housing. The authors conclude that there is a need for researchers to embark upon the use of visual tools to expand the life and use of visual productions, and in particular to ensure meaningful participation of communities in social change.

Introduction

How to influence community dialogue and the policy-making process itself is of ongoing concern for researchers, especially those working in participatory visual research in such areas as health and education. It is a legitimate concern and aspiration, given the significant investment of time and commitment of communities and individuals in participating in projects which seek to challenge inequalities in education, healthcare, food security, access to clean water and sanitation, and, as we take up in this article, safety and security in relation to housing. There has been increased recognition in the research literature on the significance of participatory visual research involving those most affected by inequalities – most often children and young people, using visual arts-based methodologies as photo-voice (Delgado, 2015), drawing (Theron, Mitchell, Smith, & Stuart, 2011), comparative mapping (Hallman, Kenworthy, Diers, Swan, & Devnarain, 2015), digital storytelling (Gubrium & Harper, 2013), participatory video (Milne, Mitchell, & De Lange, 2012), and cellphilms (MacEntee, 2015). Such approaches have been shown to be effective in altering some of the typical power dynamics related to the researched/researcher and to ensuring spaces for marginalised populations to both speak about and then 'speak back'

(Mitchell De Lange, & Moletsane, in press) through interactive workshop sessions addressing (and changing) social conditions. At the same time the products in these projects – photo exhibitions and screenings of video productions, for example – are ideally suited to be seen by many different audiences (including different community groups and policymakers) (see also Mitchell, 2015). As Rist (2003) observes:

> There is no broad-based and sustained tradition within contemporary social science of focusing qualitative work specifically on policy issues, especially given the real time constraints that the policy process necessitates. Yet it is also clear that the opportunities are multiple for such contributions to be made. (p. 641)

But what tools and approaches can ensure that the products of these participatory methods contribute to community and policy dialogue? How can digital technology itself be used to advance this work? And how might these approaches serve to maximise the potential for participant voice and minimise what could be regarded as tokenistic in relation to participatory processes?

Researcher-led video production: a review of the literature

At the centre of this article is a consideration of the development and use of researcher-generated digital productions that draw together visual and related data for the purposes of engaging participants and various audiences as part of participatory generation of data, analysis, knowledge translation, and knowledge mobilisations. A number of publications such as Burt and Code's (1995) *Changing Methods: Feminists Transforming Practice*, Schratz and Walker's (1995) *Research as Social Change: New Opportunities for Qualitative Research*, Kapoor and Choudry's (2010) *Learning from the Ground Up: Global Perspectives on Social Movements and Knowledge Production*, and Gubrium, Harper, and Otañez's (2015) *Participatory Visual and Digital Research in Action* have considered the potential (and limitations) of participatory methods for policy and community dialogue, although it is an area that remains under-studied, particularly in relation to the participation of children. Mitchell (2011) describes the ways in which researchers can work with video as a tool in visual research for outreach, separate from the processes of participatory video, and as a genre in itself. This work can range from ethnographic film as has been seen in the work by Ruby (2000) and Pink (2013), through to the documentary style work applied in health settings in, for example, Katerina Cizek's productions as part of the film maker in residence programme at St Michel's hospital in Toronto or Gary Bitel's *Living with Kidney Failure* (see Mitchell, 2011). At the other end of the spectrum are the 'composite' videos, video production that might include process footage of participatory video or a photo-voice project, as well as the actual creations produced by participants (see also De Lange & Mitchell, 2012). More recently this work also includes other types of digital productions such as digital animation (Pithouse-Morgan, Van Laren, Mitchell, Mudaly, & Singh, 2015). Contributing to an emerging body of literature that makes the production process (and not just the actual production) and the screening of such productions the focus, is the work of researchers such as the following: Mak (2006, 2012) who writes about the making and screening of *Unwanted Images*, on children's drawings of gender-violence. In addition we note Thompson, MacEntee, and Fikreyesus (2014) who describe and reflect on the production and screening of *Gender and Enset* in their work with women farmers and *enset* production in Ethiopia; and the work of De Lange and Mitchell (2012) who describe and reflect on the co-production with a small group of teachers in rural South Africa of a 'video of videos', *Youth-led Community Research to Address Gender Violence*. Much of this work on researcher-led video production in participatory visual research highlights the significance of post-data collection as a critical feature of the research itself (see, e.g. De Lange & Mitchell, 2012; Mitchell, 2011).

Framed within what might be termed a pedagogy of screenings, several researchers have made reflexivity in relation to audience response a critical feature of this work. MacEntee and Mandrona (2015), for example, describe a series of screenings organised by a group of rural teachers in relation to the cellphilms they produced on the topic of youth sexuality and HIV and AIDS. The authors pose the notion of 'discomfort' as theorised by Boler (1999) and others, as a way to consider what happens during the screenings. While not theorised directly as discomfort but no less discomforting, Mitchell (2006) similarly offers an analysis of screening the video production *Fire + Hope*, a video made with a group of young HIV activists in Cape Town to several groups of rural youth in KwaZulu-Natal who offer a critical reading of the documentary. As Mitchell (2006) observes, one of the first things they ask the research team made up primarily of white people is 'why are there no white people in the film?' (p. 231). Another group of rural youth '… want to know why it is so hard to understand the Western Cape accent. They don't quite get the gangsterism of Khayelitsha. But they too want to know where the white people are' (p. 232). In a related way Pithouse-Morgan et al. (2015) describe the production and screening of their digital animation *Take a Risk: It's as Easy as ABC* that they created based on their research on integrating HIV and AIDS into the curriculum of Higher Education in South Africa. For them the discomfort is screening the digital animation to other academics and professional colleagues working in the area of HIV and AIDS. In the same vein, Mudaly, Pithouse-Morgan et al. (2015) describe the screening of this same digital animation to a group of tech-savvy young people.

These studies of researcher-led video production (and the screenings of such productions) help to set the stage for our discussion of *More Than Bricks and Mortar*, a seven-minute digital production of the drawings, maps, and photos of 'feeling safe and not so safe' produced by children in eight informal settlement or slums in and around Nairobi. They also set the stage for tracking audience responses in the screening history of a particular video tool. As Wheeler (2012) observes in relation to a study of the policy engagement process through community-produced participatory videos, 'a single space for debate is not enough – there needs to be ongoing pressure on different fronts' (p. 376). There has been, to date, little focus on the implications for policy dialogue at either the stage of production or the tracking of follow-up actions following the screening of such productions.

The context

The focus of the participatory work with children described here addresses issues of safety, security, health, and well-being in relation to housing in a two-year study that took place in eight slum communities in and around Nairobi, Kenya.[1] As the UN Habitat (2006) study noted, it is estimated that the level of deprivation among slum dwellers is equivalent to and can be much greater than that experienced by the rural poor, often resulting in intertwined problems in relation to health, education, safety, and security. Indeed, as various studies have highlighted, the global trends towards urbanisation are often characterised by growing poverty and health inequalities (see Agarwal, 2011; Madise et al., 2012). To date, however, few studies in the Global South focusing on social inequalities in urban environments have taken into consideration the perspectives of children. As a research team working closely with an international non-governmental organisation (NGO) focusing on micro-finance and housing, we were interested in the views of children on issues of safety, security, and well-being in relation to housing. As we describe elsewhere, the study was conducted in two phases (Chege, Maina, Mitchell, & Rothman, 2014a).[2]

Phase 1: arts-based workshops

In the first phase of the study (year 1) 100 children (most ranging between the ages of 8 and 13) and from 8 communities participated in arts-based workshops in which they drew images, created maps, and took photographs in response to the prompt 'feeling safe and not so safe'. The data collection was carried out by masters and doctoral students enrolled in the School of Education, Kenyatta University. All of the data collectors participated in a week-long training session on participatory visual research with children. The initial data set was made up of more than 100 drawings, 100 maps, and several hundred photos.[3]

As researchers, we saw that the drawings, maps, and photos that the children produced made a compelling argument for why researchers and policy-makers need to consult with children in social research. Indeed as we describe elsewhere (Chege, Maina, Mitchell, & Rothman, 2014b), the 'not so safe' issues were comparatively many and their messages compelling. We offer here (Table 1) a sampling of the various issues in order to provide a backdrop for the development of the digital dialogue tool based on the children's visual representations and comments.

Many of the actual photos and drawings produced by the children could be described as Sontag (2004) suggests, as haunting, and while it is beyond the scope of this article to offer an in-depth analysis of the images (see Chege et al., 2014a), it is important to acknowledge their impact on the research team itself and our commitment to ensuring that adults in the community engage with them.

Phase 2: data analysis

In the second year of the study (and the focus of this article), our interest was in taking the data back to the children who had participated in the initial data collection. In particular, we wanted to ensure children would have a chance to not only validate the data they helped to generate but also see their own visual creations (maps, photos, and drawings on feeling safe and not so safe) as part of the 'bigger picture of housing' of how children in the region were perceiving the issues, and also as part of seeing what solutions they would suggest. We also, however, wanted to ensure that the children's productions would be taken seriously by adults. As Bober (2010) writes, children's visual productions are too often appreciated for their decorative function in, for example, a report focusing on children and not necessarily treated as data that could actually inform policy dialogue. At the same time, we were also motivated to address certain technical concerns. For example, we were aware that there could be physical challenges in setting up an exhibition in

Table 1. Children's quotes describing their drawings and photos on relevant issues.

Environmental Issues	This place is not safe and – because – this place is near school and some children may come here and play and they may – they may catch germs. And if they want to eat something, they can't wash their hands. And if they eat with their dirty hands, they become sick … (I am not safe because all over is dirty). (Boy, 11 years old)
	The river has been polluted by people who live near there. When they go to the toilet, the waste goes straight into the river. That is why you see the river is dirty. (Girl, 10 years old)
Domestic Violence	The drawing talks about a child being abused by the mother – by the stepmother. She is supposed to do the laundry, fetch water daily. And she is thoroughly beaten when she does n't – when she doesn't do the work. (Girl, 13 years old)
	I have drawn a child being beaten by their mother who does n't love them. She does not love her child. She beats the child at night and gets her to sleep on the floor […] She tells the child that if they come into the house she will kill them. The child does not want to be killed so they sleep in the tree. (Boy, 8 years old)
Gangs	The unsafe place is the shortcuts – the railway road and the road heading to Darajani. When you pass through that road at night, you can be robbed by the robbers and you might be killed. (Girl, 13 years old)
	My photo [a photo of a brick wall] means that here there gangsters crowded at seven p.m. They smoke bhang cigarettes and they do drugs like khat, cocaine, and alcohol. (Boy, 12 years old)
Child Labour	My drawing is talking about the violence against children. Here the what – the employer, she is trying to abuse the child. She used her as a shopkeeper and she doesn't pay her and she doesn't give her food. (Girl, 13 years old)
	My drawing talks about this girl is being abused by her step-mother. She is being told to do all the child chores. Sometimes she does n't complete her homework and she goes to school dirty. Some times the stepmother denies her food. (Girl, 13 years old)
Sexual Violence	So, this picture is talking about a man threatening to rape a girl. And that is common in our neighbourhood. It is common in our neighbourhood. (Boy, 14 years old)
	My drawing says that a father forcing a daughter to have sex with her. If not, he will beat her until death. I heard it. With my – I was told by my friends. The girl sweet-talked her father and then escaped never to be seen again. Yes (she ran away). Yes (until now her whereabouts are unknown). (Girl, 13 years old)
Toilets	At the toilet people will threaten you with a knife to force you (to do things you do n't want to do). Yes, I fear the toilet. I usually go with my mother (to the toilet). She waits outside. I would never go alone there. (Girl, 12 years old)
	I fear because when you go to that public toilet, you find some other strangers or thieves and so you have to be afraid. Not everyday (I don't go there everyday). (Girl, 14 years old)

informal settlements. And overall we wanted to leave behind a tool that local communities might use (and re-use) as part of the 'beyond engagement' dissemination process more broadly. In the sections below, then, we consider the methods for producing and screening *More Than Bricks and Mortar*, our findings on its use with several audiences, and a discussion of critical issues related to replicability and ethics.

Methods: producing and screening a digital dialogue tool

In the initial data collection, it was difficult for us to imagine how to get the community members (parents and community leaders) to actually view (and take seriously) the children's productions, let alone policy-makers. At the same time there were few opportunities for children to consider solutions, or to see how their own visual images fit into the bigger picture. Thus, drawing on the development of a 'digital dialogue tool' – a short digital production (sound and image) that draws together and organises visual data for the purposes of engaging participants and various audiences (communities and policy-makers), facilitated us to embark upon exploring how digital technology could be used to go 'beyond engagement' and, in particular, contribute to ensuring that the children's voices (through their visual productions) are heard (and seen) by the adults in the community and by policy-makers. In this section, we describe our methods and procedures for producing and screening *More Than Bricks and Mortar*, a seven-minute digital production of the children's drawings, maps, and photos of 'feeling safe and not so safe'.

Part 1: *producing* **More Than Bricks and Mortar**

Building on a preliminary analysis of the visual images produced by the children, the team worked with a filmmaker to create a storyboard that would frame the production of a short digital dialogue tool. The video production itself might be analysed both denotatively and connotatively. Denotatively, the video follows a fairly straight-forward storyline, including information about the participants and what they were asked to do (through the voice-over of a local broadcaster speaking in Kiswahili), along with still images of the children engaged in drawing and taking photos (see Figure 1). It is then organised into seven thematic areas, each of which includes the sub-title of the thematic areas, followed by samples of the drawings, maps, and photos. Six of these centre on 'feeling not so safe' (child labour, domestic violence, sexual violence, toilet safety, environmental security, and gangs), with one main theme on 'feeling safe' (especially inside homes and through images of churches and mosques) as seen through the eyes of children.

Connotatively, the video is meant to be emotive. In the production of the digital dialogue tool we were seeking anything but non-neutrality and regarded audience engagement (especially the engagement of adults) as critical and deliberate. We did not want audiences to walk away without being moved by the children's visual productions. It opens with footage of Kenyan children about the same age as the participants running along rural footpaths, which appear to be safe. We hear the pure clear voice of a child singing in the background. Following this musical opening, we see the title frame (Figure 1).

In the final scenes of the video the music increases in volume as the rolling credits appear. The addition of a musical soundtrack in this kind of production is not without its controversy. In our view, the music can help to set the mood and in and of itself be cathartic. Pauwels (2002) in his analysis of researcher-led or researcher-produced videos queries the use of music in researcher-led academic productions. As he writes:

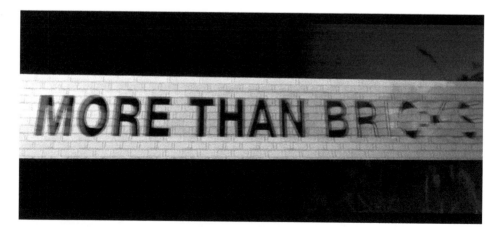

Figure 1. Screen shot from title frame of *More Than Bricks and Mortar*.

Music, unless it actually is performed during the recording and is thus an integral part of the reality conveyed (i.e. synchronic sound), indeed can have a disrupting effect on the process of knowledge transfer. Sound that is added afterward can set a particular mood and thus impose a certain interpretation upon the viewer, for which there may be no scientific grounds whatsoever. Or it will at least distract some of the viewer's attention, which otherwise would be focused on the actual material. Likewise, whether the use of commentary may be guiding or not, remains a hotly debated aspect of audio visual productions by social scientists. (Pauwels, 2002, p. 126)

Whether the absence of a soundtrack contributes to non-neutrality is an interesting question within broader studies of audience research and viewer response. Given that *More Than Bricks and Mortar* was meant to serve double and triple roles makes the engagement factor a particularly compelling one in community-based research (Figure 2).

Part 2: screening and tracking More Than Bricks and Mortar

A total of 5 participatory workshops were held with children from the participating communities, many of whose members belonged to various community-based housing organisations attached to a corporate NGO of housing cooperatives. Child participants first viewed the *More Than Bricks and Mortar* video and as we describe below, had an opportunity to talk about and produce drawings about their ideas on ways to improve safety and security in their homes and communities. In total, more than 300 children participated in these screenings. Wherever possible, efforts were made to assemble the same children who had participated in the original visual data collection workshops. This was not always possible and it is estimated that approximately a third of those who had participated in data collection workshops participated in the screenings. In some cases, the number of

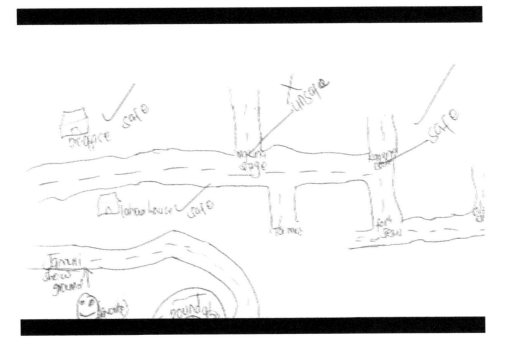

Figure 2. Screen shot from *More Than Bricks and Mortar*.

participants in each group was the anticipated 25–30 children, while in other cases, more than 120 children participated.

Three screenings were held with adults. These included a half-day workshop with approximately 30 executive committee members of the 8 communities who viewed *More Than Bricks and Mortar*, listened to a presentation on the preliminary findings of the research, and had an opportunity to work in small groups to offer their responses to the findings and video, and also to consider how they might address the findings. A second workshop involved senior managers/executive at the NGO responsible for the housing programme through which community members received loans and support for their houses. A third session was held with the masters and doctoral students who had participated as data collectors in arts-based workshops and interviews.

Findings

Children engage in dialogue on challenges and solutions

Perhaps the most dramatic impact of screening *More Than Bricks and Mortar* to the various groups of children was their immediate reaction to seeing their ordinary lives depicted so vividly in technologies with which they have seldom interacted. Perhaps in view of this, they were moved to take extraordinary actions to find solutions. While the research team had originally planned to facilitate these sessions simply as discussions, it was clear that one of the tools for engaging them in the first place (drawing and mapping) was also an important tool for follow-up with children insisting on drawing their solutions. The children were, in a sense, 'speaking back' (Mitchell & De Lange, 2013) to the issues they had highlighted in the original data collection workshops. Each workshop session included an opportunity for the older children present to also talk about their drawings and ideas in group settings. In some cases, their suggestions high-lighted what they themselves could do. For example, the children acknowledged that they could improve the sanitation of toilets by cleaning them themselves and by picking up litter around the toilets. At the same time they also highlighted the significance of the collective action of children and young people, something that can be seen in Figure 3 below their depiction of the Kibera Youth Development project.

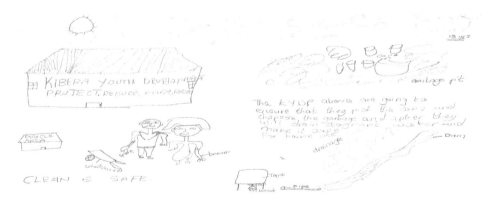

Figure 3. Collective action in the Kibera youth development project.

The children's 'speaking back' drawings also addressed such issues as sexual abuse and the need to try to address these issues in the community through education. As one child wrote as part of her drawing (Figure 4): 'The whole family is being taught. We can control child labour and abuse by educating parents.'

Finally, it is worth noting that the drawings also spoke to their hopes and dreams: as one girl wrote alongside a very prominent light bulb: 'I would like to be having a beautiful house like this for my mother.' Another child wrote alongside a drawing of a very prominent water tap: 'Our house. Our tap.' One child drew and wrote about the significance of education:

> We as children from the slums long for good education which other more privileged children get just because their parents can afford it. For us due to our parents' financial situation we are just forced to go to public school where there is no good education.

Community dialogue: adults 'reawakening' to the realities of children's lives

Adult community members who participated in validation workshops where they had an opportunity to view *More Than Bricks and Mortar* were asked two main questions: (1) As a matter of a housing cooperative, what role are you planning to play in regard to the safety of children? And (2) What support would you require to do this? The participants were both moved and surprised by the voices of children on issues surrounding their safety and security in the informal settlements when they viewed *More Than Bricks and Mortar*. The digital dialogue tool containing drawings, maps, photos, and quotes from the interviews with children proved to be powerful tools in both raising stark awareness among adults of 'their' children's daily realities in the slums, and to evoke concern. Some of the situations depicted by children were a surprise to adults who had not thought, for example, of the cumulative impact of the threats to safety experienced by

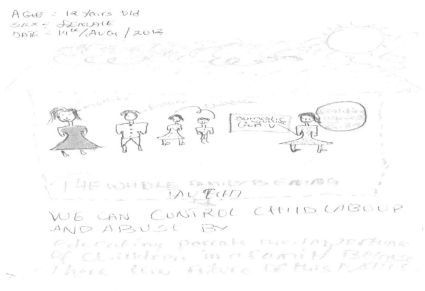

Figure 4. 'Educating parents'.

girls when they queue for water in the neighbourhood several times a day. Other concerns, such as prostitution and drugs, were well known to all participants, but seeing the issues depicted through children's eyes brought their impact into clear focus. During the follow-up, almost all participants spoke of the need to build protection mechanisms in the community. These included efforts to build trust between neighbours and to support community unity. Some participants spoke about the importance of cleaning up the community, parental education, improved access to counselling services and building more community infrastructure (a community hall, shopping centres, schools, and churches). Almost all groups spoke of the need to build a perimeter wall around the community. The idea of addressing the community itself was taken up, and especially talking with neighbours and uniting the community. Several spoke of the importance of building play-grounds and of consulting with children themselves. Less was said however about what resources would be needed to make the communities safer. At the same time, some of the discussion during the workshop was directed more towards what the housing NGO could do in terms of helping the urban poor with savings and loans that are affordable and that could enable them to relocate to safer neighbourhoods.

Dialogue with policy-makers

In the section above we draw attention to the role of adults in the community, especially parents and neighbours. The idea of policy dialogue beyond the community is more challenging. One of the groups most directly related to policy at least at a local level was the executive board of the national housing NGO since that institution has responsibility for micro-loans and also for developing policies and practices governing the overall implementation of the housing plan. Ten members of the executive board had an opportunity to participate in a validation workshop in which they viewed *More Than Bricks and Mortar* and then were given a presentation on the preliminary findings of the study. Most of the participants in the validation workshop were clearly moved by the images. Several commented that they thought it would be important to come up with ways to incorporate the voices of children, including in the design of houses since one aspect of their work is on ensuring appropriate and cost effective designs. Child safety – as seen through the eyes of children – was, they said, a new angle on the work. But there are, of course, other policy players. The initial data collection drew on focus group interviews with various adult groups including police, social workers, and teachers; hence, a key concern was to reach these groups with *More Than Bricks and Mortar*.

Dialogue beyond the community: data collectors

The graduate students from Kenyatta University who led the data collection and who later viewed *More Than Bricks and Mor*tar had a different set of perspectives on the digital dia-logue tool, in part because, for some of them at least, the fieldwork setting was the first time they had visited the slums and it was an eye-opener. As one of the graduate students observed:

> ... the most important as well as interesting aspect of my participation in this study was the opportunity to work with children. This was very important to me in the sense that it gave me

a rare opportunity to work with children at a very personal level and in their capacity not just as passive recipients of information but as active generators of knowledge through creative methodologies such as photo-voice and drawing scenarios of aspects of their life from their own experiential perspectives. (Cited in Chege et al., 2014a, p. 81)

Their experiences in the slum settlements were also terrifying at times. In the end, youth 'gate keepers' from the communities were employed to ensure the safety of the data collectors. Indeed, one of the recommendations that came out of this study, and as informed by the data collectors themselves related to adequate funds and planning to carry out work that seeks to study violence in violent settings. The screening of *More Than Bricks and Mortar* to this group was a reminder, as one participant put it, that 'it was worth it'. At the same time, these are all educators pursing masters and doctoral research in a country and region where not that many people have the advantage of accessing higher education. Many will themselves become senior officials, academics, and key actors in the policy-making process. A critical follow-up study would be to look at the impact of participating in this study in terms of research agendas and career choices over the long term.

Discussion

Clearly there are many issues – technical and ethical – that arise in this type of project and that go beyond the already complex issues associated with participatory visual research involving children, as Akesson et al. (2014) highlight. A key question coming out of this study is one of replicability: Is *More Than Bricks and Mortar* just a 'once off' initiative or can researchers build this type of production into their research from the beginning, and if so, what are the implications? In the section on 'Producing and Screening', we have tried to give a sense of the genre of the digital dialogue tool. As highlighted by Mudaly, Pithouse-Morgan, Van Laren, Singh, and Mitchell (2015) in their discussion[4] of a digital animation dialogue tool, there are a number of key features of this type of work that make it easily replicable. Their first point is that it is cheap (as in cost effective), particularly given the increasingly easy access to digital technology for participants and researchers alike to use tools such as digital storytelling, cellphilming (videos through cellphones), and other forms of participatory video. It also becomes less expensive to produce other videos associated with follow-up projects. For example, in the production of a digital dialogue tool that is very similar in length and format to *More Than Bricks and Mortar*, Mitchell, Nguyen, and Twang (2015) co-produced *Picturing Inclusion: Voices of Girls with Disabilities*. This digital dialogue tool is based on participatory visual research with girls with disabilities living in Vietnam (Nguyen, Mitchell, De Lange, & Fritsch, 2015). Once there is a structure, it is relatively straightforward to adapt to other research projects. A second and related point is that it is convenient to produce digital dialogue tools since the raw material drawings, photos, or maps already exist. Most researcher teams have the technical tools to create short digital productions. Mudaly et al. (2015) suggest that a third feature is collaboration. In the case of *More Than Bricks and Mortar*, the production reflects the collaborative work of the research team across two country contexts, although there was still room to adapt the version that the children viewed in the community screenings. Indeed, a set of questions we always asked included the following: What did you like or dislike about the video? Is there anything you would like to change? Who should see the video? In the case of *Picturing Inclusion: Voices of Girls with Disabilities*, the girls had an opportunity to view the rough cut and offer suggestions for modification. Mudaly et al. (2015) also refer to the significance of creativity. In research using arts-based methodologies, there is an additional level of integrity if researchers as well as participants engage artistically with the data (Mitchell et al., in press).

Finally, we consider some of the ethical issues. When caregivers or parents give consent and children offer their assent to engage in participatory visual research, we need to consider any ethical issues that pertain to the re-use of visual data as is the case in digital dialogue tools. In *More Than Bricks and Mortar*, the ethical consent forms included reference to exhibiting the images in a variety of outlets (articles, exhibitions in public spaces, conference presentations). In that production, the focus was on the images produced by the children and not on images of the children themselves, although we do include several process photos of children 'in action' taking pictures and creating drawings. None of these images are directly associated with any specific drawing or photograph however. This is an important consideration given that the focus of the study is on violence in the community, and there is the possibility that someone who views the video could be a perpetrator. In *Picturing Inclusion: Voices of Girls with Disabilities*, all of the girls (and their parents) had an opportunity to view the rough cut, so it was possible to re-negotiate the consent process. Only one girl did not agree to have her picture or her drawing in the video and so these were removed. But there are other ethical issues associated with displaying (and re-using) child-generated visual data, as Akesson et al. (2014) point out, particularly in relation to questions such as 'whose interpretation?' and 'who owns the data?' Taking *More Than Bricks and Mortar* to children first for their input (and letting them know that they were viewing it before any adults in the community) was a modest gesture towards addressing these questions, but it is clearly an area that requires further study.

Conclusion

We posed the question at the beginning of this article on how digital technology itself can be used to go 'beyond engagement' and in particular, how might it contribute to policy dialogue in relation to safety, security, well-being and housing. We would like to offer 'proof' of change in evidence that the adults in the community who viewed *More Than Bricks and Mortar* have actually done something to create a safer environment for children. One possible follow-up that we could have done as a research team would have been to have had community leaders go back to their respective communities with a copy of *More Than Bricks and Mortar* and the PowerPoint presentation of preliminary findings so that there could be a type of 'roll out' and accountability built into participation.

At another level, we argue that the idea of 'beyond engagement' itself warrants further theorising in relation to participatory visual research. Given the vast body of research on participation and participatory process, and the plethora of work that seeks to critique tokenistic participation (see, e.g. Kapoor & Jordan, 2009), it is incumbent on the research community to extend the possibilities in research. Thus, we offer this notion of 'beyond engagement' as a new pathway for community dialogue and policy influence in health research with a strong social agenda. The areas it could cover might include critical implications for research ethics boards, and implications for funding in terms of what is required to sustain this work from engagement to beyond engagement. Overall, 'beyond engagement' could be a powerful concept in terms of refocusing the agenda of health research and social change to frame anew the point of participatory visual research. As Pauwels (2002) observes, visual research has the potential to draw more effectively on the use of the visual at all levels of the research. *More Than Bricks and Mortar* is just one example of how this might be done to extend participatory visual work into community and policy dialogue.

Notes

1. This study looked at the safety and security issues confronting children in relation to housing in eight primary housing cooperatives in slums and informal settlements in Nairobi (including Kinyago-Kanuku; Makina-Kibera; Razaak; Soweto East; Huruma and Kawangare). This study was carried out under the Evaluation Challenge Fund – Children & Violence – in order to test out the following evaluation hypothesis: improved tenure security, housing and living conditions, and coop/community development activities contribute to reducing family stressors and the risk of violence to children through better physical security of the dwelling, larger and separate living spaces for children, safer access to external facilities such as toilets and lighting, improved family savings and livelihoods, as well as more sustainable communities. The evaluation provided the resources to test these assumptions, which emerged from experience and anecdotal testimonies on previous National Cooperative Housing Union of Kenya (NACHU) programming efforts. The evaluation was supported under Category 3 of the Evaluation Challenge Fund, which targets 'specific components of programmes not directly designed to prevent violence but potentially having an impact in terms of violence prevention for children.'
2. The study was conducted in a partnership with Rooftops Canada and NACHU a national NGO focusing on micro-finance organisation to support low-income housing. Masters and doctoral students at Kenyatta University participated in conducting the arts-based workshops with children and also helped to conduct interviews and focus group with community leaders and youth.
3. These approvals included ethical clearance from McGill University, Canada, and research permit issued by the Kenya National Council for Science and Technology as the constitutional body mandated to oversee all research in the country.
4. See, for example, *Picturing Inclusion: Voices of Girls with Disabilities* which can be viewed on YouTube (https://www.youtube.com/watch?v=K7R2z0_DcOo).

Acknowledgements

We are grateful to Fatima Khan and Lukas Labacher for their assistance in preparing this manuscript.

Disclosure statement

No potential conflict of interest was reported by the authors.

References

Agarwal, S. (2011). The state of urban health in India: Comparing the poorest quartile to the rest of the urban population in selected states and cities. *Environment and Urbanization, 23*(1), 13–28. doi:10.1177/0956247811398589

Akesson, B., D'Amico, M., Denov, M., Khan, F., Linds, W., & Mitchell, C.A. (2014). 'Stepping back' as researchers: Addressing ethics in arts-based approaches to working with war-affected children in school and community settings. *Educational Research for Social Change, 3*(1), 75–89.

Bober, L. (2010). Visualizing justice: The politics of working with children's drawings. In L. Theron, C. Mitchell, A. Smith, & J. Stuart (Eds.), *Picturing research: Drawing as visual methodology* (pp. 63–75). Rotterdam: Sense.

Boler, M. (1999). *Feeling power: Emotions in education.* New York, NY: Psychology Press.

Burt, S., & Code, L. (Eds.). (1995). *Changing methods: Feminists transforming practice.* Ontario, CA: Broadview Press.

Chege, F., Maina, L., Mitchell, C., & Rothman, M. (2014b). A safe house? Girls' drawings on safety and security in slums in and around Nairobi. *Girlhood Studies, 7*(2), 130–135. Retrieved from http://search.proquest.com/docview/1700287813?accountid=12339

Chege, F., Maina, L., Mitchell, C., & Rothman, R. (2014a). *Evaluating the potential for improving child safety and security through housing and human settlements programming in Kenya.* Brussels: Rooftops Canada, Children & Violence Evaluation Challenge Fund.

De Lange, N., & Mitchell, C. (2012). Building sustainability into work with participatory video. In E. J. Milne, C. Mitchell, & N. De Lange (Eds.), *Handbook of participatory video* (pp. 318–330). Lanham, MD: AltaMira Press.

Delgado, M. (2015). *Urban youth and photovoice: Visual ethnography in action.* New York, NY: Oxford University Press.

Gubrium, A., & Harper, K. (2013). *Participatory visual and digital methods.* Walnut Creek, CA: Left Coast Press.

Gubrium, A., Harper, K., & Otañez, M. (Eds.). (2015). *Participatory visual and digital research in action.* Walnut Creek, CA: Left Coast Press.

Hallman, K. K., Kenworthy, N. J., Diers, J., Swan, N., & Devnarain, B. (2015). The shrinking world of girls at puberty: Violence and gender-divergent access to the public sphere among adolescents in South Africa. *Global Public Health, 10*(3), 279–295. doi:10.1080/17441692.2014.964746

Kapoor, D., & Choudry, A. (Eds.). (2010). *Learning from the ground up: Global perspectives on social movements and knowledge production.* New York, NY: Palgrave Macmillan.

Kapoor, D., & Jordan, S. (Eds.). (2009). *Education, participatory action research, and social change: International perspectives.* New York, NY: Palgrave Macmillan.

MacEntee, K. (2015). Using cellphones in participatory visual research to address gender-based violence in and around rural South African schools: Reflections on research as intervention. *Agenda: Empowering Women for Gender Equity, 29*(3), 22–31. doi:10.1080/10130950.2015.1045339

MacEntee, K., & Mandrona, A. (2015). From discomfort to collaboration: Teachers screening cell-philms in a rural South African school. *Perspectives in Education, 33*(4), 42–56.

Madise, N.J., Ziraba, A.K., Inungu, J., Khamadi, S.A., Ezeh, A., Zulu, E.M., … Mwau, M. (2012). Are slum dwellers at heightened risk of HIV infection than other urban residents? Evidence from population-based HIV prevalence surveys in Kenya. *Health and Place, 18*(5), 1144–1152. doi:10.1016/j.healthplace.2012.04.003

Mak, M. (2006). Unwanted images: Tackling gender-based violence in South African schools through youth artwork. In F. Leach & C. Mitchell (Eds.), *Combating gender violence in and around schools* (pp. 113–124). Sterling, VA: Trentham.

Mak, M. (2012). Visual post-production in participatory-video processes. In E. J. Milne, C. Mitchell, & N. De Lange (Eds.), *The handbook of participatory video* (pp. 194–207). Lanham, MD: AltaMira Press.

Milne, E. J., Mitchell, C., & De Lange, N. (2012). *Handbook of participatory video.* Lanham: Alta Mira Press.

Mitchell, C. (2006). Visual arts-based methodologies in research as social change. In T. Marcus & A. Hofmaenner (Eds.), *Shifting the boundaries of knowledge* (pp. 227–241). Pietermaritzburg: UKZN Press.

Mitchell, C. (2011). *Doing visual research*. London: Sage.

Mitchell, C. (2015). Looking at showing: On the politics and pedagogy of exhibiting in community based research and work with policy makers. *Educational Research for Social Change, 4*(2), 48–60. Retrieved from http://search.proquest.com/docview/1734621552?accountid=12339

Mitchell, C., & De Lange, N. (2013). What can a teacher do with a cellphone? Using participatory visual research to speak back in addressing HIV & AIDS. *South African Journal of Education, 33* (4), 1–13. Retrieved from http://www.scielo.org.za/scielo.php?pid=S025601002013000400010&script=sci_arttext&tlng=pt

Mitchell, C., De Lange, N., & Moletsane, R. (in press). Poetry in a pocket. In K. MacEntee, C. Burkholder, & J. Schwab-Cartas (Eds.), *What's a cellphilm?* Rotterdam: Sense.

Mitchell, C., Nguyen, X., & Twang, T. (2015). *Picturing inclusion: Voices of girls with disabilities* [Video production]. Halifax, NS: ACDC, Mount Saint Vincent.

Mudaly, R., Pithouse-Morgan, K., Van Laren, L., Singh, S., & Mitchell, C. (2015). Connecting with pre-service teachers' perspectives on the use of digital technology and social media to teach socially relevant science. *Perspectives in Education, 33*(4), 23–41.

Nguyen, X. T., Mitchell, C., De Lange, N., & Fritsch, K. (2015). Engaging girls with disabilities in Vietnam: Making their voices count. *Disability & Society, 30*(5), 773–787. doi:10.1080/09687599.2015.1051515

Pauwels, L. (2002). The video-and multimedia-article as a mode of scholarly communication: Toward scientifically informed expression and aesthetics. *Visual Studies, 17*(2), 150–159. doi:10.1080/1472586022000032224

Pink, S. (2013). *Doing visual ethnography* (3rd ed.). Thousand Oaks, CA: Sage.

Pithouse-Morgan, K., Van Laren, L., Mitchell, C., Mudaly, R., & Singh, S. (2015). Digital animation for 'going public' on curriculum integration of HIV and AIDS in higher education. *South African Journal of Higher Education, 29*(2), 237–259.

Rist, R. (2003). Influencing the policy process with qualitative research. In N. Denzin & Y. Lincoln (Eds.), *Collecting and interpreting qualitative materials* (pp. 619–644). London: Sage.

Ruby, J. (2000). *Picturing culture: Explorations of film and anthropology*. Chicago, IL: University of Chicago Press.

Schratz, M., & Walker, R. (1995). *Research as social change: New opportunities for qualitative research*. London: Routledge.

Sontag, S. (2004). *Regarding the pain of others*. New York, NY: Picardor.

Theron, L., Mitchell, C., Smith, A., & Stuart, J. (Eds.). (2011). *Picturing research: Drawing as a visual methodology*. Rotterdam: Sense.

Thompson, J., MacEntee, K., & Fikreyesus, S. (2014, April). *Intention, constraints and possibilities: Exploring the logistical landscape of a documentary film project about gender and 'the false banana tree' in the context of Higher Education policy reform in Ethiopia*. Paper presented at the annual American Educational Research Association conference, Philadelphia, PA.

UN-HABITAT (2006). *State of the world's cities 2006/2007*. Retrieved from http://www.csun.edu/~vasishth/UN-State_of_the_World%27s_Cities_2006_07.pdf

Wheeler, J. (2012). Using participatory video to engage in policy processes: Representation, power and knowledge in public screenings. In E. J. Milne, C. Mitchell, & N. De Lange (Eds.), *Handbook of participatory video* (pp. 365–379). Lanham: Alta Mira Press.

'People like me don't make things like that': Participatory video as a method for reducing leprosy-related stigma

R. M. H. Peters[a], M. B. M. Zweekhorst[a], W. H. van Brakel[b,c], J. F. G. Bunders[a] and Irwanto[d]

[a]Athena Institute, Faculty of Earth and Life Sciences, VU University Amsterdam, Amsterdam, The Netherlands; [b]Netherlands Leprosy Relief, Amsterdam, The Netherlands; [c]Disability Studies in Nederland, Metamedica, VUmc, Amsterdam, The Netherlands; [d]Centre for Disability Studies, Faculty of Social and Political Sciences, Universitas Indonesia, Depok, Indonesia

ABSTRACT

The Stigma Assessment and Reduction of Impact project aims to assess the effectiveness of stigma-reduction interventions in the field of leprosy. Participatory video seemed to be a promising approach to reducing stigma among stigmatized individuals (in this study the video makers) and the stigmatisers (video audience). This study focuses on the video makers and seeks to assess the impact on them of making a participatory video and to increase understanding of how to deal with foreseeable difficulties. Participants were selected on the basis of criteria and in collaboration with the community health centre. This study draws on six qualitative methods including interviews with the video makers and participant observation. Triangulation was used to increase the validity of the findings. Two videos were produced. The impact on participants ranged from having a good time to a greater sense of togetherness, increased self-esteem, individual agency and willingness to take action in the community. Concealment of leprosy is a persistent challenge, and physical limitations and group dynamics are also areas that require attention. Provided these three areas are properly taken into account, participatory video has the potential to address stigma at least at three levels – intrapersonal, interpersonal and community – and possibly more.

Introduction

The woman quoted in the title of this paper is 26 years of age and lives in Cirebon District, Indonesia. She married a couple of years ago and has a daughter. She has been affected by leprosy and has completed multi-drug therapy (MDT). She is cured and has no impairments or visible signs but nevertheless feels insecure and ashamed because of having been infected by the disease. Health-related stigma is an important problem in the field of public health as it affects the lives of those who experience it and plays a role in the control and management of stigmatised conditions. Leprosy is the archetypal stigmatised health condition, but stigma also plays a role in other diseases such as HIV and AIDS, tuberculosis, a range of mental illnesses, Buruli ulcer, lymphatic filariasis, onchocerciasis and leishmaniasis (Atre, Kudale, Morankar, Gosoniu, & Weiss, 2009; Person, Bartholomew, Gyapong, Addiss, & van den Borne, 2009; Rafferty, 2005; Root, 2010; Rüsch, Angermeyer, & Corrigan, 2005; Weiss, 2008).

Leprosy continues to affect millions of people in large parts of Asia, Africa and Latin America. In 2013, 215,656 new leprosy cases were reported worldwide (WHO, 2014). Indonesia – with 16,856 new cases in 2013 – ranks third after India and Brazil as having the highest number of recorded new cases (WHO, 2014). Of the 34 provinces in Indonesia, 12 have detection rates of new cases in excess of 10/100,000 population and West Papua has a rate above 100/100,000 (Ministry of Health Indonesia, 2012). Stigma can result in delaying the presentation of symptoms and thus delaying the diagnosis of leprosy (Heijnders, 2004a; Nicholls, Wiens, & Smith, 2003). This prolongs the period of infectiousness and undermines control and management of the disease in general. Delayed treatment also increases the risk of disability, which in turn increases the risk of experiencing stigma.

The Stigma Assessment and Reduction of Impact (SARI) project aims to develop and assess the effectiveness of three stigma-reduction interventions in Cirebon District, Indonesia. VU University Amsterdam and Universitas Indonesia started the project in 2010. The SARI project adopted the interactive learning and action (ILA) approach, an action–research methodology, the key principles of which are participation, inclusion and transdisciplinarity. These principles were reflected in the recruitment of the research assistants, some of whom are affected by leprosy or have a disability.

There have been a number of studies on efforts to combat stigma (Brown, Macintyre, & Trujillo, 2003; Heijnders & van der Meij, 2006) and leprosy-related stigma in particular (Benbow & Tamiru, 2001; Cross & Choudhary, 2005; Ebenso et al., 2007; Floyd-Richard & Gurung, 2000; Gershon & Srinivasan, 1992). The SARI project focuses on counselling, socio-economic development and contact. 'Contact' was selected because it has shown promise in other fields, in particular mental health and HIV and AIDS (Brown et al., 2003; Heijnders & van der Meij, 2006). Contact is described as 'all interaction between the public and persons affected, with the specific objective to reduce stigmatising attitudes' (Heijnders & van der Meij, 2006, p. 359). This interaction may be direct, for instance when a stigmatised person speaks to an individual or group, or indirect, most commonly through the use of a video (Brown et al., 2003).

Participatory video involves using a set of techniques with the aim of helping people to explore the issues they face and voice their concerns (Lunch & Lunch, 2006). Positive outcomes of participatory video include building confidence, fostering empowerment and enabling advocacy, activism and thus social change (Lunch & Lunch, 2006; Milne, Mitchell, & de Lange, 2012; Shaw & Robertson, 1997; White, 2003). Both the process of developing a video and the final product have their own purposes and potential outcomes or applications. This makes participatory video promising as part of a contact intervention to address the challenges of stigma both for people who experience it (the video makers) and for those who express it (video audience). In this paper, we focus on the video makers. The impact on the stigmatisers is also very important and will be addressed elsewhere (work in progress).

There is very limited experience of using participatory video as an approach to reducing stigma, and we are aware of only one study in the field of mental health (Buchanan &

Murray, 2012). In the field of leprosy – the focus of this study – there are three foreseeable difficulties, which might also be relevant for other stigmatised conditions. First, people affected by leprosy sometimes choose to conceal their illness (Heijnders, 2004b; Kaur & Ramesh, 1994). This raises the question of their willingness to participate in the process. Second, physical limitations such as leprosy-related impairments to the hands might make it hard to use the equipment. Third, internalised stigma might influence individuals' willingness to participate and group dynamics in general. This study aimed to demonstrate the impact of the participatory video process on video makers who are affected by leprosy and to increase understanding of how to deal with the foreseeable difficulties. We hope thereby to contribute to the practice of and research on reducing stigma and to broaden the applications of participatory video.

Stigma

The body of theory and research on stigma has been developed over 50 years since its original conceptualisation. Goffman (1963) referred to stigma as an 'attribute that is deeply discrediting' (p. 3) and that reduces the bearer 'from a whole and usual person to a tainted, discounted one' (p. 3). The usefulness of Goffman's conceptualisation for understanding health-related stigma has been questioned. For example, it is inappropriate in the context of cross-cultural research and its emphasis on social interactions to the exclusion of attention to structural social elements such as class, gender and ethnicity has also been highlighted (Scambler, 2006; Weiss, Ramakrishna, & Somma, 2006). New definitions and conceptualisations of health-related stigma have since been developed (Bos, Pryor, Reeder, & Stutterheim, 2013; Corrigan, Kerr, & Knudsen, 2005; Link & Phelan, 2001; Parker & Aggleton, 2003; Weiss et al., 2006). For instance, Link and Phelan (2001) define stigma as the co-occurrence of five components – labelling, stereotyping, separation, status loss and discrimination – and underline the importance of power. Weiss (2008) described different types of stigma prevalent among the stigmatised and stigmatisers, including internalised, anticipated and enacted stigma. The definitions of stigma vary, mainly because the concept has been applied to an array of circumstances and because research on stigma is multidisciplinary (Link & Phelan, 2001), which results in conceptual ambiguity. Recently, Staples (2011) argued that stigma 'can become a lazy shortcut for multiple "social aspects" of leprosy' (p. 91) and Tal (2012) even questioned whether it was time to retire the concept. Although these propositions make it tempting to reject the concept of stigma, the overall consensus is that it should not be disregarded. Staples (2011) calls for more critical interrogation: bringing diverse disciplines together and subjecting 'the experience of leprosy to more rigorous, ethnographic examination' (p. 96).

Connecting the stages of participatory video to the levels of stigma reduction

Participatory video encompasses a wide variety of practices, purposes and philosophies. High, Singh, Petheram, and Nemes (2012) state that it is a 'mistake to treat participatory video as though it is unitary: as a single methodology, approach or movement' (p. 45). Due to the action-oriented nature of participatory video, one of its more common applications is as a methodology for action–research (Mitchell, Milne, & de Lange, 2012). One way of looking at the participatory video process in action–research is through the three non-linear 'stages' identified by Shaw (2012). Stage A is concerned with the interaction between participants (video makers), referred to as 'opening in-between communication spaces'. Stage B is concerned with expression, reflection and building agency, during which participants share and reflect on their experiences and concerns, and perhaps reframe assumptions and build agency. Stage C is concerned with exercising this agency and beyond to what Shaw calls 'social becoming'. The three stages, including the building blocks, are illustrated in Table 1. Shaw's work in particular draws attention to the gap between the potential and ideals of participatory video, and the reality of practice, and underlines the importance of acknowledging the possible tensions, limitations and constraints. The framework was built 'for future critical investigation of actuality' (p. 225). In this paper, we look at each stage of a participatory video process and use Shaw's building blocks as a guide to describe the impact on the participants.

We asked ourselves: How does participatory video affect stigma and at which level does the change – if any – take place? The five levels of stigma on which interventions to reduce it may operate are the 'intrapersonal', 'interpersonal', 'community', 'organisational or institutional' and 'governmental or structural' (Heijnders & van der Meij, 2006). Table 2 illustrates these levels and shows what stigma-reduction interventions aim to achieve, such as increasing knowledge and self-esteem or establishing relationships.

Methods

In 2011, the SARI team and stakeholders selected *kabupaten* Cirebon (Cirebon District) as the area of research and project implementation. Cirebon District is located in Indonesia on the north coast of West Java, bordering Central Java. It has a relatively high number of new leprosy cases each year and – according to national experts – more leprosy-related stigma than in other districts, and no other initiatives to address this. Administratively, Cirebon District consists of 40 *kecamatan* (sub-districts). This study looks at the processes of the making of two participatory videos. The first participatory process took place in Kedawung sub-district between May and August 2012. The SARI project research assistants selected this sub-district because of the relatively high number of new leprosy cases. After successfully screening the first video during 'contact events' in the villages of selected sub-districts in Cirebon District and a generally positive internal evaluation, the SARI team decided to organise the second participatory video process. The SARI project

Table 1. Stages and building blocks in a participatory video process.

Stages and aim	Building blocks
A: Opening in-between communication spaces	• Engaging participants • Increasing individual confidence, capacity and sense of 'can do' • Establishing inclusive and collaborative group dynamics
B: From expression to group reframing and agency	• Motivating social dialogue focused on participants' lives and concerns • Developing critically: group reflection and reframing • Building collective agency: group identity and purpose
C: Beyond exercising agency: performing and becoming	• Group communication action through video production • Social influence: showing video in wider forums • New social becoming

Source: Shaw (2012, p. 232).

Table 2. Stigma-reduction strategies at different levels.

Levels of stigma reduction	Stigma-reduction interventions at this level aim to:
Intrapersonal	Change individual characteristics such as knowledge, attitudes, behaviour and self-concept; improve self-esteem, coping skills, empowerment and economic situation
Interpersonal	Establish relationships between members of the patient's interpersonal environment (family, work environment and friendship network)
Community	Increase knowledge regarding health conditions and stigma, increase community development skills and develop support networks within specific community groups
Organisational and institutional	Change to modify health and stigma-related aspects of an organisation
Governmental and structural	Enforce the protection of rights of people affected with a stigmatising illness

Source: Heijnders and van der Meij (2006).

research assistants felt there were still many potentially damaging misconceptions in the community about leprosy-related impairments to be addressed. It was thought that a video made by people who have such impairments would bring added value to the events. The second process therefore took place in the sub-districts of Astana Japura and Lemang Abang, selected for similar reasons, from July 2013 to November 2013. All the participants in the second process had a leprosy-related impairment. In total, 91 'contact events' in which the videos, and also comics, testimonies and an interactive presentation on leprosy, were part of the programme organised in Cirebon District. Not every contact event incorporated all of the methods; a selection was based on the available time, venue and interest of the audience. Figure 1 shows Cirebon District, the 3 sub-districts where the participatory videos were made and the 16 sub-districts where contact events were organised. A paper on the effect of these 'contact events' is in progress.

The team responsible for the participatory video process comprised a Dutch researcher (first author) and nine local research assistants who were trained in social research, community-based rehabilitation, leprosy and counselling. The team was divided into two sub-teams, team A facilitated the first process and team B the second. The research assistants divided the four main roles – facilitator, networker, researcher and editor/technical support – among themselves.

The participatory video process started with training the research assistants. The 'Insights into Participatory Video: Handbook for the Field' by Lunch and Lunch (Bahasa Indonesia version) was used as a guideline (2006). There was a meeting of all the research assistants and the first author to discuss the potential strengths and challenges in the project context.

The plan for the first process was to work with a group of about 6–10 people, heterogeneous in terms of sex, age and impairments. For the second video, all participants were to have a leprosy-related impairment and, as this is less common, the team agreed on a group size of four to six people. Criteria for participation were sufficient proficiency in *Bahasa Indonesia*, commitment to the process and living relatively near each other. The SARI project research assistants selected and approached potential participants affected by leprosy, in close collaboration with the leprosy workers at the *puskesmas* (community health centre). The research assistants met about 600 people affected by leprosy during the course of the project, who were asked whether they would like to join the SARI project's activities. Only those who had agreed or (newly diagnosed) persons recommended by the leprosy worker were approached.

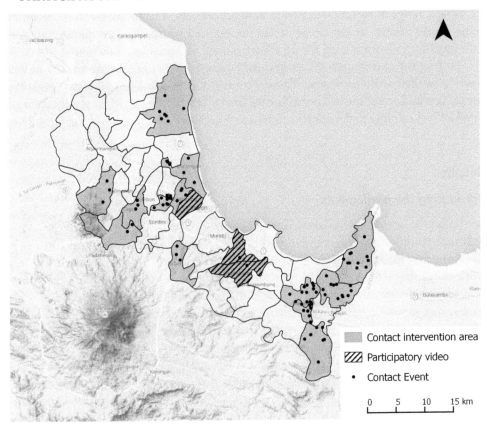

Figure 1. Sub-districts where participatory videos were made and contact events were organised (made with Quantum – Geographic Information System).

The teams and participants jointly agreed on the aim of the video – to clarify public misconceptions about leprosy and reduce public stigma. The facilitators selected games and activities based on the needs of the group (including the 'Significant Dates'[1] exercise) from Lunch and Lunch (2006) and allotted these to the sessions. The aim was to acquaint the participants with the equipment and with making a video. Minor changes were made in the selection of games and activities for the second participatory video process. During the sessions the participants' filming skills were brought to a level that they considered sufficient. The participants selected interesting themes for the final video and made story-boards that showed what needed to be filmed, including testimonies and interviews. A research assistant edited the final videos, with input from the participants. Evaluation meetings to discuss the strengths, challenges and possible solutions were held with the research assistants after each video process.

The study drew on six qualitative methods: (i) semi-structured interviews with the participants before and after the process; (ii) informal discussions with participants during the process; (iii) (participant) observation, with a focus on the participants, the process and areas for improvement; (iv) photos and videos of the process; (v) notes of the initial and evaluation meetings with the research assistants and (vi) written reflections by the research assistants on challenges and opportunities, among other topics. Triangulation by using a range of methods helped to enhance validity. The interviews were recorded, transcribed verbatim or comprehensively summarised with important quotes translated into English. NVivo was used for data management and analysis.

The relevant government offices granted ethical approval for the study. The participants gave their written consent. There were two forms: one before the start regarding the process and one at the end regarding the final product. The participants were compensated for lost earnings and made their own decisions about how to share or use this money.

Results

Introducing the participants

For both processes, the networkers visited 11 persons affected by leprosy (for the second only those with impairments) and invited them to join the process. Eight consented to do so for the first video and 4 for the second, while 10 declined. Reasons for declining were work obligations outside town, harvest season, unforeseen problems (fire) at the plantation, unexpected family situation that needed attention, old age and poor health, pregnancy, one mother's hesitations because her son was shy and a husband's denial of permission for his wife to participate. The participants represented a mix of age, sex, marital status, employment and level of impairment.

From initial interviews it became clear that leprosy influenced the lives of the participants in many ways. The three different types of stigma – internalised, perceived and enacted – emerged from the interviews. There were also themes such as the challenges posed by impairments and a range of responses – support versus exclusion – from family and community members. Some participants were still struggling with their leprosy (history) and/or impairments, whereas others had overcome them (see also Peters et al., 2013). The following quotes give some impression of leprosy-related perceptions and experiences in participants' lives before the process started:

> At that time many customers bought our yellow rice at school. But there was a gossip ... that made that people did not buy our rice. But I never give up. ... Even though the food was left over, next day I kept selling the food. The gossip came again, but I kept selling the food. ... I sold my bicycle, my hens, I sold everything but I never give up, sir ... if I had stopped that meant that I had lost. ... Finally, I could sell the food. Things went back to normal. I think if I had given up at that time, I would not have been selling food anymore. (Man, aged 59)

> I am the one who feels ashamed. My friends treat me as usual. They do not feel disgusted ... . but I cannot help feeling ashamed. I am afraid they will avoid me. (Woman, aged 43)

> When people are gathering and chatting, and I come over, those who do not like me will stride off. (Woman, aged 43)

> I felt hopeless. If God had taken my life at that time, I would have accepted it gladly. (Man, aged 39)

All participants joined the participatory video process from beginning to end, selecting the locations of meetings and arranging their schedule. For the first process, there were 12 group sessions and 22 in the second. In general, the meetings were held at participants' homes, apart from one meeting at SARI's office. The length of the sessions varied from an hour to a whole day. The two final videos told the stories that the makers wanted to tell the community, entitled *'Pastikan badai sirna'* ('Surely the storm has vanished') and *'Empat sahabat yang selalu berbagi'* ('Four friends who always share').

Impact on the participants

Stage A

Engaging participants. All participants were very engaged in the process. This was demonstrated by their high attendance, willingness to meet late at night and at the weekend, the food they brought to the meetings so they could eat together, spouses who joined and a small party organised by the first group. The participants emphasised what fun they had. One said, 'I became a happy person during that time.'

Increasing individual confidence, capacity and sense of 'can do'. Some participants were surprised that they had been asked to join, and one said, 'people like me do not make things like that'. Throughout the process their confidence, capacity to handle the equipment, which they had often never used before, and communication skills all grew. Learning new things was stressful and demanding but also joyful:

> I had a lot of fun. I gained a lot of experience. Really. I could even shoot someone climbing a tree. I was truly happy. (Man, aged 39)

> I was happy, but I was also shaking because I had never done that [interviewing a leprosy officer] before ... I was shaking like leaves but happy [laughs] (Woman, aged 26)

Establishing inclusive and collaborative group dynamics. There was a clear sense of togetherness that emerged between the group members and facilitators. Some participants joined because they were keen to meet their peers, with whom they did not have to worry about their condition and no longer felt alone. According to one participant the relationship both with peers and with the facilitators was important. For example, facilitators were not afraid of being associated with people affected by leprosy or of catching the disease:

> I wanted to socialise with my friends [peers]. I wanted to know whether I was the only one suffering from leprosy or if there were others out there. It turned out that I was not the only one who is like this [showing his impaired hand]. (Man, aged 61)

> At first, I felt so insecure, but the feeling is gone. ... Maybe it is because ... I also socialise with healthy ... people. ... This handsome young [research assistant] is willing to get along with someone like me [laughs] and ... [this other research assistant] does not mind drinking from the same glass with me. (Man, aged 61)

Participants supported each other in multiple ways. At one point, the facilitators and participants heard that a fellow participant had been fired from his job. There had been a conflict between a participatory video meeting and the participant's work and he had chosen to attend the meeting instead of his job. Although surprised that this had happened, all group members and facilitators discussed and tried to solve the problem together. A few days later a new job was arranged. Another participant thought about leaving because her boyfriend was unhappy about her participating in the activity. Again group members gave support. In the end she decided to stay because she felt the experience was good for her. Another participant who had joined a self-care group initiative (at the community health centre) had learnt how to use a stone to take care of and prevent wounds, and brought a stone for another participant. Another participant encouraged another to continue the MDT treatment so that his then minor impairment would not worsen. Facilitators were surprised by the closeness between participants. One wrote:

> The effect of making the participatory video is the proximity between the participants, a sense of caring, knowing each other better and the togetherness. This is a good first step for my friends who have had leprosy. (Reflection by research assistant)

Stage B

Motivating social dialogue focused on participants' lives and concerns. There were dialogues about leprosy and experiences of having leprosy, sometimes stimulated by exercises such as the Significant Dates exercise and sometimes spontaneously. Simply sharing basic knowledge about leprosy was key. Several participants did know the basics about their illness.

Developing critically: group reflection and reframing. Some participants just had a fun time, made friends and gained new knowledge about the disease, but there the impact more or less stopped. For others, the elements of Stage B were important, whereas for one participant Stage C was most important. Two participants said that they found the Significant Dates exercise the most valuable as it helped them to reflect on their own lives and reframe their experiences by putting them into perspective. Three participants who displayed an exceptional spirit, commitment and attitude to life were role models for others:

> I learn about perseverance from him [other participant]. Regardless his impaired condition, he keeps up his spirit, and his wife is very supportive. ... It inspires me. He inspires me to do this and that ... He does not feel insecure, neither does he worry that no one will buy his chips. (Man, aged 61)

Building agency: purpose. Group members became clearer about their purpose during the process. Some felt a desire to change community perspectives, increase knowledge and call for inclusion as shown by these quotes:

> I want the community to change their opinion and attitude so that the affected people do not feel insecure. I hope community can accept us. Really. (Woman, aged 26)

> I want people to know that regardless my imperfect physical state, I do not hide myself and keep doing what I can do. I want that people who watch the video see that people like me cannot do some work, on the contrary, I can do many kinds of work. (Man, aged 61)

> I realised that there are many other people, in many areas who suffer from the same disease as I did. People who are isolated by the community. I was touched, and I was determined to share my knowledge about leprosy to these people. ... That was the sole objective in my mind. ... In the past, I did not even go out of my house because every time people saw me, they turned away from me. I felt ashamed of myself. I hope no more people will have such an experience. (Man, aged 39)

Of course, expressing a desire for change does not necessarily mean that the participants will take action to achieve it in real life. It was not possible to follow up on these comments to see what these participants did subsequently.

Stage C

Group communication action through video production. In various ways, the video production led to unplanned awareness-raising activities beyond the screening. The neighbours of one participant in the second process were concerned about the intentions of the SARI project and hence with his participation. He shared this with the group and proposed to organise a gathering to explain the aim of the video process and the SARI project to his family, neighbours and friends. The research assistants and group members agreed. Contrary to what the research assistants expected, more than 25 neighbours and friends came to the participant's home. According to the research assistants, the neighbours listened 'enthusiastically' to the explanation, supported the video process and even offered their help. Other participants realised that it would be worth organising a similar gathering with their own neighbours and one was set up for each of the four members of this group.

Social influence: showing the video in wider forums. The SARI project screened and discussed the video content during 91 village 'contact events', attended by over 4440 community members (paper in progress). One participant suggested helping to organise the contact events by giving testimonies. After the first event he shared his initial doubts, but also said that he felt happy:

> This is the first time I delivered a testimony in front of many people. I was rather doubtful at first whether I can do it or not, but after the testimony when people started raising questions, I felt happy. I want to keep giving testimonials. (Man, aged 39)

New or restored social identity. First, the video process had an impressive impact on the self-esteem of several participants. Sometimes participants said that the internalised stigma disappeared, some others said it had lessened:

> I know more about leprosy now, and if you are asking me about my insecurity, I think there is only a very small part of it left in me. The knowledge I have recently gained made me more confident. I am positive that I have recovered. (Man, aged 21)

> After video activity, I feel full of spirit. When people say something bad, I do not let it bother me. We have our private life. As long as I do not cause trouble for other people, I have nothing to worry. [laughs] ... I have recovered now, so let people talk! I feel free these days. Nobody stops me from going here and there or from doing this or that. (Woman, aged 26)

Second, some participants describe the normalised relationship with their neighbours:

> I do not feel shy towards my neighbours any more. I chat with my neighbours and friends. Things have gone back to normal. (Woman, aged 26)
> When someone talked evil about leprosy or an affected person, I lectured him/her even in front of many other people. (Man, aged 39[2])

Third, what stands out in terms of social identity is the renewed focus on others. One participant said that before the process he cared only about his family and his business and that now he cares about the community again. Others had similar experiences. One participant offered to volunteer and help to start up a self-care group in a new area; two participants found new potential leprosy cases and directed them to the community health centre.

Understanding difficulties

Concealment

Even before the process began, the research assistants raised the key challenge of conceal-ment. The teams realised the need to go through an entire process in order to understand how it was influenced by concealment. Most of the participants had disclosed their illness (or at least others knew about it), but a few had not.

One participant in the first process had partially disclosed his illness but had experi-enced several difficulties. On the one hand, he really enjoyed participating in the process. More than all of the other participants he most seemed to enjoy handling the camera and shooting film and it made him proud. On the other hand, there was the con-stant worry. He was afraid that acquaintances would learn about his own leprosy history and would then avoid him. He decided not to appear in the final video, but remained involved in the sessions.

Another participant in the second process decided halfway through that she wanted to inform her neighbours about her illness, partly because she was afraid they would in any case find out. She discussed this with the research assistants and co-participants. A gather-ing was organised where the participant told them, the first final video was broadcast and basic information was shared about leprosy, such as the cause and the fact that leprosy is no longer infectious once medication is taken. The participant said that her neighbours subsequently treated her normally and that nobody talked 'bad' about her, but rather that neighbours were interested and asked about the progress of making the video.

The final videos tell the stories of seven participants. Most were happy or even eager to screen the video in the area where they live. For 4 of the 12 participants, however, screen-ing in their own village or sub-district was a step too far. Some were worried about the screening and possible responses of the audience for themselves ($n = 2$), for other partici-pants ($n = 1$) or for their family ($n = 1$). For example, a young woman who appears in the video did not object to broadcasting it, but another, an older man, objected to her being in the video. He was worried about her future as a labourer and as an unmarried woman. He said: 'her future is still long'. One woman was embarrassed not because of her illness but because she was not fluent in Bahasa Indonesia. The next quote illustrates the anxiety felt by one participant regarding the possible response of relatives:

> I do not mind the video being played anywhere because people have known my real con-dition. There is nothing I can do about it. However, I am afraid that my husband and other relatives object to the idea. I want people to know about this, but I am worried about my family's reaction. (Woman, aged 43)

Due to concerns about disclosure expressed by four participants, the participants asked the SARI team not to broadcast the videos in their own sub-districts. As a result, the partici-pants were unable to benefit from the potential impact of screening the video in their neighbourhood. For one participant the screening element was very important, perhaps even his sole reason for participating, but his wish could not be realised. Screening the videos outside their own sub-district was not a problem and was in fact encouraged by the video makers. Participants' ownership of the finished videos is a cornerstone of most participatory processes. To prevent involuntary disclosure by screening the videos in the participants' sub-districts the project decided not to distribute the videos to the participants. The videos are in the hands of a local disabled people's organisation, Forum Komunikasi Difabel Cirebon (FKDC), where some of the SARI project research assistants work and to which some of the video makers belong. Any questions regarding screening and distribution of the videos will go through FKDC.

Physical limitations

Some participants were worried about the impact of making the video on their physical condition. For those whose hands were impaired, it was challenging to learn to operate the devices, in particular zooming and keeping the camcorder stable. There was a need for more than the anticipated number of sessions to acquire the basic skills. Participants and the team jointly found creative solutions, such as an enlarged pin in the tripod to make it easier for the participants to operate the device unassisted. Although the process was challenging and time-consuming, ultimately all participants could use the equipment:

> My problem is my physical limitation. I felt tired quickly, but thanks to God, I could stay in the process until the end. I was afraid of getting sick because of the activity because I usually get sick when I am too tired. (Man, aged 61)

> You see the condition of my arms and hand. It is not easy to shoot with this kind of arm. However, everything is possible if we are willing to learn. I am happy because I finally could do it. (Man, aged 39)

Behaviour caused by internalised stigma

Most participants seemed reasonably confident during the process and only a few felt insecure and ashamed. As expected, internalised stigma played a role. Some participants needed a bit more time to get familiar with the activities and support from the facilitators:

> At first, I felt insecure and ashamed. I cannot tell you how, but that was what I felt … After I knew the activity better, I felt comfortable doing it. I could meet many people and we could share with each other. (Man, aged 21)

Discussion

This paper has explored the impact of a participatory video process on participants affected by leprosy. It focused on three difficulties: concealment, physical limitations and behaviour caused by internalised stigma. The stages outlined by Shaw (2012) were helpful in analysing the impact on the participants. We made two changes in the names of the building blocks; individual rather than collective agency seemed more relevant to this study and a new or restored 'social identity' was chosen rather than 'social becoming', which was a better fit with the context of stigma. In terms of reducing stigma and the levels identified by Heijnders and van der Meij (2006), the impacts described in Stages A and B operate at the intrapersonal level, whereas the impacts in Stage C operate at the 'interpersonal' and 'community' levels. Although not explored in this project, it is also possible to broadcast the video at organisational, institutional and governmental levels, making it potentially a multi-level stigma-reduction strategy,

This paper also showed that participatory video is a process from which the participants can benefit in many ways. The diversity of impacts also makes it complex and difficult to pinpoint what exactly contributes to reducing stigma and for whom. This corresponds with the experience of Blazek and Hraňová (2012) who wrote that 'our experience shows that participatory video is an immensely complex activity because of the range of relationships and positionalities that various actors bring to the collaborative process' (p. 164). Similar to Buchanan and Murray (2012), the suggestion of Howarth (2006) is relevant and demonstrated 'in action':

> Howarth (2006) has suggested that by coming together in dialogue, debate and critique, members of a stigmatised group can become aware of themselves as agents not objects. She emphasised that alone the individual cannot develop the confidence and emotional strength to challenge stigma but can do so in combination with others. (Buchanan and Murray, 2012, p. 41)

We will try to grasp and make explicit the dynamics of the process that contributed to reducing stigma: (i) getting accustomed to the devices and in particular a sense of 'can do'; (ii) increased self-confidence; (iii) having fun; (iv) a sense of family and caring; (v) not feeling alone with the disease or impairment; (vi) greater knowledge and self-awareness; (vii) seeing other ways of thinking and behaving in role models; (viii) finding a new purpose; (ix) seeing the possibility of becoming an agent of change and an increased capacity to act; (x) new ways of communicating with others and (xi) a new or restored social identity.

Concealment was a key difficulty. It put some participants in a difficult position, balancing their desire to participate with anxiety about disclosure and possible negative effects. Ultimately, four participants objected to screening the final video in their own sub-district, which created the challenges described. The issue of concealment is also prominent in Buchanan and Murray (2012), but is reflected only in a reluctance to participate. We cannot say that participants in our study were reluctant to participate since the reasons given for declining participation seem very common. In future initiatives, it may be possible to reduce the risk of negative effects due to disclosure, for instance by meeting and filming outside the area in which the participants live. It might also be possible to encourage participants to prepare a video that they would all be content to screen in their own area – but this might undermine the benefit of all participants being able to participate in whatever way they wish without having to consider the aspect of broadcasting. Exploring ways to film anonymously might be interesting, but should be addressed in games and activities early in the participatory video process. Concealment remains a major challenge and should be carefully considered in similar initiatives.

We are aware of two other studies where people who are labelled 'disabled' – physically or mentally – made a participatory video: Buchanan and Murray's study on mental health (2012) and Capstick's study on dementia (2012). Due to their impairments, participants in this study needed extra time to become familiar with the equipment, but they all succeeded, which gave a real confidence boost to each participant. In this way, an initial challenge became an opportunity. It is important to be aware of the participants' physical condition. A slower pace and flexibility to adapt the process to the participants' needs and desires are even more important than usual. We agree with Capstick (2012) that more attention and reflection is needed on how participatory video can be made more inclusive and accessible for people who are labelled 'disabled'.

The challenge of involving people who have internalised stigma is, to our knowledge, not described elsewhere. The potential to increase self-esteem through the participatory video process is described by others (Buchanan & Murray, 2012; Lunch & Lunch, 2006; Shaw & Robertson, 1997). In our study, internalised stigma was a minor but relevant challenge only for a few participants. Solutions included allowing more time and having well-trained facilitators with a thorough understanding of leprosy and counselling skills. In addition, the local facilitators allowed us to benefit from:

> Research being led by community researchers meant that they could navigate the cultural norms and rules so as to create relatively safe spaces for community members to participate and reflect on their experiences. (Wheeler, 2009 p. 14)

This was also beneficial in view of some of the challenges (e.g. the participant who was fired) and inequalities among participants (e.g. the man who rejected screening the film because a young unmarried woman participated in it, whereas she was happy to do so) that arose.

Aspects that were not addressed in depth here include (i) high expectations, responsibility and dependence on the research assistants (as one research assistant said, 'what if our spirit had dropped?'); (ii) the dynamics between participants and research assistants; (iii) how to foster an environment to make a long-term or sustainable impact on reducing stigma; (iv) illiteracy, unfamiliarity and practical challenges with some exercises in the handbook (something simple as throwing a die was difficult for those with hand impairments) and (v) a more participatory editing process. It is also important to note that stigma-reduction interventions can, inadvertently, foster stigma. Interventions' emphasis on leprosy and associated stigma could temporarily reinforce or amplify them. There were no indications that this happened during these processes, but it is important to be aware of the possibility, look for any signs of it and take appropriate action when it occurs. Heijnders and van der Meij also emphasised this danger (2006).

Participatory video as a stigma-reduction strategy is a new field and we therefore have many ideas for further research and practice. First and most important is maximising the communication potential and understanding of the impact of screening the video on community-level stigma. Mistry, Bignante, and Berardi (2014) emphasise the importance of motivation and say that the surfacing of individuals' motivations should be stimulated in order to ensure better outcomes. In retrospect, this is relevant in our context and seems worth exploring in the future. It might also be worth studying how stigmatised identities intersect with other aspects of identity (such as sex, age or socio-economic status) and how this influences group (power) dynamics. In addition, it would be interesting to see specific groups develop participatory videos, such as children, adolescents, family members, those cured of but with reactions to leprosy, and others including newly diagnosed persons, health workers, family members and policy-makers at the Ministry of Health. In particular, we would encourage a greater involvement of participants in the organisation of screening activities. In our case, there was some involvement, but perhaps less than might have been desirable, due to overall project objectives and time limitations.

Conclusion

Despite some important challenges, participatory video has the potential to address stigma at least at three levels — intrapersonal, interpersonal and community — and possibly more

This is all very promising, but the proof of its impact will be whether demonstrable effects on community stigma are achieved by screenings of the videos. The intervention seems easily replicable and thus scalable. Gradual implementation elsewhere is recommended provided there are well-trained facilitators and with an emphasis on learning and reflection so that the approach can better respond to the challenges posed by concealment, the participants' physical condition and group dynamics.

Notes

1. Exercise described in the handbook (Lunch & Lunch, 2006) where participants get to know each other by sharing life events, in our case some related to leprosy.
2. This participant also joined the SARI project's counselling intervention.

Acknowledgements

We would like to thank all participants and research assistants of the SARI project. We thank Mike Powell and Deborah Eade for their comments on an earlier draft. We also express our gratitude to the District Health Office in Cirebon, the West Java Provincial Health Office and the Sub-Directorate for Leprosy and Yaws of the Ministry of Health for facilitating this study.

Disclosure statement

No potential conflict of interest was reported by the authors.

Funding

We thank the organisations that provide financial support to the SARI project: Netherlands Leprosy Relief (NLR), American Leprosy Missions (ALM), Sasakawa Memorial Health Foundation (SMHF) and effect:hope (formerly TLMC).

References

Atre, S., Kudale, A., Morankar, S., Gosoniu, D., & Weiss, M. G. (2009). Gender and community views of stigma and tuberculosis in rural Maharashtra, India. *Global Public Health*, 6(1), 56–71. doi:10.1080/17441690903334240

Benbow, C., & Tamiru, T. (2001). The experience of self-care groups with people affected by leprosy: ALERT, Ethiopia. *Leprosy Review*, 72(3), 311–321. Retrieved from http://www.ilep.org.uk/fileadmin/uploads/Documents/Infolep_Documents/Leprosy_Articles/Articles_2001/BENBOW2001.pdf

Blazek, M., & Hraňová, P. (2012). Emerging relationships and diverse motivations and benefits in participatory video with young people. *Children's Geographies*, 10(2), 151–168. doi:10.1080/14733285.2012.667917

Bos, A. E. R., Pryor, J. B., Reeder, G. D., & Stutterheim, S. E. (2013). Stigma: Advances in theory and research. *Basic and Applied Social Psychology*, 35(1), 1–9. doi:10.1080/01973533.2012.746147

Brown, L., Macintyre, K., & Trujillo, L. (2003). Interventions to reduce HIV/AIDS stigma: What have we learned? *AIDS Education and Prevention*, 15(1), 49–69. doi:10.1521/aeap.15.1.49.23844

Buchanan, A., & Murray, M. (2012). Using participatory video to challenge the stigma of mental illness: A case study. *International Journal of Mental Health Promotion*, 14(1), 35–43. doi:10.1080/14623730.2012.673894

Capstick, A. (2012). Participatory video and situated ethics: Avoiding disablism. In E.-J. Milne, C. Mitchell, & N. de Lange (Eds.), *Handbook of participatory video* (pp. 269–282). Plymouth: AltaMira Press.

Corrigan, P. W., Kerr, A., & Knudsen, L. (2005). The stigma of mental illness: Explanatory models and methods for change. *Applied and Preventive Psychology, 11*(3), 179–190. doi:10.1016/j.appsy.2005.07.001

Cross, H., & Choudhary, R. (2005). STEP: An intervention to address the issue of stigma related to leprosy in Southern Nepal. *Leprosy Review, 76*(4), 316–324.

Ebenso, B., Fashona, A., Ayuba, M., Idah, M., Adeyemi, G., & S-Fada, S. (2007). Impact of socio-economic rehabilitation on leprosy stigma in Northern Nigeria: Findings of a retrospective study. *Asia Pacific Disability Rehabilitation Journal, 18*(2), 98–119.

Floyd-Richard, M., & Gurung, S. (2000). Stigma reduction through group counselling of persons affected by leprosy – a pilot study. *Leprosy Review, 71*(4), 499–504.

Gershon, W., & Srinivasan, G. R. (1992). Community-based rehabilitation: An evaluation study. *Leprosy Review, 63*(1), 51–59.

Goffman, E. (1963). *Stigma: Notes on the management of spoiled identity.* New York, NY: Simon & Schuster.

Heijnders, M., & van der Meij, S. (2006). The fight against stigma: An overview of stigma-reduction strategies and interventions. *Psychology, Health & Medicine, 11*(3), 353–363. doi:10.1080/13548500600595327

Heijnders, M. L. (2004a). Experiencing leprosy: Perceiving and coping with leprosy and its treatment. A qualitative study conducted in Nepal. *Leprosy Review, 75*(4), 327–337.

Heijnders, M. L. (2004b). The dynamics of stigma in leprosy. *International Journal of Leprosy and Other Mycobacterial Diseases, 72*(4), 437–447. doi:10.1489/1544-581X(2004)72<437:TDOSIL>2.0.CO;2

High, C., Singh, N., Petheram, L., & Nemes, G. (2012). Defining participatory video from practice. In E.-J. Milne, C. Mitchell, & N. de Lange (Eds.), *Handbook of participatory video* (pp. 35–48). Plymouth: AltaMira Press.

Howarth, C. (2006). Race as stigma: Positioning the stigmatized as agents, not objects. *Journal of Community & Applied Social Psychology, 16*, 442–451. doi:10.1002/casp.898

Kaur, H., & Ramesh, V. (1994). Social problems of women leprosy patients: A study conducted at 2 urban leprosy centres in Delhi. *Leprosy Review, 4*(65), 361–375.

Link, B. G., & Phelan, J. C. (2001). Conceptualizing stigma. *Annual Review of Sociology, 27*, 363–385. doi:10.1146/annurev.soc.27.1.363

Lunch, C., & Lunch, N. (2006). *Insights into participatory video: A handbook for the field.* Oxford: InsightShare.

Milne, E.-J., Mitchell, C., & de Lange, N. (Eds.). (2012). *Handbook of participatory video.* Plymouth: AltaMira Press.

Ministry of Health Indonesia. (2012). *Annual Leprosy Statistics Indonesia 2011.* Jakarta: Author.

Mistry, J., Bignante, E., & Berardi, A. (2014). Why are we doing it? Exploring participant motivations within a participatory video project. *Area.* doi:10.1111/area.12105

Mitchell, C., Milne, E.-J., & de Lange, N. (2012). Introduction. In E.-J. Milne, C. Mitchell, & N. de Lange (Eds.), *Handbook of participatory video* (pp. 1–18). Plymouth: AltaMira Press.

Nicholls, P. G., Wiens, C., & Smith, W. C. S. (2003). Delay in presentation in the context of local knowledge and attitude towards leprosy – the results of qualitative fieldwork in Paraguay. *International Journal of Leprosy and Other Mycobacterial Diseases, 71*(3), 198–209.

Parker, R., & Aggleton, P. (2003). HIV and AIDS-related stigma and discrimination: A conceptual framework and implications for action. *Social Science & Medicine, 57*(1), 13–24. doi:10.1016/S0277-9536(02)00304-0

Person, B., Bartholomew, L. K., Gyapong, M., Addiss, D. G., & van den Borne, B. (2009). Health-related stigma among women with lymphatic filariasis from the Dominican Republic and Ghana. *Social Science & Medicine, 68*(1), 30–38. doi:10.1016/j.socscimed.2008.09.040

Peters, R. M. H., Dadun, L. M., Miranda-Galarza, B., van Brakel, W. H., Zweekhorst, M. B. M., Damayanti R., … Irwanto. (2013). The meaning of leprosy and everyday experiences: An exploration in Cirebon, Indonesia. *Journal of Tropical Medicine.* doi:10.1155/2013/507034

Rafferty, J. (2005). Curing the stigma of leprosy. *Leprosy Review, 76,* 119–126.

Root, R. (2010). Situating experiences of HIV-related stigma in Swaziland. *Global Public Health, 5* (5), 523–538. doi:10.1080/17441690903207156

Rüsch, N., Angermeyer, M. C., & Corrigan, P. W. (2005). Mental illness stigma: Concepts, consequences, and initiatives to reduce stigma. *European Psychiatry: The Journal of the Association of European Psychiatrists, 20*(8), 529–539. doi:10.1016/j.eurpsy.2005.04.004

Scambler, G. (2006). Sociology, social structure and health-related stigma. *Psychology, Health & Medicine, 11*(3), 288–295. doi:10.1080/13548500600595103

Shaw, J. (2012). Interrogating the gap between the ideals and practice reality of participatory video. In E.-J. Milne, C. Mitchell, & N. de Lange (Eds.), *Handbook of participatory video* (pp. 225–239). Plymouth: AltaMira Press.

Shaw, J., & Robertson, C. (1997). *Participatory video: A practical approach to using video creatively in group development work.* London: Routledge.

Staples, J. (2011). Interrogating leprosy 'stigma': Why qualitative insights are vital. *Leprosy Review, 82*(2), 91–97.

Tal, A. (2012). Is it time to retire the term stigma? *Stigma Research and Action, 2*(2), 49–50. doi:10. 5463/SRA.v1i1.18

Weiss, M. G. (2008). Stigma and the social burden of neglected tropical diseases. *PLoS Neglected Tropical Diseases, 2*(5), 237. doi:10.1371/journal.pntd.0000237

Weiss, M. G., Ramakrishna, J., & Somma, D. (2006). Health-related stigma: Rethinking concepts and interventions. *Psychology, Health & Medicine, 11*(3), 277–287. doi:10.1080/13548500600 595053

Wheeler, J. (2009). 'The life that we don't want': Using participatory video in researching violence. *IDS Bulletin, 40*(3), 10–18. doi:10.1111/j.1759-5436.2009.00033.x

White, S. A. (2003). *Participatory video: Images that transform and empower.* Thousand Oaks, CA: Sage Publications.

WHO. (2014). Global leprosy update, 2013; reducing disease burden. *Weekly Epidemiological Record, 89*(36), 389–400.

Supporting youth and community capacity through photovoice: Reflections on participatory research on maternal health in Wakiso district, Uganda

David Musoke[a], Rawlance Ndejjo[a], Elizabeth Ekirapa-Kiracho[b] and Asha S. George[c]

[a]Department of Disease Control and Environmental Health, School of Public Health, Makerere University College of Health Sciences, Kampala, Uganda; [b]Department of Health Policy, Planning and Management, School of Public Health, Makerere University College of Health Sciences, Kampala, Uganda; [c]Bloomberg School of Public Health, Johns Hopkins University, Baltimore, MD, USA

ABSTRACT

This paper reflects on the experiences of using photovoice to examine maternal health in Wakiso district, Uganda. The project involved 10 youth aged 18–29 years old, who were diverse in education, occupation, and marital status and identified by community leaders with researchers. By taking photos and sharing images and experiences in monthly meetings over five months, youth reported becoming more knowledgeable. They realised that they had common experiences but also reflected on and reinterpreted their circumstances. While they acquired self-confidence and enhanced their communication skills, they also initially faced community resistance regarding consent and lack of trust in their motives. Ethical practice in photovoice goes beyond institutional approval and individual consent. It includes extensively discussing the project with community members and building relationships with them. In certain instances, photos needed not to identify community members, or not be taken at all. Through these relationships and with improved capacity, youth engaged in individual instances of health education and advocacy, as well as spurred further local action through community dialogues. Researchers supporting photovoice must be open to learning alongside participants, flexible regarding study focus and processes, sustain interest and manage logistics, all while being reflective about the balance of power in such partnerships.

Introduction

Photovoice is a community-based participatory research approach by which taking and discussing photos supports a process through which people identify and reflect on particular issues relevant to their well-being (Wang & Burris, 1997). In certain instances, it also supports participants in changing their circumstances, with further reflection on the effects of such efforts to initiate change. In this sense, photovoice can contribute to empowering participants by assessing community needs and assets, reflecting on identified

163

issues, and taking action in the community (Strack, Magill, & McDonagh, 2004; Wang & Burris, 1997).

Youth are a neglected stakeholder in community-based research initiatives, despite being a substantial demographic group in most low- and middle-income country contexts (Sankoh et al., 2014). Previous photovoice initiatives have worked with children and youth to record their community's strengths and concerns, promote critical dialogue and knowledge about community issues (Hergenrather, Rhodes, Cowan, Bardhoshi, & Pula, 2009; Lal, Jarus, & Suto, 2012), and reach policy-makers (Wang, 2006). Such initiatives can enable youth to develop individually, which is important in building social competency and becoming positive agents within their communities. Photovoice has also been noted as an appealing experience for youth because it is more accessible to them, gives the opportunity to advance their personal and social identities, and is fun (Moletsane et al., 2007; Strack et al., 2004).

Although several studies exist in Uganda on maternal health regarding the health of women during pregnancy, childbirth, and postpartum period, they mainly use conventional quantitative and qualitative research methods (Mayora et al., 2014; Okal et al., 2013). In addition, there is limited experience of using photovoice for maternal and other health fields in the country. Photovoice projects elsewhere show promising experiences in informing public health practice and policy (Mohammed, Sajun, & Khan, 2013; Van Oss, Quinn, Viscosi, & Bretscher, 2013). Considering the scope for learning about photovoice in the Ugandan context, this article reflects on the experience of youth collaborating with researchers through photovoice to examine maternal health in rural communities in Wakiso district, Uganda. It provides information that could be used by others in Uganda and beyond on photography as a participatory research method. We discuss the experiences of the youth photographers in the project and the lessons we learned as researchers while facilitating the photovoice project.

Methods

Study design

Photovoice was undertaken as community-based participatory research over five months in 2013, during which researchers and youth engaged in dialogue with the aid of photography to explore how youth can contribute to maternal health in rural communities. Discussions explored how youth themselves framed maternal health priorities in their communities, supported dialogues with other community stakeholders to share learning, and spurred local actions to address identified maternal health problems. The project was participatory in the sense that youth themselves chose what photos to take, which photos were prioritised for discussion, and analysed them jointly in the discussion sessions. Concurrently, we as researchers also recorded these discussions as a way of documenting the process and to qualitatively analyse the changes reported by the youth. Further reflection and analysis was done by the researchers alone and forms the basis of this article. The researchers comprised a team with expertise in maternal health and qualitative research, including use of photovoice. In particular, the lead researcher had worked with the communities regarding other public health fields and wanted to use this opportunity to explore maternal health concerns more holistically.

Study context and area

Globally, over 250,000 maternal deaths occur every year mainly in low- and middle-income countries (Lozano et al., 2011; WHO, 2012). In Uganda, the maternal mortality rate is 438 deaths per 100,000 live births (Uganda Bureau of Statistics [UBOS], 2012), far higher than the country's target of 131 deaths per 100,000 live births by 2015 (Government of Uganda [GoU], 2010). Several challenges constrain improvements in maternal health in Uganda. These challenges include those related to the supply of services, such as limited access to health services, shortage of skilled health workers, and stock out of medical supplies and drugs (Khan, Wojdyla, Say, Gulmezoglu, & Van Look, 2006), as well as on the demand side, such as lack of health knowledge, low male involvement, and poverty (Okal et al., 2013). Increasingly, communities are engaged in measures that address both these supply and demand side elements of maternal and child health (Marston, Renedo, McGowan, & Portela, 2013). One important element of community engagement is including those whose contributions are often neglected, such as those of youth.

The photovoice study with youth to explore their perspectives and contributions to improving maternal health was carried out in five villages in Bulwanyi parish, Ssisa sub-county (68,900 people in 2012) (UBOS, 2011), Wakiso district, a rural area in the central region of Uganda. These villages have similar social, economic, and demographic characteristics, with livelihoods based on crop farming, animal husbandry, petty trading, stone quarrying, brick making, and sand mining. Bulwanyi parish experienced maternal health-related challenges typical of rural areas in the country and was therefore purposively selected for the study.

Study participants and training

The study started by researchers consulting local leaders about the proposed photovoice initiative in their communities, and discussed with them the ideal profile of participating youth photographers. Community leaders were members of local village council committees, which consist of between 5 and 10 members, who are mainly, but not entirely, male. Community leaders were chosen to recommend youth participants because they are knowledgeable about youth in their communities, are key gate-keepers in the area, and would help to further build local relationships, and ensure societal relevance.

The final list of 10 recommended youth photographers was developed jointly by community leaders and researchers to ensure that selected participants met the set criteria. Youth participants were aged between 18 and 29 years old. Although youth can be categorised as aged 15–29 years old (Eurostat, 2009; International Labour Organization [ILO], 2012), those under 18 years were excluded due to concerns about their ability to independently consent to participate in the photovoice project. Further consideration was given to their social context to ensure diversity with regard to education, economic, occupation, and marital status. From each of the five villages in the parish, two youth (one male and one female) were selected. Among the participants, six had children, two were community health workers, and three carried out agriculture as their main source of income.

A meeting was held between the selected youth and researchers during which the purpose of the study was clearly explained to the participants so that they could make an informed decision regarding their participation. This meeting did not involve community leaders and therefore enabled youth to decide on their own whether they wanted to participate in the study, separately from being recommended by community leaders.

After the youth confirmed their interest and availability to participate, researchers conducted a training workshop for them. The five-hour training covered aspects of use and care of cameras, ethics in photography, and use of photography in research. To minimise potential risks to youth participants, the training discussed several issues including how to approach and inform community members about the photovoice initiative, and how to seek consent before taking pictures. General maternal health issues regarding pregnancy, child birth, and postpartum care were also discussed. During the workshop, facilitators first assessed the level of participants' knowledge on maternal health by asking them pre-listed questions, then afterwards provided them with more in-depth information.

Photography assignment

Study cameras were loaned to youth photographers for a period of five months. The participants were encouraged to take as many photographs as they could and were also provided with notebooks to record their experiences, reflections and situations of interest, which may not be captured on camera. Notebooks were used especially in scenarios where consent to take photos was not granted.

A follow-up meeting with the researchers two weeks after commencement of taking photos helped to answer questions and solve any problems related to the participants' use of cameras, as this was a new technology for the youth photographers. The follow-up meeting also helped ensure that the youth understood the photovoice methodology. Initially, a few youth photographers literally focused on the theme of maternal health by taking portraits of pregnant women that removed them from their social context. An ongoing dialogue was required to support the overall purpose of undertaking the photovoice study: to unpack youth and community perspectives on maternal health issues in their communities by understanding maternal health in its social context and explore how youth can contribute to improving maternal health.

Discussing photos and data analysis

During the photovoice project, five monthly meetings were convened between the researchers and youth photographers to review progress and discuss photographs. The meetings, which involved all the participants and two researchers, lasted for three to four hours during which the participants talked about the photographs taken and discussed what they meant to them. A projector was used to display the photographs on a wall to facilitate the group discussions.

The discussions created opportunities for mutual learning and encouragement, as well as laying a foundation for developing a collective voice and mobilising for unified action regarding maternal health. The SHOWeD guidelines were used in the discussion of each photograph, which involved answering the following questions: What do you see here? What's really happening here? How does this relate to our lives? Why does this problem/condition/situation/strength exist? Who could the image educate? What can we do about it? (Wallerstein, 1987).

Participatory analysis during the monthly meetings involved participants identifying the concerns that were most pertinent to maternal health in their community and how they could contribute in improving the situation. All participants were involved in the participatory analysis both for their own photos and those taken by colleagues. For example, the youth photographer who had taken a photograph discussed it first, which provided a foundation for other participants to also contribute and ask questions. Pertinent issues on maternal health that were not captured on camera and were written in participants' notebooks were also raised and discussed during the meetings. Issues that had been raised in previous meetings were also discussed in later meetings, but with less time dedicated to them, with emphasis on newly emerging concerns identified by the participants.

A research assistant did note taking to keep a record of all discussions during the meetings, which was key in tracking the evolution of changing perceptions, and challenges in the research. All discussions from the meetings were also audio recorded and transcribed verbatim in *Luganda*, the main local language used in central Uganda. While notebooks themselves were not analysed by researchers, the discussions of issues recorded in them were audio recorded, transcribed, and analysed by researchers, together with the discussions about the photos. Validation of the transcripts involved consulting youth participants, who provided clarity on issues that were ambiguous to the researchers. Typed narratives were then translated into English and verified for accuracy by the researchers. Researchers developed a set of codes initially based on what youth identified as priorities and then reviewed the transcripts several times to undertake thematic content analysis (Graneheim & Lundman, 2004). Transcripts were coded and managed using Atlas ti version 6.0.15 qualitative data analysis software.

Dissemination

After completion of five discussion meetings with participatory analysis of the photos taken, youth and researchers worked together to share key findings with community members. Following the suggestions of youth participants, three community workshops were convened, which involved various stakeholders, including community leaders, health officials, researchers, journalists, and community members. During the workshops which lasted between two and three hours, a selection of photographs reflecting the main issues emerging from the research were presented by the youth photographers themselves, who shared their findings, stories, and recommendations to the wider community. The photographs used during the dissemination were selected by both the participants and researchers. Youth did the first round of selection, but as not all photos they selected could be used for dissemination, a further round was done by researchers based on what the youth had selected.

Ethical considerations

Ethical approval to conduct the study was obtained from Makerere University School of Public Health Higher Degrees, Research and Ethics Committee, and Uganda National Council for Science and Technology. Researchers initially faced difficulty with ethical approval of the study as photovoice was a new methodology that had not previously been encountered by university reviewers. This led to several questions being asked by the Institutional Review Board (IRB) mainly related to ethics in use of photography in research, such as how consent before taking pictures would be guaranteed. This led to delays in the review process as it required further dialogue and revisions before the approval was granted.

Participation in the study was voluntary and participants were informed about ethical issues including concerns in the use of photography in research, such as getting people's consent before taking their photos. Being recommended by the local leaders did not automatically make the youth participate in the study. Youth participants discussed their participation with researchers independently of community leaders. They individually provided written informed consent after they had received a clear explanation of what the research entailed, including the anticipated risks and potential benefits of participating before they took part. No photograph identifying an individual was released or used for any form of dissemination without the written consent of both the photographer and the identified person.

Results

We first review the experiences of the youth photographers in the project, before reflecting on the lessons we learned as researchers while facilitating the photovoice project. The youth experiences are presented under acquisition of knowledge; recognition and interpretation of experiences; gaining new skills, confidence, and community exposure; and eliciting trust from community members; contributing towards improving maternal health at a community level. The researchers' experiences are presented under flexibility in study objectives and processes, sustaining interest, and handling logistics.

Experiences of youth photographers in photovoice

Acquisition of knowledge

Youth came from diverse backgrounds and had no previous background in health, with the exception of two, who were also community health workers. Apart from the orientation provided at the beginning of the photovoice process, discussing the issues raised from the photos enabled participants to gain further understanding organically about maternal health in discussion with others. The photovoice process created a safe group atmosphere where youth could ask questions related to maternal health and learn from each other and researchers over time. Topics explored included contraception, nutrition, pregnancy, and male responsibility. For example, one youth participant reflected:

> From this research, I have got more knowledge on family planning. I learnt that when you go to a health centre for family planning services, you need to see a health worker to explain to you the various options before you make an informed decision on the choice of method to use. (Photographer 2, male, 25 years)

Recognition and interpretation of experiences

Youth participants also shared with researchers how the discussions they were involved in not only added new technical knowledge, but also endured realisation of important commonalities regarding life experiences shared among them. They felt that the sharing enabled them to learn from each other, question and validate existing experiences, and inspire them to be role models for others. Youth participants noted:

> We have been in this research and it has just been like a seminar which has involved a lot of learning. There were many instances when my colleagues brought up situations that I would realize related to my personal life. It was such a great learning experience and I am going to put whatever I learnt into practice and become a role model in my community. (Photographer 9, male, 29 years)
> Through this research, I have met more people. It has also helped me change as a person, as I am now supposed to be an example to inspire others. I have realized that I did not treat my wife very well when she was pregnant and have now understood what I should do the next time she is expecting, after giving birth and during breastfeeding. (Photographer 2, male, 25 years)

Gaining new skills, confidence, and community exposure

While youth photographers did learn photography skills, they also reported benefiting more broadly by gaining self-confidence, enhanced community exposure, and learning how to speak in public. Several participants reported that the process of meeting regularly and discussing first in a small group, enabled them to build confidence and self-esteem that enabled them to speak more openly in public.

> I have got many benefits from this research. I did not know everyone in the research team but now they are all my friends. I also did not know how to use a camera but now I have learnt. I have also become more responsible and spend time thinking about what I need to do in order to benefit my community. The research has certainly made me more generous because we are volunteers for something that will benefit the whole world. (Photographer 7, female, 24 years)
> Before I got involved in this research, I used to have the fear of speaking in public. I could not explain my ideas to people and even when I did, I would look down fearing to face them directly. This has since changed because of my involvement in the research as I always got a chance to speak in our monthly meetings, which helped me build my confidence and improve communication skills. In fact nowadays, I can face community leaders and talk about our community concerns. (Photographer 10, female, 20 years)

The youth said knowledge gained through discussions was beneficial to them as individuals and also useful for enhancing their engagement at a community level, as through their discussions they reached a better understanding of community problems and how they could be acted upon. At the end of the project, youth participants were able to individually present findings from the research to the community during dissemination (Figure 1).

Through being well known in the community due to participation in the research, several participants were able to create new friends and networks. Some said that this would give them political leverage in the future and enable them to contest for political positions, while others thought that they would get more customers for their businesses, find more work opportunities, and engage in other research.

Eliciting trust from community members

Despite increased confidence and popularity in communities due to their participation in photovoice, this process was not without its challenges. Community members at the beginning did not trust their motives, and expected direct returns after taking their photographs as shown below:

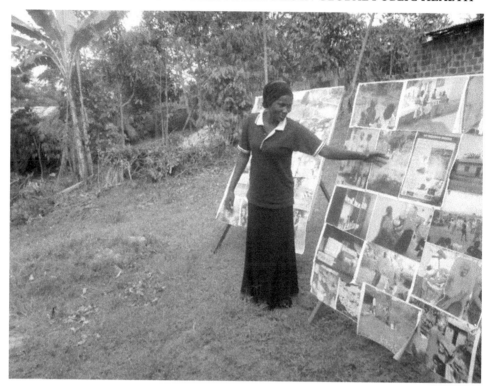

Figure 1. One of the youth photographers presenting photos during a community dissemination workshop.

> The challenge I had at the start of the research was how to convince people to take their photos as some could claim that we had been paid a lot of money and would sell the pictures to developed countries. However, I later fully understood the essence of the research and would comfortably explain to them why I was taking their photos. (Photographer 4, male, 24 years)
>
> There was a hardship requesting to take peoples' photos as some would even lay down tough conditions before consenting. For example, a few people would ask for money and other kinds of help before they could allow you take their photo. (Photographer 6, female, 25 years)

The youth photographers used a number of approaches to overcome these challenges including being introduced as researchers in village meetings and clearly explaining the context, aims, and benefits of the study to community members. Part of gaining trust was learning how to seek consent of those they wanted to photograph and learning to use judgement on what should be photographed ethically. In some instances, youth photographers noted down the scenarios that could not be captured on camera, or took photos that would not identify community members by not capturing faces or taking photos from a distance (Figure 2). The quotations below show how the youth overcame some of the challenges they faced while taking photos:

> Taking photos required a lot of creativity thus one needed to think about a situation and decide whether they need the photo for the research or not. In case a situation was suitable, but I was unable to capture it on camera, I would just note it down in the notebook provided and share it in the monthly meetings. (Photographer 9, male, 29 years)

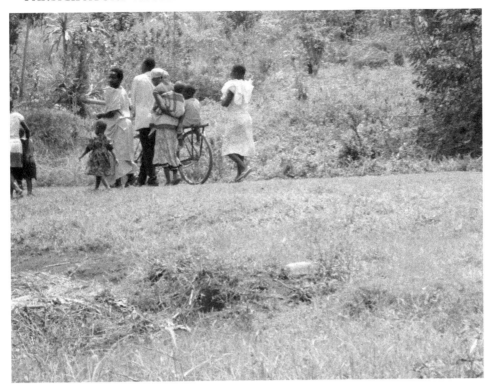

Figure 2. A photo taken from a distance showing a couple with other family members taking a child to a health centre for immunisation.

> Nowadays, I have learnt to take photos from a distance. In this way, I am able to capture several situations without bothering any person. I have also learnt to explain to the people what the research is about before they accept to take their photos. (Photographer 10, female, 20 years)

Contributing towards improving maternal health at community level

Based on the information gained and confidence from the group discussions, youth subsequently sought opportunities to share health information with community members through one on one sensitisation, as well as through the use of drama. Drama sessions conducted by the youth (Figure 3) ensured that many community members listened to the health promotion messages developed by the participants.

In the reflections shared by youth participants, below they detail individual instances of providing advice or advocacy within their communities.

> In this photo is a pregnant woman who told me about the side effects of the family planning method that she previously used until she abandoned it hence conceiving when she did not want to. I advised her to visit the bigger health centre in the area where they offer several options to choose from so as to prevent any other unwanted pregnancies in future. (Photographer 9, male, 29 years)
> The lady in this photo was heavily pregnant and stood at that shop for a very long time waiting to be served. I went and spoke to the shop attendant to come and attend to her first, which he did. We as youth need to advise the community to always give priority to

171

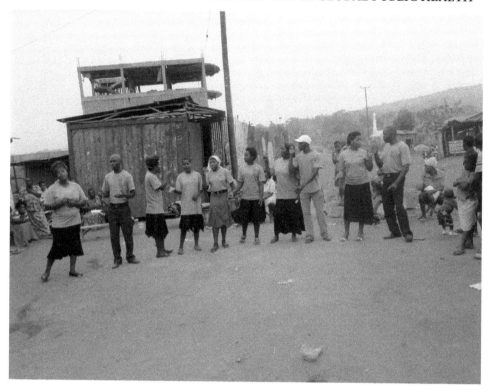

Figure 3. Youth taking part in drama to health educate the community.

expectant women when they visit their businesses or in need of any other service. (Photographer 6, female, 25 years)

By organising community dialogues based on their photos, youth and researchers enabled various stakeholders to appreciate the challenges that affected maternal health in the area. These challenges included poor transport to health facilities, and socio-determinants affecting maternal health such as nutrition, income generation, and alcoholism. After the dialogues, youth and community members worked together to address some of the challenges identified. For example, the community mentioned that there was need to address the problem of late arrival of health workers at facilities. As such, the youth participants became involved, and suggested that selected community members including some youth could intervene in the government-run health facilities to ameliorate this specific situation. In addition, when the issue of teenage pregnancies featured in the dialogues, health workers were subsequently invited to counsel adolescents in the community.

Researchers' experiences with photovoice

Flexibility in study objectives and process

Although the researchers had initiated the photovoice study, they had to adapt themselves to the community context and be flexible in changing their expectations and the purpose of the study in various ways. At the start of the study, the researchers had planned to explore the role youth could play in improving access to maternal health services. As the study evolved, youth photographers expanded the scope of the study by taking photographs focusing on maternal health as a broad theme and not merely on access to maternal health-care services. They took photographs highlighting several socio-determinants and other multi-sectoral concerns, which affected maternal health in their communities which were initially not anticipated by the researchers. For example, water and sanitation was an important issue in the community, including pregnant women having to collect water on their own for domestic use (Figure 4).

The researchers had also planned a series of specific topics for discussion, linking it to themes that they had planned for youth photographers to focus on each month. These topics were health service delivery, access to information, use of technology, and integration of maternal health services with existing programs. In practice, the study focus expanded organically and in unanticipated ways since the situations captured were dictated by the actual contexts encountered by the youth photographers. Such openness and flexibility by the researchers was needed for the photography assignment, and also during monthly discussions and participatory analysis with the youth.

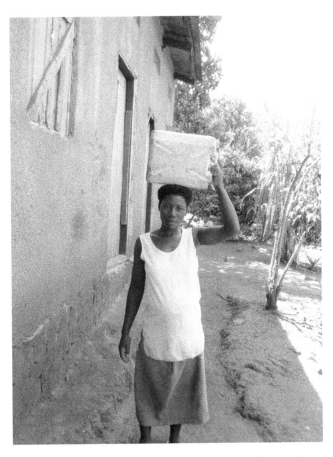

Figure 4. A pregnant woman returning home after collecting water from a distant source for household use.

Sustaining interest

During the course of the study, 1563 photographs were taken among which 903 were relevant to the research and discussed as a group, averaging to about 18 photographs per youth participant per meeting. The photographs relevant to the research hence discussed were identified by the participants before commencement of monthly meetings. Over time, the number of photos taken reduced as participants were not finding new topics to document. This was discouraging to the youth photographers who were always eager to share photos on new themes in every meeting. The researchers assured the participants that it was normal for topics to be repeated and the number of new images to reduce as the study progressed.

Handling logistics

Other challenges faced by the research team were related to the infrastructural constraints of working in remote areas, including electricity cut-offs leading to power outages, which led to delays in charging cameras, and occasionally the non-use of the projector. As a result, in some of the meetings the group resorted to participants converging around a laptop so that they could all view and discuss the photos (Figure 5), despite the absence of electricity.

Convening effective meetings also took some flexibility and facilitation. Initially, youth photographers at times arrived late or had trouble participating in meetings due to their own health problems or other livelihood commitments. Subsequent consultations led to

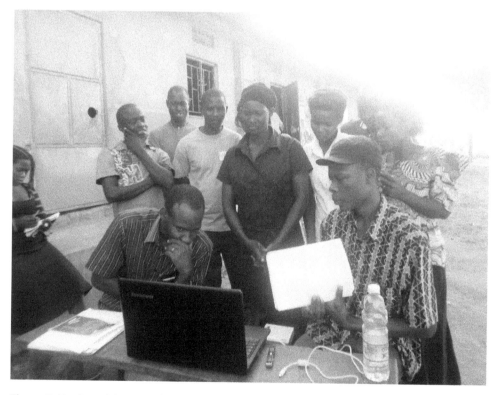

Figure 5. Youth participants and researchers converge around a laptop to view photos when a projector could not be used.

organising the meetings on days and times that were more convenient for the youth photographers. This ensured their high attendance in the monthly discussions. The youth photographers were also continuously encouraged to keep time so as to ensure that everyone could participate in the discussions.

Discussion

With limited use of photovoice in sub-Saharan Africa in the past (Catalani & Minkler, 2010), it was not surprising that our research protocol delayed getting ethical clearance due to minimal prior exposure to the methodology by the reviewers. We hope that our article contributes, along with others, to increase the existing knowledge base on the methodology and inform others interested in future application of photovoice in similar settings about its purpose, procedure, and ethical concerns.

It is vital for researchers to establish rapport and good working relationships with the community in photovoice undertakings. Establishing key partnerships between researchers, community, and other key stakeholders such as local authorities is very instrumental for the success of any photovoice project (Streng et al., 2004). Involvement of local leaders from the start of a study is the beginning of respectful engagement, which along with ongoing trust building and dialogue ensures community ownership and support, which is crucial for any community participatory research such as photovoice.

One of the challenges faced by youth photographers was receiving consent from community members before being photographed. It is important that photovoice participants fully understand the research procedures, objectives, benefits, and other pertinent information about the study including ethics (Wang, 2006). This would enable them to explain the research purpose to the community and also equip them with information and interpersonal skills necessary to ask for consent respectfully before taking photographs. Training done among participants before photovoice research therefore requires a component of ethics (Catalani & Minkler, 2010). In situations where consent is not feasible, encouraging youth to write down the issues they see in their notebooks, taking photos without revealing the identity of the participants or not taking photos at all need to be supported. In all instances, respect for those photographed and permission to use their images needs to be emphasised.

The reducing number of photos taken by participants over time indicated that a point of saturation had been reached as noted in several qualitative studies (Anderson, Hure, Kay-Lambkin, & Loxton, 2014; O'Brien, Finlayson, Kerr, & Edwards, 2014; Paul, Sossouhounto, & Eclou, 2014). When saturation has been reached, usually no new ideas are generated. In our study, data saturation was observed by the researchers and participants at the end of the fifth month as the photographs taken were related to the issues identified earlier with no new data generated. It is therefore important that the duration of photovoice discussions and research processes are carefully thought through to be adequate for each study. This would avoid a photovoice project being longer than necessary so as not to burden photographers and community members with volunteering for photographs that are of declining utility to them. Although our study was carried out for five months, a review of photovoice literature showed that community participation in previous studies ranged from two weeks to several years with a median of three months (Catalani & Minkler, 2010) depending upon the objectives of each project.

An important learning was flexibility of the researchers to let the study evolve over time and give space for initiative and creativity to emerge among photovoice participants as they understand better the situations that exist in their communities (Tomar & Stoffel, 2014). Community members are a vital source of expertise and what researchers consider important may not be the same with the photographers (Wang & Burris, 1997). While our photovoice project was undertaken primarily as a study headed by researchers, a key part of participatory research is balancing power with community participants (Cornwall & Jewkes, 1995).

Through the photovoice process, we found that youth were eager to learn about maternal health. In addition to their own individual learning, they gained new skills and experiences that led them to support change to improve maternal health in their communities. Previous studies have shown the potential of youth in health promotion through development of their personal abilities and subsequent involvement in education of communities (Birkhead, Riser, Mesler, Tallon, & Klein, 2006; Garcia, Minkler, Cardenas, Grills, & Porter, 2014; Powers & Tiffany, 2006; Strack et al., 2004). After reflecting on their own learning and experiences, photovoice participants usually decide how best to share the acquired knowledge to inform and educate others (Wang & Burris, 1994). A study done in Baltimore, USA, found that youth felt more empowered and did things differently such as raising their concerns to policy-makers to effect change in the community after a photovoice project due to the realisation that their opinions and thoughts mattered (Strack et al., 2004). Although the study carried out in the USA was in a different setting, similarity with our study was observed regarding improvements in youth knowledge and skills enhancement, development of self-confidence, and legitimisation of their perspectives.

Conclusion

This paper discusses key issues in using photovoice which could inform researchers intending to employ the methodology elsewhere. In our experience, by using photovoice, youth were able to explore, discuss, and reflect on issues that they associated with maternal health within their communities. The resulting discussions among their peers, with those photographed and in subsequent community dialogues, not only built their own capacity, but also spurred local community actions in support of maternal health as defined by local participants. When considering photovoice as a research process, researchers need to sustain ethical processes to go beyond institutional approval and individual consent to ethically representing those photographed; remaining open to learning alongside photographers, being flexible about the study processes and focus, sustaining youth interest and managing study logistics to ensure fair viewing and discussion of the photos, all while being reflective about the balance of power in such partnerships.

Acknowledgements

We thank the youth photographers for their time, dedication, commitment, and contribution to the research. We also thank the local leaders of the communities for the support offered during the course of the study. Special appreciation goes to the youth mobilisers who were critical in linking the researchers and the participants during all stages of implementation. The entire community of the five villages is also acknowledged for contributing towards the success of the study.

Disclosure statement

No potential conflict of interest was reported by the authors.

Funding

This work has been undertaken as part of the research for the Future Health Systems Research Consortium, which is supported by the UK Department for International Development (DFID).

References

Anderson, A. E., Hure, A. J., Kay-Lambkin, F. J., & Loxton, D. J. (2014). Women's perceptions of information about alcohol use during pregnancy: A qualitative study. *BMC Public Health, 14*(1), 1048. doi:10.1186/1471-2458-14-1048

Birkhead, G. S., Riser, M. H., Mesler, K., Tallon, T. C., & Klein, S. J. (2006). Youth development is a public health approach: Introduction. *Journal of Public Health Management and Practice, 12*(6), S1–S3.

Catalani, C., & Minkler, M. (2010). Photovoice: A review of the literature in health and public health. *Health Education & Behavior, 37*, 424–451. doi:10.1177/1090198109342084

Cornwall, A., & Jewkes, R. (1995). What is participatory research? *Social Science & Medicine, 41*, 1667–1676. doi:10.1016/0277-9536(95)00127-S

Eurostat. (2009). *Youth in Europe. Statistics explained.* Retrieved from http://epp.eurostat.ec. europa.eu/statistics_explained/index.php/Youth_in_Europe

Garcia, A. P., Minkler, M., Cardenas, Z., Grills, C., & Porter, C. (2014). Engaging homeless youth in community-based participatory research: A case study from skid row, Los Angeles. *Health Promotion and Practice, 15*(1), 18–27. doi:10.1177/1524839912472904

Government of Uganda (GoU). (2010). *National development plan (2010/11–2014/2015).* Kampala: Government of Uganda.

Graneheim, U. H., & Lundman, B. (2004). Qualitative content analysis in nursing research: Concepts, procedures and measures to achieve trustworthiness. *Nurse Education Today, 24*, 105–112.

Hergenrather, K. C., Rhodes, S. D., Cowan, C. A., Bardhoshi, G., & Pula, S. (2009). Photovoice as community-based participatory research: A qualitative review. *American Journal of Health Behavior, 33*(6), 686–698.

International Labour Organization (ILO). (2012). *Youth statistics: A global database on youth labour market indicators.* Retrieved from: http://www.youthstatistics.org

Khan, K. S., Wojdyla, D., Say, L., Gulmezoglu, A. M., & Van Look, P. F. (2006). WHO analysis of causes of maternal death: A systematic review. *The Lancet, 367*, 1066–1074. doi:10.1016/S0140-6736(06)68397-9

Lal, S., Jarus, T., & Suto, M. J. (2012). A scoping review of the Photovoice method: Implications for occupational therapy research. *Canadian Journal of Occupational Therapy, 79*(3), 181–190. doi:10.2182/cjot.2012.79.3.8

Lozano, R., Wang, H., Foreman, K. J., Rajaratnam, J. K., Naghavi, M., Marcus, J. R., ... Murray, C. J. (2011). Progress towards millennium development goals 4 and 5 on maternal and child mortality: An updated systematic analysis. *The Lancet, 378*, 1139–1165. doi:10.1016/S0140-6736(11)61337-8

Marston, C., Renedo, A., McGowan, C. R., & Portela, A. (2013). Effects of community participation on improving uptake of skilled care for maternal and newborn health: A systematic review. *PLoS One, 8*(2), e55012. doi:10.1371/journal.pone.0055012

Mayora, C., Ekirapa-Kiracho, E., Bishai, D., Peters, D. H., Okui, O., & Baine, S. O. (2014). Incremental cost of increasing access to maternal health care services: Perspectives from a demand and supply side intervention in Eastern Uganda. *Cost Effectiveness and Resource Allocation, 12*(1), 14. doi:10.1186/1478-7547-12-14

Mohammed, S., Sajun, S. Z., & Khan, F. S. (2013). Harnessing photovoice for tuberculosis advocacy in Karachi, Pakistan. *Health Promotion Internastional, 30,* 262–269. doi:10.1093/heapro/dat036

Moletsane, R., de Lange, N., Mitchell, C., Stuart, J., Buthelezi, T., & Taylor, M. (2007). Photo-voice as a tool for analysis and activism in response to HIV and AIDS stigmatisation in a rural KwaZulu-Natal school. *Journal of Child and Adolescent Mental Health, 19*(1), 19–28. doi:10. 2989/17280580709486632

O'Brien, J., Finlayson, K., Kerr, G., & Edwards, H. (2014). The perspectives of adults with venous leg ulcers on exercise: An exploratory study. *Journal of Wound Care, 23,* 496–509.

Okal, J., Kanya, L., Obare, F., Njuki, R., Abuya, T., Bange, T., … Bellows, B. (2013). An assessment of opportunities and challenges for public sector involvement in the maternal health voucher program in Uganda. *Health Research Policy and Systems, 11*(1), 38. doi:10.1186/1478-4505-11-38

Paul, E., Sossouhounto, N., & Eclou, D. S. (2014). Local stakeholders' perceptions about the intro-duction of performance-based financing in Benin: A case study in two health districts. *International Journal of Health Policy and Management, 3,* 207–214. doi:10.15171/ijhpm.2014.93

Powers, J. L., & Tiffany, J. S. (2006). Engaging youth in participatory research and evaluation. *Journal of Public Health Management and Practice, 12*(6), S79–S87.

Sankoh, O., Sharrow, D., Herbst, K., Whiteson Kabudula, C., Alam, N., Kant, S., … Clark, S. J. (2014). The INDEPTH standard population for low- and middle-income countries, 2013. *Glob Health Action, 7*(1), 23286. doi:10.3402/gha.v7.23286

Strack, R. W., Magill, C., & McDonagh, K. (2004). Engaging youth through photovoice. *Health Promotion Practice, 5*(1), 49–58. doi:10.1177/1524839903258015

Streng, J. M., Rhodes, S. D., Ayala, G. X., Eng, E., Arceo, R., & Phipps, S. (2004). Realidad Latina: Latino adolescents, their school, and a university use photovoice to examine and address the influence of immigration. *Journal of Interprofessional Care, 18,* 403–415. doi:10.1080/13561820400011701

Tomar, N., & Stoffel, V. (2014). Examining the lived experience and factors influencing education of two student veterans using photovoice methodology. *American Journal of Occupational Therapy, 68,* 430–438. doi:10.5014/ajot.2014.011163

Uganda Bureau of Statistics (UBOS). (2011). *UBOS projections 2011. Wakiso district population estimates.* Kampala: UBOS.

Uganda Bureau of Statistics (UBOS). (2012). *Uganda demographic and health survey 2011.* Kampala, Uganda; Calverton, Maryland: UBOS, ICF International Inc.

Van Oss, T., Quinn, D., Viscosi, P., & Bretscher, K. (2013). PHOTOVOICE: Reducing pedestrian injuries in children. *Work, 44*(1), S83–S93. doi:10.3233/WOR-121495

Wallerstein, N. (1987). Empowerment education: Freire's ideas applied to youth. *Youth Policy, 9* (11), 11–15.

Wang, C., & Burris, M. A. (1994). Empowerment through photo novella: Portraits of participation. *Health Education Quarterly, 21*(2), 171–186.

Wang, C., & Burris, M. A. (1997). Photovoice: Concept, methodology, and use for participatory needs assessment. *Health Education and Behavior, 24,* 369–387. doi:10.1177/109019819702400309

Wang, C. C. (2006). Youth participation in Photovoice as a strategy for community change. *Journal of Community Practice, 14*(1–2), 147–161. doi:10.1300/J125v14n01_09

World Health Organization (WHO). (2012). *Trends in maternal mortality 1990-2010: WHO, UNICEF, UNFPA and The World Bank Estimates.* Geneva: WHO.

Using participant-empowered visual relationship timelines in a qualitative study of sexual behaviour

Tamar Goldenberg[a,b], Catherine Finneran[c], Karen L. Andes[c] and Rob Stephenson[a,b]

[a]Department of Behavior and Biological Sciences, University of Michigan School of Nursing, Ann Arbor, MI, USA; [b]Center for Sexuality and Health Disparities, University of Michigan, Ann Arbor, MI, USA; [c]Hubert Department of Global Health, Rollins School of Public Health, Emory University, Atlanta, GA, USA

ABSTRACT
This study examines how the use of participant-empowered visual relationship timelines adds to the quality of an ongoing qualitative data collection in a case study examining the influence of emotions on sexual risk-taking and perceptions of HIV risk among men who have sex with men. Gay and bisexual men ($n =$ 25) participated in a 10-week, three-phase study. During a baseline in-depth interview, participants created a visual timeline using labelled stickers to retrospectively examine their dating/ sexual histories. Participants then completed three web-based quantitative personal relationship diaries, tracking sexual experiences during follow-up. These data were extracted and discussed in a timeline-based debrief interview. The visual cues assisted with data collection by prompting discussion through the immediate identification of patterns, opportunities for self-reflection, and rapport-building. The use of flexible data collection tools also allowed for a participant-empowered approach in which the participant controlled the interview process. Through this process, we learned strategies for improving a participant-empowered approach to qualitative research, including: allowing visual activities to drive the interview, using flexible guidelines to prompt activities, and using discrete imagery to increase participant comfort. It is important that qualitative data collection utilise more participatory approaches for gains in data quality and participant comfort.

Introduction

Gay, bisexual, and other men who have sex with men (MSM) experience a disproportionate burden of new HIV infections. In 2011, MSM accounted for 62% of new HIV infections, despite only comprising 2% of the population (Centers for Disease Control and Prevention, 2012). To address this, decades of research have examined biomedical and behavioural interventions to prevent and treat HIV among MSM, including condom use, HIV testing and counselling, antiretroviral therapy, and pre-exposure prophylaxis (Centers for Disease Control and Prevention, 2014, 2015; Sullivan et al., 2012). Much research has also examined sexual risk-taking among MSM, especially condomless anal intercourse (CAI), a primary biological risk for HIV transmission; this research has addressed societal and structural factors (Finneran & Stephenson, 2014), relationship characteristics (Blashill, Wilson, O'Cleirigh, Mayer, & Safren, 2014; Davidovich, Wit, & Strobbe, 2006; Hoff, Chakravarty, Beougher, Neilands, & Darbes, 2012; Mustanski, Newcomb, & Clerkin, 2011; Newcomb, Ryan, Garofalo, & Mustanski, 2014), and individual cognitive processes (Rogers & Prentice-Dunn, 1997; Rosenstock, 1974; Weinstein, 1988). While some research has examined perceptions of HIV risk and the ways in which it influences sexual risk-taking and the uptake of HIV interventions (including condom use) (Belcher, Sternberg, Wolitski, Halkitis, & Hoff, 2005; Carballo-Diéguez & Bauermeister, 2004; Carballo-Dieguez & Dolezal, 1996; Cox, Beauchemin, & Allard, 2004; Kellerman et al., 2002; MacKellar et al., 2005, 2007; Suarez & Kauth, 2001; Suarez & Miller, 2001), few studies have addressed how emotions influence perceptions of HIV risk and sexual risk-taking among MSM. This is an important area to consider because the influence of emotions on perceptions of HIV risk could influence sexual decision-making and the utilisation of HIV interventions.

Traditional research methods

While some research has examined the influence of emotions on perceptions of HIV risk among MSM, it has been mostly quantitative, often using scales to measure emotional experiences (Bauermeister, Carballo-Diéguez, Ventuneac, & Dolezal, 2009; Bauermeister, Leslie-Santana, Johns, Pingel, & Eisenberg, 2011; Bauermeister, Ventuneac, Pingel, & Parsons, 2012; Berg, 2009; Carballo-Dieguez & Dolezal, 1996), with fewer studies using traditional qualitative methods (like standard individual in-depth-interviews) to examine emotions and sexual decision-making among MSM (Carballo-Diéguez et al., 2011). While these previous studies have been useful in understanding MSM's experiences of emotions, in order to understand the complexities and nuances of how emotions are experienced within a larger context of relationship dynamics, innovative qualitative methodologies are useful. While traditional qualitative methods are intended to capture contextual meaning, using open-ended questions to answer research questions (Patton, 2005), these methods lack a dialogical process because the researchers still rely on their own assumptions of the research problem and lived experiences of the community (Montoya & Kent, 2011). Alternatively, research methods that promote dialogue generate a co-learning experience between the community and the researcher, rather than building on preconceived notions of the researcher (Montoya & Kent, 2011).

Participatory research methods

Participant-empowered research – defined as research that uses elements of community-based participatory research (CBPR) – presents a potential alternative for capturing complex and nuanced data. To address the limitations of static research, in which participants answer fixed questions created by researchers, and to ground research within communities, there has been a growth of CBPR (Cornwall & Jewkes, 1995; Macaulay et al., 1999). Traditionally, CBPR involves collaboration with communities to incorporate the community members as active researchers, allowing them to develop research questions, play an active role in data collection, and make decisions about the research process

(Green et al., 1995; Israel, Eng, Schulz, & Parker, 2005; Israel, Schulz, Parker, & Becker, 1998; Minkler & Wallerstein, 2010). CBPR is especially useful when addressing health disparities and examining social and environmental determinants of health because it allows the community to be actively involved in identifying and addressing the problems that concern them (Cacari-Stone, Wallerstein, Garcia, & Minkler, 2014; Israel et al., 1998; Minkler, 2010; Viswanathan et al., 2004; Wallerstein & Duran, 2010). However, true CBPR methods are challenging to achieve. CBPR requires the capacity to develop and sustain community partnerships (Israel et al., 2006; Israel, Schulz, Parker, & Becker, 2003). This poses some challenges for public health funding; CBPR requires that funding agencies offer flexibility for the timing of project completion, take a passive role in the research process, and offer evaluation measurement instruments that match the needs of the community (Minkler, Blackwell, Thompson, & Tamir, 2003). Using CBPR methods can also raise ethical concerns because it is difficult to attain a true community-driven agenda with an equal partnership between the researcher and the community (Minkler, 2004, 2005).

Some researchers have examined how to overcome the challenges that CBPR poses through successful partnerships with communities (Ahmed, Beck, Maurana, & Newton, 2004; Israel et al., 2003, 2006; Minkler, 2005). However, in some circumstances, alternatives to CBPR may be appropriate; these alternative participant-empowered approaches deviate from classical researcher-driven methods through the utilisation of some elements of CBPR without facing the same challenges that occur when building community partnerships through a traditional CBPR approach. In this paper, we use the term 'participant-empowered' to describe a data collection process that includes action-oriented activities (e.g. social mapping, body mapping, pile sorting, and photo voice) in order to engage participants in qualitative research methods. These activities are commonly used within CBPR research (Bourey, Stephenson, Bartel, & Rubardt, 2012; Israel et al., 2005; White & Stephenson, 2014) and are meant to engage participants because they allow the participant, rather than the researcher, to guide the collection of data. These participant-empowered activities often include visual elements of research (e.g. maps, diagrams, timelines); the activities are often guided by prompts from the researcher, but ultimately allow for participants to build their own visual representation of data.

Many of these activities also involve the production of visual representations of public health problems or use visual cues in order to guide the interview process. These visual-based activities often include a set of prompts or guidelines from the researcher, but ultimately the participant is expected to build their own visual representation of data, thus allowing for a data collection process that engages the participant to actively consider the public health problem or research question. Furthermore, qualitative activities involving visualisations can be useful to convey depth and detail that expand beyond verbal expression (Bagnoli, 2009; Guest, Namey, & Mitchell, 2012). Visual aids can include drawings, photography, film, etc. and can be used in qualitative research as data, to elicit additional data, to provide feedback or documentation of the research process, or as a form of data interpretation (Prosser & Loxley, 2008). Previous research suggests that incorporating participatory, visual activities into focus group discussions or individual in-depth interviews (IDIs) helps to enhance the complexities and nuances of the data (Bourey et al., 2012; White & Stephenson, 2014).

Life-history calendars

One method for creating visual cues is the life-history calendar (LHC) (Axinn, Pearce, & Ghimire, 1999; Martyn & Belli, 2002), an instrument that has been previously used to examine HIV and sexual health (Kabiru, Luke, Izugbara, & Zulu, 2010; Luke, Clark, & Zulu, 2011). The LHC is an instrument that provides a calendar-based context to improve recall in retrospective studies through an increase in autobiographical memory (Belli, 1998). The cues help participants to visually and mentally relate to the data (Freedman, Thornton, Camburn, Alwin, & Young-DeMarco, 1988) and facilitate recall with greater precision of timing (Belli, 1998; Fisher, 2012; Yoshihama, Clum, Crampton, & Gillespie, 2002). LHCs are traditionally created in the form of calendars, graphs, or tables with cues for important domains and timing of events to visually illustrate a sequence of events that occurred over a period of time (Axinn et al., 1999; Belli, 1998; Freedman et al., 1988). Currently, we do not understand how LHCs or visual timelines can be used in combination with other instruments to create a visual and participant-empowered approach for prospective qualitative data collection. In this paper, we use a case study examining the influence of emotions on sexual risk-taking and perceptions of HIV risk among gay and bisexual men (GBM) in order to describe an innovative participant-empowered timeline method and to examine how the use of participant-empowered visual relationship timelines during IDIs can add to the quality of ongoing qualitative data collection.

Methods

Building and designing the method

This study was approved by the Emory University Institutional Review Board. The purpose of this study was to design a methodological approach to examine the complexities and nuances of how emotions influence perceptions of HIV risk and sexual decision-making among GBM. In order to conceptualise emotions, it was necessary to deviate from traditional qualitative approaches (e.g. standard qualitative IDIs, focus group discussions). However, at the same time, building community partnerships using traditional CBPR methods was not appropriate because the researcher had already established a research question. Therefore, as an alternative, this study employed some participatory action-based activities to allow the participant to guide the interview process.

This study also aimed to capture data over time; however, instead of using classical longitudinal methods, applying the same tool on multiple occasions, this study administered three separate research tools in an ongoing qualitative data collection over 10 weeks. Thus, different forms of data are collected from the same research participant over a 10-week period; the data are therefore dynamic and not longitudinal. We used three different methods that sequentially built upon each other to capture different aspects of emotions and to understand the patterns of emotions and sexual risk-taking over time. First, participants completed a timeline-based IDI in order to understand participants' sexual and relationship histories. This first method provided a foundational background in understanding participants' general perceptions of relationships. The timeline activity in the baseline IDI allowed participants to guide the interview by actively building the timeline, using stickers and prompts from the interviewer as a guide. Next, participants completed three web-based quantitative personal relationship diaries (PRDs), one every three weeks (at weeks three, six, and nine). Though the PRDs were not a participatory activity, they served the purpose of collecting data about sexual behaviours over the 10-week study period. For the final research tool, the researchers extracted data from the PRDs and used them in another timeline-based debrief IDI to understand participants' ongoing experiences with emotions and sexual behaviours over the 10-week study period. In total, we conducted 25 baseline IDIs, 75 PRDs, and 25 debrief IDIs with 25 participants.

Study population and recruitment

Recruitment occurred from November 2012 to February 2013. All participants had pre-viously taken part in cohort studies at Emory University and were interested in participat-ing in additional research. All potential participants were contacted via email to complete a screening survey. All eligible and interested participants were then contacted by phone to schedule an interview. Participants were eligible for this study if they self-identified as a gay or bisexual man, were aged ≥18, lived in the Atlanta metropolitan area, and had CAI within the three months prior to being screened for the study. After 20 baseline IDIs were completed and summarised, the data were reviewed to assess saturation and variation in participant demographics. The final five participants were recruited based on age and race to ensure saturation in each age/race category.

Baseline interview

Upon enrolment, all participants completed a baseline IDI, which used a visual relation-ship timeline using stickers to develop an overview of each participant's dating and sexual history. The baseline IDIs followed a step-by-step process with seven discrete steps where participants placed stickers on the timeline in response to questions about relationship dynamics and sexual experiences (Table 1). Probes and follow-up questions addressed specific domains of interest for each step.

To construct the timeline, participants added non-identifying nicknames for five 'sexual and/or romantic partners' who were 'significant or memorable' to the participant in some way; participants defined for themselves what 'significant or memorable' meant. The timeline began with the age of when the participant first met the earliest partner and ended at the current age. Lines were added to show when and how long each relationship occurred. Participants were given flexibility on how to draw the lines in order to best represent the timeline of their relationship history (e.g. participants could choose to use different types of lines to represent different parts of the relation-ship, lines could stop and start again, lines for different people could overlap over the same time period).

Participants then answered a series of questions on each relationship through a process that involved participants applying stickers with predetermined labels to the timelines. All labels were created with input from various GBM of different races and ages in order to develop a representative and appropriate list of terms; blank stickers were also provided so participants could write in their own terms if none of the predetermined labels were

Table 1. Outline of baseline IDI timeline tool.

	Stickers/instructions	Questions	Objective	Domains of interest
Step 1: Build the timeline	Add nicknames, Write ages, Include lines and arrows	In your experience, what makes someone more significant or memorable?	Warm up the interview with a general, non-threatening question; Build the basic outline of the timeline	N/A
Step 2: Relationship definitions	As many 'Relationship Tags' that the participant finds appropriate for each partner	How did you define your relationship with this person when you were together?	Understand relationship characteristics, definitions, development, transitions, and rules	Exclusivity, Commitment, Trust, Intimacy, Desire
Step 3: Emotions	Up to five 'Emotion/ Attribute Tags' for each partner	How did you feel about this person when you were together?	Examine negative and positive emotions associated with each partner	Intimacy, Affection, Lust/Desire, Trust, Commitment
Step 4: Love	A read heart on partners with whom participants were (or are) in love.	What did it mean to be in love with this person?	Identify partners with whom participants identified being in love	Intimacy, Affection, Support, Understanding, Openness
Step 5: Anal sex experiences	As many purple and green dots to describe anal sex with each partner; there were three different sizes of purple (CAI) and green (anal sex with condom) stickers to describe frequency	How did you make decisions about condom use?	Understand sexual decision-making, self-efficacy with condom use, HIV/STI risk behaviours and risk reduction	Exclusivity, Trust, Intimacy, Desire, Passion, Love
Step 6: HIV/STI risk	HIV/STI risk ranking stickers from 1 (most risky) to 5 (least risky)	How do you define HIV/STI risk? Why did you choose these rankings?	Examine perceptions of HIV/STI risk	Exclusivity, Trust, Intimacy, Love
Step 7: Overview	N/A	Do you see any patterns here?	Summarise relationship history	N/A

appropriate. Building the timeline with stickers allowed for an action-oriented process where the participant had control over what the timeline would look like through the placement of the stickers and the creation of a visual representation of data.

Participants first used 'relationship tag' stickers with definition terms (e.g. partner, boyfriend, friends with benefits). Participants then answered the question, 'How did you feel about this person when you were together?' by adding up to five positive and/or negative 'emotion tags' for each partner (e.g. trusting, loved, disrespected, not myself). Then, participants added red hearts to each participant with whom they experienced feelings of love. All placement of stickers was followed up with questions and prompts to elaborate on the meanings of the stickers and the relationships.

After discussing the emotional aspect of each relationship, participants were asked to describe their sexual experiences with each partner using purple and green dots; purple dots represented CAI and green dots represented anal intercourse with a condom. There were three different sizes for each colour to represent frequency; smaller dots were less frequent and larger dots were more frequent. Participants were then asked to rank each partner on a one to five scale based on how 'risky' they thought each participant was for HIV or STIs, with one being the most risky and five being the least risky. Participants were asked how they defined risk in this context and were asked to explain why they chose their rankings, focusing on the most risky and the least risky partners.

Personal relationship diaries

During the nine weeks after enrolment, each participant completed three PRDs (at weeks three, six, and nine). The PRDs were quantitative web-based surveys created through SurveyGizmo (SurveyGizmo, Boulder, Colorado), a HIPAA compliant, secure, web-based survey-building software. The PRDs asked questions about participants' sexual and dating experiences over the follow-up period. Participants reported the number of sexual partners that they had during the previous three weeks (anal and/or oral sex) and then answered questions about each partner. If a participant had more than three partners, he was asked to choose only three to discuss. Participants were then asked about their commitment to each partner, how they knew each partner, how long they knew each partner, how many sexual encounters they had with each partner (stratified by type: oral, penetrative anal, receptive anal), how frequently condoms were used, and how they ranked each person on a scale from one to five based on how well they knew the partner, emotional risk, and HIV/STI risk. Participants were also asked to choose applicable statements from a list of 26 'hotspot' statements that demonstrated a variety of emotions/relationship characteristics (e.g. 'I don't know the first thing about him,' 'I am or was in love with him,' 'I am afraid that talking about safer sex with him will make him like me less,' 'I get jealous when he flirts with other people,' 'I trust him a lot,' 'We have an agreement that we will not see other people.'). Participants who did not have any sexual encounters over the time period were asked questions about romantic partners with whom they did not had sex, seeking sex, and any reasons why they did not seek sex (if applicable).

Debrief IDIs

Data from PRDs were extracted and demonstrated to participants using visual timelines in the debrief IDI. The purpose of the debrief IDI was to discuss the PRD extractions and learn about day-to-day sexual and romantic encounters within a 10-week time period in order to further understand emotions and sexual decision-making in both casual and formal relationships. Each debrief IDI was tailored to participant responses in PRDs, with slightly different interview guides for participants with multiple sexual partners, participants with one sexual partner, participants who discussed romantic interests who were not sexual partners, and participants who did not discuss any romantic interests or sexual partners. Data were presented to participants on a separate timeline for each partner, signifying changes between each PRD three-week period. Participants followed a systematic, participatory process in which they were asked to qualitatively describe previously reported PRD answers, which were represented on the timelines with stickers. Similar to the baseline IDI, the debrief IDI also followed a step-by-step process to understand how relationships were defined, the emotions that were present, and the sexual experiences that occurred (Table 2). Participants described why they chose their answers and how they interpreted different statements and questions. During the interview, participants also added new information about each partner, using predetermined labels to answer questions; similarly to the baseline IDIs, all labels were created with input from GBM and blank stickers were provided to allow participants to include their own words. Additional questions in the debrief IDIs addressed relationship definitions (e.g. partner, boyfriend, friends with benefits), sexual decision-making processes

Table 2. Outline of debrief IDI timeline tool for multiple sexual partners.

	Stickers/instructions	From PRD?	Questions	Objective	Domains of interest
Step 1: Relationship definitions	One 'Relationship Tags' for each PRD	No	How would you define this relationship?	Understand relationship characteristics, definitions, development, and rules	Exclusivity, Commitment, Trust, Intimacy, Desire
Step 2: Commitment	A gold star to represent commitment	Yes	What does it mean that you were/are committed to this partner?		Exclusivity, Commitment, Love
Step 3: Hotspots	List of all chosen 'Hotspots' from the 27 options on the PRD	Yes	Why did you choose this statement?	Examine general feelings for sexual partner	Love, Intimacy, Trust, Commitment, Desire, Lust
Step 4: Sexual experiences	Colour-coded dots to represent each incident of oral sex (blue), anal sex with a condom (green), and CAI (purple)	Yes	What kinds of decisions did you make when you had sex with this partner? How did you make these decisions?	Understand sexual decision-making, self-efficacy with condom use, HIV/STI risk behaviours and risk reduction	Typical?, Self-efficacy, conversations about sex, control, safety, trust
Step 5: Sex descriptions	One 'Sex Description Tag' for each PRD	No	How would you describe the sex that you had?	Understand how participant perceived sexual encounter	Affection, Love, Intimacy, Trust, Commitment, Desire, Lust
Step 6: Sex feelings	Up to three 'Emotion Tags' for each PRD	No	How did you feel at the time that you had sex with this partner?	Examine feelings associated with sexual activities	Love, Intimacy, Trust, Desire, Lust
Step 7: Rankings	Ranking of 1–5 for how well participant knows partner, Emotional Risk, HIV/STI Risk (1 = least, 5 = most)	Yes	Why did you choose this ranking? How did you define emotional risk? How did you define HIV/STI risk?	Examine perceptions of HIV/STI risk and emotional investment	Vulnerability, Love, Trust, Security, Commitment
Step 8: Comparisons	N/A	No	What kinds of patterns do you see? Who is the most risky/ least risky in terms of HIV/STIs?		N/A

(e.g. decisions about condom use, penetrative vs. receptive intercourse, relationship agreements), terms used to describe sex (e.g. making love, hooking up), and emotions associated with sexual encounters (e.g. comfortable, into it, insecure, bored).

Data analysis

Innovative research methods required innovative analytical techniques. Data collection generated two types of qualitative data, including textual data from qualitative interviews and visual data from the timelines. Most data were in the form of qualitative transcripts, which were analysed in a two-step process, using a more traditional thematic analysis in addition to a more innovative case-based analysis. Analysis of visual data also required unique analysis approaches and supplemented an analysis of textual data to increase the understanding of each participant's experiences.

Textual data: a traditional approach to qualitative analysis

All IDIs were audio-recorded and transcribed verbatim by an outside organisation that conducts transcription services. Research analysts checked the quality of transcriptions, comparing them to audio-recordings at randomly selected moments during the interviews. All inaudible recording was marked with a time stamp in the transcript. All of these time stamps were double-checked by analysts to determine if the audio-recording could be understood. Textual analysis was conducted using MAXQDA, version 10 (Verbi Software, Berlin, Germany). A team of six analysts conducted a thematic analysis, examining patterns of themes across participants. This thematic analysis entailed the consistent application of a set of codes to all verbatim transcripts in order to examine how themes were discussed across participants and between groups of participants. A preliminary codebook was created based on a close reading of several transcripts, incorporating explicit domains from interview guides as well as pervasive, unanticipated themes that were emergent across various transcripts. Provisional definitions were given to each code and six analysts applied the codes to a single transcript. The six versions of the coded transcript were merged for comparison and all instances of disagreement were discussed among the analysts. Codes and definitions were revised based on these discussions and the process was repeated until consistent agreement was attained among all coders; three baseline IDIs and one debrief IDI were coded in this way.

Once the final codebook was established, these codes were applied to all 50 baseline and debrief IDI transcripts, with at least 2 analysts coding each transcript. A consensus approach was used; the coding was merged and compared for each transcript, after which the study coordinator reconciled all differences to determine final code application and how much context to include in each text segment. A focused reading of coded text allowed analysts to develop thick descriptions for each theme. These descriptions identified common concepts, patterns, and unique statements that appeared in the transcripts. Data were also compared between demographics; for the purpose of data retrieval by theme, types of respondents were grouped together based on age, race, relationship status, and relationship development (e.g. relationships that developed from casual to serious or relationships that transitioned from serious to casual).

Textual data: an innovate analysis approach

In addition to a thematic analysis, a case-based analysis was also conducted to analyse textual data as individual life-stories. After multiple close readings, data analysts created detailed descriptions characterising each participant, summarising his relationships and identifying his relationship style, patterns of condom use, and risk definitions. One analyst created each description and then descriptions were discussed among a group of six analysts, with revisions being made if necessary. The case-based descriptions enabled analysts to preserve the context of each participant's experiences and each relationship while conducting the thematic analysis.

Visual data: an innovative analysis approach

Visual timelines were analysed separately during the case-based analysis. These data were used to supplement textual data and better understand relationship experiences. Using these timelines, analysts were able to create detailed descriptions of each relationship, based solely on the information provided in the visual timeline; one analyst wrote each description, but descriptions were discussed among six analysts and revised when necessary. Visual timelines enabled analysts to visually identify patterns that occurred for each participant and patterns that occurred across participants; these patterns were described in each detailed description. For example, visual timelines enabled analysts to easily identify relationships that developed from casual to serious. Visual timelines also enabled analysts to identify participants' patterns across partners (e.g. multiple casual partners with condom use or non-condom use, multiple partners with emotional attachments, multiple partners with one committed partner). The timelines were especially useful for analysts to visually understand the relationships between partners, sexual activities, and perceptions of risk. These visual representations also enabled analysts to have a clearer understanding of the context of each relationship, ensuring that the contextual nuances of the relationship were considered as analysts conducted a thematic analysis.

Results

The visually focused and participant-empowered approach used in this study proved to be successful in gathering thick and in-depth data on relationships and sexual experiences among GBM. Among the 25 participants, we had 100% retention in this study; each participant enrolled at baseline completed all three PRDs and a debrief IDI. Both types of IDIs generated a great amount of thick data, with interviews ranging from 45 minutes to 3 hours, depending on the participant's experiences and the number of partners discussed in each interview.

Demographics at baseline (age, race, sexual orientation, relationship status) are described in Table 3. In the baseline IDIs, participants provided retrospective dating and sexual histories for between three to five partners in each interview. A total of 125 PRDs were completed by 25 participants, including details on 76 sexual partners, ranging from 1 to 7 partners per participant over 9 weeks; all of these partners were discussed in the debrief IDIs.

Data represented in-depth discussions of dating and sexual histories, with a variety of both inductive and deductive themes. Participants described multiple types of relationships and experiences, capturing a wide range of expected and unexpected data. Multiple components of these data collection methods proved to be most successful in producing data depth, especially the use of visual cues for data collection and a participatory process that enabled flexible interaction between the participants and the research tools.

Table 3. Participant demographics at baseline.

	Mean	Range
Age	32.2	19–50
Race	*n*	%
Caucasian/white	12	48
African-American/black	11	44
Multiple races	2	8
Sexual orientation		
Gay/homosexual	23	92
Bisexual	2	8
In a relationship at the time of baseline IDI		
Yes	6	24
No	17	68
Don't know	1	4
No answer	1	4

Note: Being in a relationship was defined as: 'being committed to someone above all others'.

Visual cues for data collection

The use of visual tools aided the interview processes by prompting discussion, enabling identification of patterns, providing opportunities for self-reflection, and building rapport.

Immediate identification of patterns

Visual cues enabled participants to identify their own dating and sexual patterns, resulting in in-depth discussions of links between the different components of the timelines and the patterns that occurred over time. In the baseline IDI, visual cues were especially useful in facilitating conversations about patterns of sexual risk-taking and perceptions of risk for participants' more significant relationships:

> P103: That's I guess kind of a nice summary of each [relationship] ... you never really understand the full impact of it until it's like if you put it in a graphical format so to speak to where you can look back.

The creation of this visual representation enabled most participants to immediately identify links between their behaviours and how they defined sexual risk in their relationships. For example, using the visual timeline (Figure 1) created during his baseline IDI, P119 recognised a pattern between the frequency of anal intercourse with and without

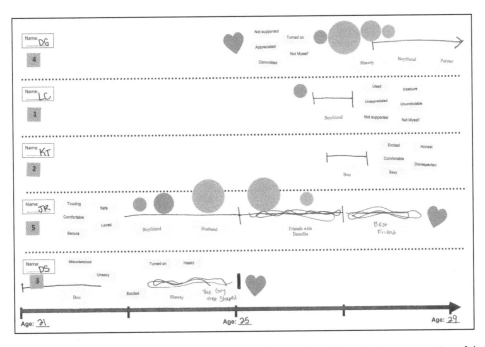

Figure 1. P119 timeline for baseline interview. Notes: For confidentiality, this is representative of data, but is not an actual baseline timeline. Key: Yellow = relationship definitions, blue = emotions experienced during relationship, hearts = experienced love, green dots = anal intercourse with a condom, purple dots = condomless anal intercourse (smaller→larger = less frequent→most frequent), pink number = HIV/STI risk ranking (5 = least risky, 1 = most risky).

condoms (represented by green and purple dots) and perceptions of HIV/STI risk rankings for each partner (pink numbers):

Interviewer: So how do you think the way that you ranked risk was related to your condom use with each of these guys?

P119: Hmm, It's funny that I, [surprised] oh yeah!, I opted to be unprotected and more so with the number, according to the number [referring to the way that he ranked HIV/STI risk on the timeline]. That's interesting.

Interviewer: Right, with the two guys, the two guys who you said were least risky were the two that you had unprotected sex with.

Participant 119. Yea. Yea. Yea.

The identification of this pattern enabled further discussion about why P119 ranked his experiences of CAI as the least risky.

In the debrief IDIs, visual cues also enabled participants to identify patterns within and between partners. Timelines in debrief IDIs visually represented the development (or lack of development) of a relationship over a nine-week period. Figure 2, based on data from P104, represents an example of a developing relationship that occurred during the PRD period; each PRD included additional stickers and stronger feelings. This visualisation enabled P104 to identify when changes occurred in his relationship and prompted anecdotes describing

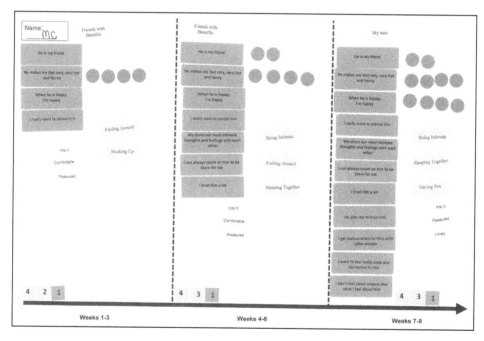

Figure 2. P104 timeline for debrief interview. Notes: For confidentiality, this is representative of data, but is not an actual debrief timeline. Key: Yellow = relationship definitions, grey = 'hotspot', blue dot = oral sex, green dot = anal sex with a condom, purple dot = condomless anal sex (1 dot = 1 incident), pink = sex descriptions, blue = emotions during sex, green number = ranking how well knew partner, yellow number = emotional risk ranking, pink number = HIV/STI risk ranking (ranking on a scale of 1–5, 1 = least, 5 = most).

how the relationship changed over time and how these changes impacted sexual decision-making:

> P104: [describing the grey stickers] Well I feel like these were all positive character-istics, for lack of better word. And it's clear that like as time went by, more things were apparent to me in our relationship, whatever that relationship was.

Participants were also able to use the timeline to point to time periods in order to chronologically explain how development occurred in their relationships. Using the time-line represented in Figure 2, P104 was able to recount an experience that occurred between the second and the third PRD in order to identify when feelings began to change for this partner. He was able to use the 'hotspot' stickers that identified feelings of jealousy in order to talk about how that played into his relationship.

In addition to facilitating the identification of patterns within a relationship, the visual timeline used in the debrief IDI also enabled all participants to identify patterns between partners. At the end of each debrief IDI, all of the timelines were laid out in front of the participant and they were asked to further discuss their dating patterns. The process of building the timeline and then examining a visual representation of all of the relationships side-by-side allowed participants to identify common and uncommon experiences that participants had with different partners. For example, when P101 examined his timelines at the end of his debrief IDI, he identified patterns that were common to most of his partners as well as characteristics unique to one partner:

> Interviewer: So now … we're going to lay these out. [lays out all of the timelines in front of P101] … So, when you look over all of these guys, do you see any patterns?
> P101: Yes. I see that I like giving blowjobs. I see that. I see also that I have a lot of friends with benefits. I see that. I also see that I don't feel comfortable a lot. I feel disrespected a lot. Not trusting. Not really into it and not in control. Only was pleasure was Panther [partner's nickname]. Or intimate. Or intimate. I'm not really seeing intimate a lot … Most of them all were hook ups or either friends with benefits. But with him I was at least feeling a little more intimate. I was fooling around. And I wasn't as uncomfortable as I was with everyone else.

Self-reflection

The immediate identification of patterns through visual cues also provided opportunities for self-reflection. Many participants described the study process as a 'lesson' or learning experience; the realisations that occurred while participants examined their own sexual decision-making provided valuable data on why behaviours occur:

> Interviewer: So before we wrap up, can you just tell me how you felt going through this whole process? …
> P102: I felt as though I learned a lot about myself because I'm always trying to self-evaluate, but I feel like my pattern, I feel like I have a pattern and I think my pattern is, is I don't wait now, I don't wait long enough to understand a person I'm dealing with and I don't understand, I don't understand the concept of affection.

Visual aids in both sets of IDIs increased participants' awareness of their own behaviours, allowing for explanations of emotional processes. For example, at the end of his debrief IDI, when all of his timelines were side-by-side in front on him, P124 put his face in his hands as he began to reflect on his own behaviours and come to terms with his behavioural patterns, expressing a great amount of discomfort with the experiences that he reported during the study period:

Interviewer: What kinds of patterns do you see when you look at this?
P124: OK, so, um, everyone I think, so there's lots of not trusting, not really into it, not trusting, not trusting. I associated, sex is associated with a lot of negative feelings, a lot of negative emotions and not safe emotions. Sex is something I think that comes [from] a not healthy, an unhealthy place for me and I've almost always associated it with that …
Interviewer: So why do you think that is?
P124: (Sighs) Um, I don't want to say that I don't know, but if I had to say it might be just from, I mean, it could go all the way back to my childhood and like growing up and coming out with my mom and feeling negative and feeling like it's something that I have to hide, feeling like I'm going to hell for it. The way that we meet other guys, the social structure of being gay, the scenarios of like, you know, social media applications and websites and the emphasis on sex and the self-reinforcing behaviour of it all, it all kind of plays in together, I think.

Other participants also recognised that they were able to reflect on and learn about their own experiences by going through the study:

Interviewer: What have you learned?
P103: Definitely about myself as far as how much an emotional risk somebody is versus the much lesser of a risk, how, in regards to the people that are in my life and who I have sex with and whatnot … It's been a very valuable learning tool, I think, for me in more ways than one. Being able to look at different risk aspects as well as just emotions all together.

Building rapport

Rapport was built when creating visual timelines through the use of nondescript stickers, which increased participants' comfort and safety. Using different coloured dots to represent sexual experiences provided a non-threatening and discrete way to demonstrate frequency of sex and condom use with each partner prior to asking questions related to decision-making about sex and condom use. One participant described how using the dots to describe sex made him feel during the interview:

This was actually very good, as far as replaying my sexual history in a different way. Because it doesn't make it looks like it's, I don't see dick and ass on the table. But it's dick and ass on the table. Literally. So it was good to actually see. (P101)

Multiple participants also expressed how the stickers made it easier to talk and created a visual that made the interview 'more fun'.

Participatory interaction

The visual timelines for the baseline and debrief IDIs provided an action-oriented activity to engage participants using a participant-empowered approach. Participants chose which partners they wanted to discuss and defined all terms. Participants were also asked to define all relationship terms that they used, all emotions that they discussed, and how they perceived HIV/STI risk. All participants completed all of the writing on the timeline and added stickers. They were encouraged to take ownership of their timelines and per-sonalise it so that it expressed their unique experience.

Flexibility with instructions

The step-by-step process of constructing the timeline was flexible; participants wrote in their own words on description labels, ripped hearts in half, used multiple hearts on part-ners to describe their experiences of love, used squiggly lines instead of straight lines to represent different stages of relationships, and found alternative, more personal ways to describe ranking for HIV and STI risk.

The flexibility to edit the rules of the timeline and interact with the tools in the way that best represented his relationships enabled P115 to continue his discussion of one of his partners, explaining why he chose to put a broken heart on the timeline:

> Interviewer: [after putting hearts on the timeline] So anything else you want to add before we move on to the next part here?
> P115: Do you want a broken heart?
> Interviewer: You can put one there if you want to.
> P115. You want a broken heart?
> Interviewer: You can put one there if you want to. Yes, tear it in half or something.
> P115. Yes, I would probably say this one. You know, he would have been a broken heart for sure because it was a fling. It was fun ... because it really could have worked out, I think, if we had been close.

For participant 119, he personalised the timeline in types of lines that he used to rep-resent the length of each relationship. He used straight lines to represent when the defi-nitions of his relationships were more straightforward and squiggly lines to represent when he the nature of the relationship was more complex (e.g. when they still had feelings for each other, but were just friends). These acts of deviating from the original instructions produced timelines that were unique and more accurate representations of each partici-pant's relationship experiences.

Discussion

Findings from this study present the benefits of using a visual and participatory-empow-ered approach to add to traditional qualitative research methods when examining the influence of emotions on sexual risk-taking behaviours among MSM. Through this unique data collection process, we learned strategies for implementing a participant-empowered visual timeline in an ongoing qualitative study, including: the success in allowing the timeline to drive the interview; the importance of having guidelines to provide prompts in the activity, but also offering flexibility to deviate from the guidelines; and the value of using discrete imagery and colloquial language to increase participant comfort.

Since the timeline was the driving activity in the interviews, each interview was conducted as a systematic step-by-step process that flowed as the timeline was built. Rather than building the timeline at the beginning of the interview and discussing it later, participants built the timeline throughout the interview process. Each step was unpacked with follow-up questions and discussed in-depth before moving on to the next piece. These sequential steps enabled a dynamic process, with each piece of the timeline building on the previous one.

Having clear, yet flexible guidelines were also useful in the building of the timeline. Instructions offered general ideas for how participants should approach building the timeline, but they were able to deviate from those instructions in order to make the timeline more accurately tell their story. Interviewers encouraged participants to take ownership of their timelines and 'make it their own'. Some participants followed the rules exactly and went through the timeline in a more systematic process, describing their feelings and experiences with each step of the timeline. However, others changed the stickers, wrote in their own labels, and chose not to follow the instructions exactly as they were given. Interviewers encouraged these deviations, especially if it helped participants to further describe their experiences.

The visual aids of the timeline assisted with prompting discussion, but it was especially important that the cues that were used added to participant comfort. When researching a sensitive topic, like sexual behaviour, it is important to use tools to increase comfort levels through rapport-building in order to facilitate disclosure of intimate information (Dickson-Swift, James, Kippen, & Liamputtong, 2007). This becomes especially important when working with disenfranchised hard-to-reach or vulnerable populations (Liamputtong, 2006). The visual cues that we had were discrete; anybody else looking at the timeline would not have understood what the dots signified. Furthermore, these cues enabled participants to first place their experiences on the timeline rather than verbally describing their sexual experiences. In addition, the labels that we used to describe relationship definitions, emotions, and sexual experiences all used informal language and some labels even included profanity; often times, interviewers would read the words out loud first so that participants would be comfortable using and saying whichever words that felt most comfortable and natural. Labels also offered a variety of definitions that were open to interpretation. Interviewers always asked for how participants defined the terms that they used, which assisted interviewers and analysts to better understand and interpret the timelines and the meanings of the timelines.

There were some limitations in this study. We only applied these methods to one population (GBM) with one topic (emotions and sexual risk-taking). Therefore, we do not know how this method would be similar or different with a different topic and among a different population. Furthermore, all research was done in Atlanta, GA and we do not know how these methods would apply in other settings, especially resource-poor settings where access to timeline supplies may not be as readily available or as easily accessible to participants. In addition, there could have been social desirability bias when reporting behaviours in the PRDs; this could have resulted in under-reporting or over-reporting of sexual behaviour and/or emotions. PRD data were collected prospectively, but the debrief IDI was a retrospective examination of that prospective data and involved the interviewer interacting with the participant as they discussed their experiences; this interaction could have also added bias when the participants reflected on their experiences.

Still, these findings demonstrate that the use of innovative participant-empowered methods that go beyond traditional qualitative research can help to generate complex and nuanced data. These methods enabled enough flexibility to assist with participant disclosure and provided guidelines to capture the complex and dynamic nuances of a sensitive research question. The visual aids proved to be useful in providing discrete prompts to increase participant comfort and ease the interview process. It is important that qualitative data collection evolve towards a more participatory approach for gains in data quality and participant comfort.

Acknowledgement

This research was conducted at the Rollins School of Public Health at Emory University.

Disclosure statement

No potential conflict of interest was reported by the authors.

Funding

Research funding was supported by the University Research Committee at Emory University and the Center for AIDS Research at Emory University [P30 AI050409].

References

Ahmed, S. M., Beck, B., Maurana, C. A., & Newton, G. (2004). Overcoming barriers to effective community-based participatory research in US medical schools. *Education for Health, 17*(2), 141–151. doi:10.1080/13576280410001710969

Axinn, W. G., Pearce, L. D., & Ghimire, D. (1999). Innovations in life history calendar applications. *Social Science Research, 28*(3), 243–264. doi:10.1006/ssre.1998.0641

Bagnoli, A. (2009). Beyond the standard interview: The use of graphic elicitation and arts-based methods. *Qualitative Research, 9*(5), 547–570. doi:10.1177/1468794109343625

Bauermeister, J. A., Carballo-Diéguez, A., Ventuneac, A., & Dolezal, C. (2009). Assessing motivations to engage in intentional condomless anal intercourse in HIV-risk contexts ("bareback sex") among men who have sex with men. *AIDS Education and Prevention, 21*(2), 156. doi:10.1521/aeap.2009.21.2.156

Bauermeister, J. A., Leslie-Santana, M., Johns, M. M., Pingel, E., & Eisenberg, A. (2011). Mr. Right and Mr. Right now: Romantic and casual partner-seeking online among young men who have sex with men. *AIDS and Behavior, 15*(2), 261–272. doi:10.1007/s10461-010-9834-5

Bauermeister, J. A., Ventuneac, A., Pingel, E., & Parsons, J. T. (2012). Spectrums of love: Examining the relationship between romantic motivations and sexual risk among young gay and bisexual men. *AIDS and Behavior, 16*(6), 1549–1559. doi:10.1007/s10461-011-0123-8

Belcher, L., Sternberg, M. R., Wolitski, R. J., Halkitis, P., Hoff, C., & the Seropositive Urban Men's Study Team. (2005). Condom use and perceived risk of HIV transmission among sexually active HIV-positive men who have sex with men. *AIDS Education & Prevention, 17*(1), 79–89. doi:10.1521/aeap.17.1.79.58690

Belli, R. F. (1998). The structure of autobiographical memory and the event history calendar: Potential improvements in the quality of retrospective reports in surveys. *Memory, 6*(4), 383–406. doi:10.1080/741942610

Berg, R. C. (2009). Barebacking: A review of the literature. *Archives of Sexual Behavior, 38*(5), 754–764. doi:10.1007/s10508-008-9462-6

Blashill, A. J., Wilson, J. M., O'Cleirigh, C. M., Mayer, K. H., & Safren, S. A. (2014). Examining the correspondence between relationship identity and actual sexual risk behavior among HIV-positive men who have sex with men. *Archives of Sexual Behavior, 43*(1), 129–137. doi:10.1007/s10508-013-0209-7

Bourey, C., Stephenson, R., Bartel, D., & Rubardt, M. (2012). Pile sorting innovations: Exploring gender norms, power and equity in sub-Saharan Africa. *Global Public Health, 7*(9), 995–1008. doi:10.1080/17441692.2012.709259

Cacari-Stone, L., Wallerstein, N., Garcia, A. P., & Minkler, M. (2014). The promise of community-based participatory research for health equity: A conceptual model for bridging evidence with policy. *American Journal of Public Health, 104*(9), 1615–1623. doi:10.2105/AJPH.2014.301961

Carballo-Diéguez, A., & Bauermeister, J. (2004). "Barebacking": Intentional condomless anal sex in HIV-risk contexts. Reasons for and against Iit. *Journal of Homosexuality, 47*(1), 1–16. doi:10.1300/J082v047n01_01

Carballo-Dieguez, A., & Dolezal, C. (1996). HIV risk behaviors and obstacles to condom use among Puerto Rican men in New York City who have sex with men. *American Journal of Public Health, 86*(11), 1619–1622. doi:10.2105/AJPH.86.11.1619

Carballo-Diéguez, A., Ventuneac, A., Dowsett, G. W., Balan, I., Bauermeister, J., Remien, R. H., … Mabragaña, M. (2011). Sexual pleasure and intimacy among men who engage in "bareback sex". *AIDS and Behavior, 15*(1), 57–65. doi:10.1007/s10461-011-9900-7

Centers for Disease Control and Prevention. (2012). *Estimated HIV incidence in the United States, 2007–2010* (HIV Surveillance Supplemental Report, Vol. 17).

Centers for Disease Control and Prevention. (2014). *Preexposure prophylaxis for the prevention of HIV infection in the United States – 2014: A clinical practice guideline.*

Centers for Disease Control and Prevention. (2015). *Effective interventions: HIV prevention that works.* Retrieved from https://effectiveinterventions.cdc.gov/

Cornwall, A., & Jewkes, R. (1995). What is participatory research? *Social Science & Medicine, 41*(12), 1667–1676. doi:10.1016/0277-9536(95)00127-S

Cox, J., Beauchemin, J., & Allard, R. (2004). HIV status of sexual partners is more important than antiretroviral treatment related perceptions for risk taking by HIV positive MSM in Montreal, Canada. *Sexually Transmitted Infections, 80*(6), 518–523. doi:10.1136/sti.2004.011288

Davidovich, U., Wit, J., & Strobbe, W. (2006). Relationship characteristics and risk of HIV infection: Rusbult's investment model and sexual risk behavior of gay men in steady relationships. *Journal of Applied Social Psychology, 36*(1), 22–40. doi:10.1111/j.0021-9029.2006.00002.x

Dickson-Swift, V., James, E. L., Kippen, S., & Liamputtong, P. (2007). Doing sensitive research: What challenges do qualitative researchers face? *Qualitative Research, 7*(3), 327–353. doi:10.1177/1468794107078515

Finneran, C., & Stephenson, R. (2014). Intimate partner violence, minority stress, and sexual risk-taking among US men who have sex with men. *Journal of Homosexuality, 61*(2), 288–306. doi:10.1080/00918369.2013.839911

Fisher, C. M. (2012). Assessing developmental trajectories of sexual minority youth: Discrepant findings from a life history calendar and a self-administered survey. *Journal of LGBT Youth, 9*(2), 114–135. doi:10.1080/19361653.2012.649643

Freedman, D., Thornton, A., Camburn, D., Alwin, D., & Young-DeMarco, L. (1988). The life history calendar: A technique for collecting retrospective data. *Sociological Methodology, 18*(1), 37–68.

Green, L. W., George, M. A., Daniel, M., Frankish, C. J., Herbert, C., Bowie, W. R., & O'Neill, M. (1995). *Study of participatory research in health promotion. Review and recommendations for development of participatory research in health promotion in Canada.* Ottawa, ON: The Royal Society of Canada.

Guest, G., Namey, E. E., & Mitchell, M. L. (2012). *Collecting qualitative data: A field manual for applied research*. Los Angeles, CA: Sage.

Hoff, C. C., Chakravarty, D., Beougher, S. C., Neilands, T. B., & Darbes, L. A. (2012). Relationship characteristics associated with sexual risk behavior among MSM in committed relationships. *AIDS Patient Care and STDs, 26*(12), 738–745. doi:10.1089/apc.2012.0198

Israel, B. A., Eng, E., Schulz, A. J., & Parker, E. A. (Eds.). (2005). *Methods in community-based participatory research for health*. San Francisco, CA: John Wiley.

Israel, B. A., Krieger, J., Vlahov, D., Ciske, S., Foley, M., Fortin, P., ... Palermo, A. G. (2006). Challenges and facilitating factors in sustaining community-based participatory research partnerships: Lessons learned from the Detroit, New York City and Seattle Urban research centers. *Journal of Urban Health, 83*(6), 1022–1040. doi:10.1007/s11524-006-9110-1

Israel, B. A., Schulz, A. J., Parker, E. A., & Becker, A. B. (1998). Review of community-based research: Assessing partnership approaches to improve public health. *Annual Review of Public Health, 19*(1), 173–202. doi:10.1146/annurev.publhealth.19.1.173

Israel, B. A., Schulz, A. J., Parker, E. A., & Becker, A. B. (2003). Critical issues in developing and following community-based participatory research principles. In M. Minkler & N. Wallerstein (Eds.), *Community-based participatory research for health: From process to outcomes* (1st ed., pp. 53–76). San Francisco, CA: Jossey-Bass.

Kabiru, C. W., Luke, N., Izugbara, C. O., & Zulu, E. M. (2010). The correlates of HIV testing and impacts on sexual behavior: Evidence from a life history study of young people in Kisumu, Kenya. *BMC Public Health, 10*(1), 412. doi:10.1186/1471-2458-10-412

Kellerman, S. E., Lehman, J. S., Lansky, A., Stevens, M. R., Hecht, F. M., Bindman, A. B., & Wortley, P. M. (2002). HIV testing within at-risk populations in the United States and the reasons for seeking or avoiding HIV testing. *Journal of Acquired Immune Deficiency Syndromes, 31*(2), 202–210. doi:10.1097/01.QAI.0000024005.76120.97

Liamputtong, P. (2006). *Researching the vulnerable: A guide to sensitive research methods*. Los Angeles, CA: Sage.

Luke, N., Clark, S., & Zulu, E. M. (2011). The relationship history calendar: Improving the scope and quality of data on youth sexual behavior. *Demography, 48*(3), 1151–1176. doi:10.1007/s13524-011-0051-2

Macaulay, A. C., Commanda, L. E., Freeman, W. L., Gibson, N., McCabe, M. L., Robbins, C. M., & Twohig, P. L. (1999). Participatory research maximises community and lay involvement. *British Medical Journal, 319*(7212), 774–778.

MacKellar, D. A., Valleroy, L. A., Secura, G. M., Behel, S., Bingham, T., Celentano, D. D., ... Shehan, D. (2005). Unrecognized HIV infection, risk behaviors, and perceptions of risk among young men who have sex with men: Opportunities for advancing HIV prevention in the third decade of HIV/AIDS. *Journal of Acquired Immune Deficiency Syndromes, 38*(5), 603–614. doi:10.1097/01.qai.0000141481.48348.7e

MacKellar, D. A., Valleroy, L. A., Secura, G. M., Behel, S., Bingham, T., Celentano, D. D., ... Thiede, H. (2007). Perceptions of lifetime risk and actual risk for acquiring HIV among young men who have sex with men. *AIDS and Behavior, 11*(2), 263–270. doi:10.1007/s10461-006-9136-0

Martyn, K. K., & Belli, R. F. (2002). Retrospective data collection using event history calendars. *Nursing Research, 51*(4), 270–274. doi:10.1097/00006199-200207000-00008

Minkler, M. (2004). Ethical challenges for the "outside" researcher in community-based participatory research. *Health Education & Behavior, 31*(6), 684–697. doi:10.1177/1090198104269566

Minkler, M. (2005). Community-based research partnerships: Challenges and opportunities. *Journal of Urban Health, 82*, ii3–ii12. doi:10.1093/jurban/jti034

Minkler, M. (2010). Linking science and policy through community-based participatory research to study and address health disparities. *American Journal of Public Health, 100*(S1), S81–S87. doi:10.2105/AJPH.2009.165720

Minkler, M., Blackwell, A. G., Thompson, M., & Tamir, H. (2003). Community-based participatory research: Implications for public health funding. *American Journal of Public Health, 93*(8), 1210–1213. doi:10.2105/AJPH.93.8.1210

Minkler, M., & Wallerstein, N. (2010). *Community-based participatory research for health: From process to outcomes.* San Francisco, CA: John Wiley.

Montoya, M. J., & Kent, E. E. (2011). Dialogical action: Moving from community-based to community-driven participatory research. *Qualitative Health Research, 21*(7), 1000–1011. doi:10.1177/1049732311403500

Mustanski, B., Newcomb, M. E., & Clerkin, E. M. (2011). Relationship characteristics and sexual risk-taking in young men who have sex with men. *Health Psychology, 30*(5), 597. doi:10.1037/a0023858

Newcomb, M. E., Ryan, D. T., Garofalo, R., & Mustanski, B. (2014). The effects of sexual partnership and relationship characteristics on three sexual risk variables in young men who have sex with men. *Archives of Sexual Behavior, 43*(1), 61–72. doi:10.1007/s10508-013-0207-9

Patton, M. Q. (2005). Qualitative research. *Encyclopedia of Statistics in Behavioral Science.* doi:10.1002/0470013192.bsa514

Prosser, J., & Loxley, A. (2008). *Introducing visual methods: ESRC National Centre for Research Methods review paper.* Leeds: National Centre for Research Methods.

Rogers, R. W., & Prentice-Dunn, S. (1997). Protection motivation theory. In D. S. Gochman (Ed.), *Handbook of health behavior research 1: Personal and social determinants* (pp. 113–132). New York, NY: Plenum Press.

Rosenstock, I. M. (1974). The health belief model and preventive health behavior. *Health Education Monographs, 2*(4), 354–386.

Suarez, T., & Kauth, M. R. (2001). Assessing basic HIV transmission risks and the contextual factors associated with HIV risk behavior in men who have sex with men. *Journal of Clinical Psychology, 57*(5), 655–669. doi:10.1002/jclp.1035

Suarez, T., & Miller, J. (2001). Negotiating risks in context: A perspective on unprotected anal intercourse and barebacking among men who have sex with men – where do we go from here? *Archives of Sexual Behavior, 30*(3), 287–300. doi:10.1023/A:1002700130455

Sullivan, P. S., Carballo-Diéguez, A., Coates, T., Goodreau, S. M., McGowan, I., Sanders, E. J., … Sanchez, J. (2012). Successes and challenges of HIV prevention in men who have sex with men. *The Lancet, 380*(9839), 388–399. doi:10.1016/S0140-6736(12)60955-6

Viswanathan, M., Ammerman, A., Eng, E., Garlehner, G., Lohr, K. N., Griffith, D., … Lux, L. (2004). Community-based participatory research: Assessing the evidence. *Evidence Report/Technology Assessment, 99,* 1–8.

Wallerstein, N., & Duran, B. (2010). Community-based participatory research contributions to intervention research: The intersection of science and practice to improve health equity. *American Journal of Public Health, 100*(S1), S40–S46. doi:10.2105/AJPH.2009.184036

Weinstein, N. D. (1988). The precaution adoption process. *Health Psychology, 7*(4), 355–386.

White, D., & Stephenson, R. (2014). Using community mapping to understand family planning behavior. *Field Methods, 26*(4), 406–420. doi:10.1177/1525822X14529256

Yoshihama, M., Clum, K., Crampton, A., & Gillespie, B. (2002). Measuring the lifetime experience of domestic violence: Application of the life history calendar method. *Violence and Victims, 17*(3), 297–317. doi:10.1891/vivi.17.3.297.33663

Regarding realities: Using photo-based projective techniques to elicit normative and alternative discourses on gender, relationships, and sexuality in Mozambique

Emily S. Holman[a], Catherine K. Harbour[b,c], Rosa Valéria Azevedo Said[c] and Maria Elena Figueroa[a,c]

[a]Department of Health, Behavior and Society, Johns Hopkins Bloomberg School of Public Health, Johns Hopkins University, Baltimore, MD, USA; [b]Children's Investment Fund Foundation, London, UK; [c]Johns Hopkins Center for Communication Programs, Johns Hopkins University, Baltimore, MD, USA

ABSTRACT
This paper argues for the methodological merit of photo-based projective techniques (PT) in formative HIV communication research. We used this technique in Mozambique to study multiple sexual partnerships (MSPs) and the roles of social and gender norms in promoting or discouraging these behaviours. Facilitators used ambiguous photographs and vignettes to ease adult men and women into discussions of sexual risk behaviour and HIV transmission. Visuals upheld a third-person perspective in discussions, enabling participants to safely project their worldviews onto the photographed characters, and indirectly share their attitudes, normative environments, personal and peer experiences, perceived risks and benefits, and theories about motivations for extramarital sex. Visually grounded storylines contained rich detail about the circumstances and interpersonal conversations that contextualise MSP behaviour and norms. The research yielded findings about conflicting social practices of public encouragement and private disapproval. Despite concerns around the verifiability of PTs, the repetition and convergence in the elicited conversations – and confirmation through subsequent campaign design and evaluation – suggest these techniques can reliably elicit information for formative public health and communication research on psychosocial and normative factors.

Introduction

> ... the only material we have at our disposal for making a picture of the whole world is supplied by the various portions of that world of which we have already had experience.
>
> (William James, *A pluralistic universe*, 1909, p. 8)

Visual projective techniques for health behaviour research

A longstanding challenge of the HIV epidemic has been 'keeping sexual behaviour at the centre of the conversation' (Timberg & Halperin, 2012) – not only in HIV policy and programmes, but also in research that informs and reforms HIV interventions. This methodological paper describes our experience using photo-based projective techniques (PT) within focus group discussions (FGDs) as part of preparatory or 'formative' research to guide the design of HIV communication programmes on multiple sexual partnerships (MSPs) in Mozambique. Findings from this formative research are described elsewhere (Said, 2008; Said & Figueroa, 2008) as are evaluation results of the communication campaign that this research informed (Figueroa & Kincaid, 2014; Figueroa et al., 2015; Figueroa, Kincaid, & Hurley, 2014). Here, we focus on describing visual PTs and the nature of data they can elicit, as we have found limited examples outlining how PTs can be used for exploratory or formative health behaviour research. We found PTs particularly suited to investigating psychosocial constructs, such as implicit attitudes and deep-seated norms, which are difficult to assess through direct questioning, especially for sensitive issues like sexual behaviour. The purpose of this piece is not to engage long and thoughtful debates on gender norms, sexual risk, and concurrent partnering, but rather to share our experience with PTs as a methodology to inform development of strategic health communication.

Reducing sexual concurrency to prevent new HIV infections in Mozambique

In late 2007, when we designed this study, 16% of Mozambique's adults were HIV-positive and incidence was rising (Conselho Nacional de Combate ao HIV e SIDA [National Council for the Combat of HIV and AIDS, CNCS], 2006).[1] Behavioural investigators linked MSP networks to the epidemic's growth (Halperin & Epstein, 2004; Luke & Kurz, 2002; Morris & Kretzschmar, 1995; UNAIDS, 2007), as did regional policymakers (SADC, 2006). In Mozambique, the National AIDS Council and HIV researchers also identified MSP behaviours, including concurrent, transactional, and cross-generational sex, to be prevalent drivers of the national epidemic (CNCS, 2006; Manuel, 2007; Pearson et al., 2007; UNAIDS, 2008).

The National AIDS Council called for communication campaigns that could change existing social norms around MSP behaviours (CNCS, 2006), especially among cohabitating adults.[2] Infection rates were highest in the provinces of Maputo (26%), Sofala (23%), and Zambézia (19%) (UNAIDS, 2008). The task was to design, implement, and evaluate evidence- and theory-based health communication programmes to reduce MSP-related behaviour and weaken social support for MSP, while avoiding a morality framing of MSP. Inventive research would be needed to thoughtfully inform these interventions.

Previous findings from Mozambique on multiple sexual partnering

Studies in Mozambique had identified inequitable sexual and gender norms and structural economic disadvantage as motivators for MSP (Aboim, 2009; Agadjanian, 2002; Bagnolle & Chamo, 2003; CNCS, 2006; Hawkins, Mussá, & Abuxahama, 2005; Karlyn, 2005; Machel, 2001; Manuel, 2007; da Silva et al., 2006). Researchers had examined drivers such as MSP-related HIV risk perception (Agadjanian, 2005; Agha, Kusanthan, Longfield, Klein, & Berman, 2002; Luke & Kurz, 2002; Prata, Morris, Mazive, Vahidnia, & Stehr, 2006), social expectations around gender and status performance in sexual partnering (Hawkins et al., 2005; Karlyn, 2005; Manuel, 2007), social beliefs about MSP prevention

(Agadjanian, 2005), and the role of sexual desire and sexual dissatisfaction (Hawkins et al., 2005; Manuel, 2005), with an understanding that MSP was more normative for men than women (Agadjanian, 2005).

Gaps remained in understanding the full range of values, motivations, attitudes, and norms supporting or challenging MSP across age groups (Kuate-Defo, 2004; SADC, 2006), the nature of family and peer influence on adult sexual behaviour (Bagnolle & Chamo, 2003), and how HIV risk was perceived across distinct MSP scenarios. There were also calls to examine how shifting gender expectations and diverse individual values might be impacting MSP, while respecting that MSP practices may be a 'functional way of life' for some communities (Manuel, 2007, p. 13).

Our paper's aims

This paper describes our use and assessment of visual PTs to elicit participant perspectives on MSP to address the gaps identified above. These methodologies were comfortable for participants, despite the delicate nature of the topic. Local facilitators learned to use the techniques with minimal training, and were not required to probe for self-disclosure about intimate topics. The methods minimised language bias and the risk that facilitators prompt participants towards parroting socially desirable responses. The study revealed emerging attitudes that questioned prevailing MSP norms, offering an opening for communication programming to address MSP-related HIV risks and the norms that support them.

Subsequent research

Since the time of our fieldwork, additional studies in Mozambique have improved understanding of MSP predictors and their contribution to HIV infection (Audet et al., 2010; Pearson et al., 2011), MSP motivations and gender issues (N'weti, 2008; Population Services International [PSI], 2010; Vera Cruz & Maússe, 2014), and pathways by which economic inequality contributes to gender differences in MSP behaviour and culpability (Bandali, 2011). Anthropological work has broadened understanding of the range of personal and family motives for sexual risk-taking and risk protection across economic classes (Groes-Green, 2009a, 2010, 2012, 2013). Authors have proposed how health and social marketing can improve to address HIV risk communication for Mozambicans, especially for community subgroups (Baltazar et al., 2015; Nalá et al., 2015), and have shed light on why some MSP communication fails to resonate with marginalised populations (Groes-Green, 2009a).

Background

Formative research for health communication about MSP

The Government of Mozambique sought to address MSP within broader HIV health promotion efforts. Health communication is a critical component of health promotion, bringing together theory and practice to activate communication processes that prompt behaviour change (Rimal & Lapinski, 2009). Successful interventions rely on rigorous formative research to design strategic messaging approaches that are relevant to the audience (O'Sullivan, Yonkler, Morgan, & Merritt, 2003). This research 'gives the audience a chance to speak first – to provide valuable information about their own situations, beliefs and values, current and past behaviour, and hopes and dreams for a better life' (Kincaid, Delate, Storey, & Figueroa, 2012, p. 306). Often, formative studies use qualitative methods such as FGDs to elicit a deeper understanding of influences at multiple levels (individual, organisational, and structural) and to identify concepts, phrases, and tone used when people talk about the behavioural practices of interest. For taboo communication topics such as HIV, formative research is most useful when it can isolate terms and metaphors that convey clear meanings across audience segments. These everyday verbal framings, when carefully selected, inform the design of health communication content that is meaningful to target groups (Kincaid et al., 2012).

Research setting requirements

We were challenged to design formative research that could overcome participants' reluctance to discuss taboo sexual opinions and practices. For this task, we favoured FGDs over individual interviews because FGDs generate a broader range of responses and a more in-depth depiction of the multi-layered normative environment (Ward, Bertrand, & Brown, 1991; Wutich, Lant, White, Larson, & Gartin, 2010). However, group members tend to silence themselves when touchy subjects come up, even when they receive positive reinforcement (Wutich et al., 2010). As sexuality researchers, we needed to 'create ... a climate of trust that [would] allow people to talk freely about intimate matters' (Groes-Green, Barrett, & Izugbara, 2011, p. 49).

Also, to elicit socially normative values about gender and sexual partnerships, it was important to have participants talking in peer groups with minimal facilitator influence on and involvement in group dialogue. The study needed to gather information not only on these dominant norms around MSP, but also on the complex *range* of these norms, including minority positions, emerging attitudes, and discordant opinions, which would be crucial for designing communication to challenge and transform harmful gender norms (MacPhail, 2003).

To run these groups, we needed facilitators who could speak local languages, were familiar with the study concepts, and had experience probing on sexuality issues (Wutich et al., 2010). Limited local researcher availability and restricted time for implementing the study made it necessary to design instruments that facilitators could learn within a weeklong workshop. We opted to employ PTs, judging they had compelling methodological potential to satisfy this complex set of group elicitation aims.

PTs: underutilised and promising

PTs are a broad set of associational psychometric tools that were organised under the term 'projective' in the 1930s (Pinto, 2014). They were originally developed for clinical psychological assessment, whereby individuals would be shown a series of pictures or incomplete phrases and then asked to explain what they see or extend the phrase. The Rorschack or 'ink blot' test is one example. PTs can include the interpretation of images, such as drawings or photographs, as well as sentence completion, word associations, and ordering activities (Donoghue, 2000; Korchin, 1976).

The traditional psychoanalytic assumption is that the past fears and inner drives of the subconscious self are 'projected' onto the patient's responses to the tools. This idea of projection later expanded beyond Freudian theory to indicate 'the dislocation of feelings, ideas and emotions that one considers positive and valuable, even conscious ones', onto an external object (Pinto, 2014, p. 140). How one understands and evaluates the outside world within one's interior mental world ('perception') is ultimately projected onto one's assessment of outside objects ('apperception'). The direction the individual takes in interpretation belies his or her broader associational pattern, which is influenced by deep-seated emotions, experiences, and memory (Pinto, 2014).

PTs fell into clinical disfavour over concerns about objectivity, and scholars questioned the methods' reliability and validity (Lilienfeld, Wood, & Garb, 2000; Pinto, 2014; Piotrowski, 2015; Soley, 2010). Researchers in marketing, agriculture, consumer research, sociology, anthropology, and cultural studies re-appropriated visual projection as a study elicitation tool (Collier, 1967; Harper, 2002; Soley, 2006). Communication and marketing authors have highlighted PTs as an under-tapped resource for social-behavioural research (Pich & Dean, 2015; Soley, 2006; Wiehagen et al., 2007), because they provide an indirect method for eliciting attitudes, behavioural evaluations, motivations, perceived social norms, and personal experience without the invasiveness or social desirability bias of more direct methods (Curry, 1986; Donoghue, 2000; Regan & Liaschenko, 2008; Soley, 2010; Wiehagen et al., 2007).

PTs offer a way to access thoughts or feelings that are cognitively distant, under-processed, or 'taken for granted' (Wiehagen et al., 2007). While these may not be quickly retrievable in direct questioning ('What are your views about cross-generational sex?'), they may be easier to articulate in response to questions about a third-party character ('What do you think about this man who is dating this adolescent?'). Participants may speak more comfortably in the third person ('he feels that ...') instead of the first ('I feel that ...'). Researchers assume that in speaking of others, participants are indirectly speaking of themselves or the world they know (Catterall & Ibbotson, 2000; Wiehagen et al., 2007). Thus, PTs offer a less-burdensome way for respondents to access their own values and experiences, by evaluating and characterising the 'other' – the projective object.

This object can take form in language, such as word associations, or visually through images or photos. Visuals are inherently polysemic (Prosser, 2006), inviting a broad range of possible interpretations. Photographic visuals are highly informative, offering a 'realistic reconstruction' of 'objects, persons, and physical and social circumstances' in one glance (Lapenta, 2011, p. 203) and triggering a deep range of feelings and memories (Harper, 2002). Photo interpretation is customarily viewed as a more collaborative research exercise than traditional interviewing (Lapenta, 2011), with images helping break down conventions held by both researchers and participants and forcing the reconstruction of a shared understanding (Harper, 2002).

We anticipated that discussion about characters in photo-based vignettes would provide a low-threat entrée to private topics of sexual mores and HIV and yield information on deep rooted gender and sexual norms.

Methods: incorporation of visual PTs into formative HIV health communication research

The research described here was conducted between November 2007 and March 2008 in the Central Mozambican provinces of Zambézia (districts of Mocuba, Morrumbala and the city of Quelimane), Sofala (city of Beira and district of Dondo), and the Southern province of Maputo (districts of Marracuene and Boane). The research encompassed in-depth interviews with key informants,[3] which are not described here, and discussion groups facilitated with PTs, which are the focus of this manuscript. The study was approved by the Johns Hopkins Bloomberg School of Public Health Institutional Review Board (IRB) and the National Bioethics Committee of the Ministry of Health in Mozambique.

Instrument design

Research staff culled ambiguous photos depicting couples and family relationship scenes from the Photoshare archive and from photonovela-style magazines published in Mozambique by N'weti Health Communication and Population Services International (PSI), who generously shared them for use in the study. We embedded photos in a four-part facilitation guide. Facilitators were instructed not to mention 'HIV' until halfway through, in hopes that its initial invocation would come from respondents, not from the research instrument.

The sessions opened with a 'talking only' discussion about characteristics of the ideal man and the ideal woman (part 1). Next, using unscripted photos (part 2), the facilitator asked participants to interpret what they thought was happening in the photo, imagine what had happened just before the moment captured in the photo, and postulate what was going to happen next.

The unscripted photos were followed by a series of scripted photos (part 3). For each, the facilitator read a one- or two-line set-up, followed by questions about each character in the script. Facilitators asked participants to describe, for example, the character's motivations or fears, how their peers viewed them, or how they might interact with their fictional spouse or extended family.

Finally, in two longer vignettes (part 4), the facilitator showed a photo and read a one-paragraph story of the character's history and current situation. One vignette was about concurrent MSP (the case of Samuel) and the other was about a transactional cross-generational MSP relationship (the case of Fatima and João). For each vignette, the facilitator asked about HIV transmission, risk perception, interpersonal communication ('Will Samuel share this problem with someone or will he keep silent, and why?'), social norms, and other factors that influence one's *ideation* or 'ways of thinking' about MSP (Kincaid, 2000, p. 724).

Field team

To accommodate linguistic differences, facilitators were trained separately for each province. Most facilitators were middle-income professionals who grew up in the province and were native speakers of both the local language and Portuguese, with prior social science research experience and academic training.

We conducted a five-day training for each regional team. Training covered health communication and psychosocial theories, research ethics, group facilitation skills, classroom simulation, and field practice. Facilitator trainees field-tested the discussion guide in local dialect. Training emphasised maintaining a natural but neutral voice tone and facial expressions, to avoid showing approval or disapproval around any of the sexual behaviours or scenarios.

Study participants and data collection

Sampling was intended to broadly represent the diversity of livelihoods and social practices in the study provinces, purposively sampling 2–3 districts per province, and within each district, a mix of urban, peri-urban, and rural neighbourhoods. Within each neighbourhood, we held separate discussion groups with young adult men (ages 25–35), older adult men (ages 35–50), and adult women (ages 25–40). A gender-matched facilitator moderated the discussion while a co-facilitator operated the audio recording device. Participants could express themselves in their native language or in Portuguese. Discussions lasted about two hours, and took place under trees, around tables, in meeting halls, or other neutral locations that were out of sight and earshot of other community members. A total of 17 group sessions were held in Zambézia, 10 in Sofala and 10 in Maputo with the combined participation of over 250 adults.

Data preparation and analysis

We used Atlas-Ti 5.2 QDA software (Gmbh, Berlin) and MS Word to analyse Portuguese transcripts translated by native speakers from the local languages. Transcript review drew on principles of discourse analysis, attending to individual statements as selectively voiced expressions of consciousness situated within the interpersonal group context (Said, 2008).

Statements within the 37 transcripts were coded according to areas of inquiry, such as gender roles or types of MSP behaviour. Within these, analysis highlighted the ideational constructs expressed (risk perception, social norms, motivations, etc.). In addition, data analysts assigned new theoretical codes *en vivo* as they identified themes and patterns. Researchers examined whether statements were challenged or reinforced as other participants within the same group 'chimed in'. We gave special attention to recurring arguments across topics and discourse attributes such as silences, interruptions, emphatic markers, unresolved ambiguities, and the omission of opinions or details about a specific topic. Thematic consistency was assessed within and across neighbourhoods, provinces, and respondents' sex.

Findings: attributes of qualitative data generated projectively

This section describes notable features of the data generated using visual PTs within group discussions. The findings regarding the attitudes and practices of MSP and other HIV risk behaviours are described elsewhere (Holman, 2008; Said, 2008; Said & Figueroa, 2008).

Projection in the unscripted photos: one image, multiple readings

The ambiguous, unscripted photos (part 2 of facilitators' guide) allowed participants to jointly craft a story to explain the character's actions and feelings. The facilitator (F) encouraged participants (P) to give multiple interpretations, creating the opportunity to agree with or refute prior contributions. For example, in response to an ambiguous photo of a man in a towel with a clothed woman in the foreground (Figure 1), distinct readings were easily proposed:

> P: It could be that the husband is returning from work and the wife has not cooked for him.
> …
> P: It could also be that the man came home late and when the woman asks, in addition to not saying where he was, he prefers to use force to shut her up.
>
> (Older men, Morrumbala, Zambézia)

Another group's members, dissecting the same photo, collaboratively created a story of marriage turned sour, possibly by an extramarital affair:

> P: In this photo I see a woman and a man beside her undressed with a towel on.
> …
> P 2: In my view a fight is about to happen.
> P 1: Perhaps the man doesn't want his wife, or the wife committed an error, or the man got another woman and is trying to throw his wife out.
> …
> F: … What happened before this?
> P: … First they fell in love and got married … and then there came a phase where loving transformed into fighting because … one of the two of them isn't behaving well.
> F: What will happen next?
> P: Next there will be divorce, or … perhaps some people can come to counsel them in their home, they can reunite through this counsel.
>
> (Young men, Quelimane, Zambézia)

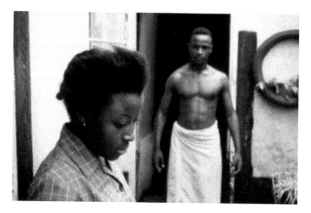

Figure 1. Unscripted photo: Man in towel. Source: ©1993 John Riber, Media for Development International (MFDI), Courtesy of Photoshare.

While the details are different, both groups project a ready familiarity with mistrust and lack of communication leading to violence between spouses – one example of how photos elicited interpretations that were diverse yet thematically convergent.

Without explicitly talking about their experiences or feelings, participants nonetheless shared personal insights. The emotional vividness of hypothetical portrayals suggested men and women were speaking from personal or closely observed experiences.

Projection in the scripted photos: expanding typical scenes

The scripted photos (part 3) were also ambiguous, but included a one- to three-line caption. Surprisingly, these captions did not limit the group to just one storyline, perhaps because at this point in the discussion, participants were ripe to volunteer additional points of view. Here, a respondent offered three possible storylines for the woman with HIV (Figure 2):

> In the case where a husband is positive and the wife is not, the wife continues to take care of the husband … but in many cases the husband forces the wife to have sex without a condom, alleging 'we are married', but if he is very sick he doesn't stand a chance, he has to accept what the wife says.
>
> (Women, Beira, Sofala)

Participants made it clear they intended their descriptions to speak not to exceptional cases, but to general social practices ('in many cases … '). They used the scripted photo as a comparison point for scenarios that were or were not typical. In contrast to concerns that PT participants generate 'fanciful' stories (Belk, 2006, p. 146), we observed participants to strive for realistic depictions.

Projection in the photo vignettes: condoning and condemning

In the photo vignettes (part 4), the visual was accompanied with the character's background and recent history. One vignette described a married adult man, João, who pursues a relationship with the adolescent Fatima. Following the story, the facilitator asked scripted questions about the characters:

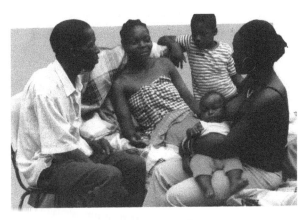

Figure 2. Scripted photo: Woman sick with HIV. Source: N'weti Health Communication.

F: Could João's wife have some problem?
P: She'll have a problem.
F: Like what problem?
P: That, my husband is now going after children, he leaves me at home with the kids and he seeks out others, other girls, teenage lovers, hmmph. ... out there where the husband is walking he is getting disease to bring back to the home, contaminating his wife in the house ... .

(Young men, Mocuba, Zambézia)

The participant indirectly projects his disapproval of cross-generational sex by using negative phrases ('going after children') and associating the relationship with disease ('contaminating'). He uses metaphor for MSP ('out there where the husband is walking').

Opining on the MSP vignette about Samuel (Figure 3), some men approved of Samuel's extramarital partner but criticised him for not having used a condom with her:

F: Could Samuel have avoided getting infected?
P1: Yes ... using a condom, being faithful to his wife, controlling his own outings.
P2: He should've tried to find out the [HIV] status of his lover before getting involved without a condom.

(Young men, Mocuba, Zambézia)

Similar statements expressing negative attitudes towards MSP, or towards certain categories of MSP, were consistent across groups and study sites. This personal disapproval of a publicly reinforced behaviour was one of several new findings incorporated into the MSP communication programme.

Nature of the data elicited using PTs

Mock dialogues and internal monologues. Participants formulated dialogue for characters in the scenes, giving insight into norms governing how sexual behaviour can be discussed – or not –within the photos' dyadic scenarios (husband-wife, youth-godmother, etc.). One female participant conveyed the sensitive nature of spousal conversations in her proposed script for a photographed wife, who refers to sex with the metaphor of eating:

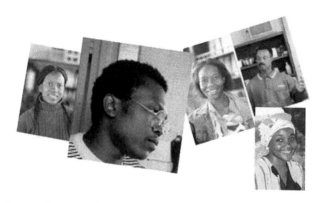

Figure 3. Photo vignette: The case of Samuel. Sources: N'weti Health Communication; ©1990, Media for Development International (MFDI), Courtesy of Photoshare and © 1994, John Riber, MFDI, Courtesy of Photoshare.

... when he 'walks around' in a way that you don't like, sometimes you can ask your husband **'And here there isn't anything to eat?'** and he gets mad at you ... he begins to insult you, then this is not a good man.   (Women, Quelimane, Zambézia)

The following mock dialogue was proposed after viewing an unscripted photo of an older woman talking to an adolescent (Figure 4):

This daughter here is in the home and went to her grandmother's house to ask for advice, and the grandmother asks, 'What is going on, my child?', and she says, 'Grandmother, I am being driven out of my home,' and she says, 'My dear granddaughter, my dear child, I always tell you to fully respect your husband and his family, because where you are it is not like here, over there you have no say and you do not decide. You have to be like me, here in the home with my husband and I always respect him.'   (Men, Boane, Maputo)

In addition to showcasing rules governing discussion of sex, these mock dialogues illustrated *how* conversation reinforces or challenges the norms that influence behavioural choices.

Frequently participants also composed inner thoughts and self-talk for depicted characters:

These men don't have this thing of seeking out another woman. He stays in good comfort and begins to think, 'If I begin to do something I'm going to contaminate my woman, my family, it's not worth the cost, better for me to sit and conserve myself.'
                                                                 (Young men, Mocuba, Zambézia)

These inner monologues presented ways men and women may rationalise their relationship actions – or inactions – and expanded understanding of motivations perceived to drive these behaviours.

Perceived rewards and judgments. Visual PTs facilitated descriptions of a range of ideational constructs sought in the study, including the perceived costs and benefits surrounding MSP:

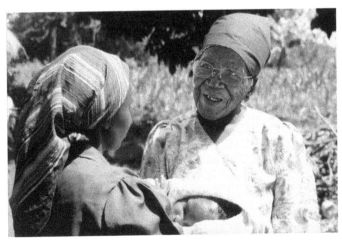

Figure 4. Unscripted photo: Young woman with old woman. Sources: © 1995, John Riber, MFDI, Courtesy of Photoshare and © 2010, Cpl. Scott Schmidt, USMC.
Note. This is an edited composite of two images created to represent the original photo used in the PT study, courtesy of PSI/Mozambique, for which the digital records have since been lost due to an electronic media malfunction. The original image did not include an infant child.

... that is why many women want men who are married, because they are well taken care of by other women's husbands, and she also does not have expenses because the wife washes that man's clothes, the wife does everything but only she (the lover) gets the money, that is why she wants her friend's husband.

(Women, Boane, Maputo)

Participants revealed their attitudes indirectly in *how* they framed responses. This participant's use of 'organised' and pejorative phrasing of MSP as being 'all over the place' suggest his admiration for fidelity:

Others are different because this is an organised couple ... in the sense that, for example, this man is with his woman at home, they are just understanding each other, the two people, you and your wife. Meanwhile there are other men who leave their own woman at home to go outside and find other women with a lot going on, they are all over the place.

(Older men, Mocuba, Zambézia)

Norms. PT conversations elicited both descriptive norms (perceived majority behaviours) and injunctive norms (perceived ideal behaviours). Here, the participant uses the man feeding the baby (Figure 5) to articulate what he believes the majority of men think:

This man is different from the majority because many men do this but it is not consistent. Many men think that they have more rights than women when in reality they have the same rights.

(Men, Dondo, Sofala)

Scripted facilitator prompts made it easy for groups to articulate multiple normative viewpoints. Here, considering normative injunctions, participants suggest youth may view MSP with an adolescent to be laudable or deplorable, depending upon which peer group you ask:

F: What do João's friends think of his behaviour?
P1: (brief pause) There are some that don't like it, and there are others that like that he has [a teenage girl], that have the same idea as João.
P2: That it is better to walk around with little girls than with his own woman.
P3: ... there are others that say 'that João is too much [older], she must be his daughter ... '.

(Women, Mocuba, Zambézia

Locally defined conceptual categories of MSP. Photo-based projection and vignettes allowed facilitators to avoid use of international health jargon, such as 'concurrency' and 'multiple sex partnerships' in favour of colloquial terms introduced by group members. Participants repeatedly used the euphemisms *andar fora* and *ir la fora* ('to walk outside/cheat' and 'to go outside') for a relationship outside the home (Holman, 2008). *Andar e se proteger –* 'walking [outside] and protecting oneself' referred to extramarital sex with a condom, which many respondents framed as consonant with fidelity because it protects the main partner from HIV and extramarital pregnancy. In contrast, the term *se espalhar* ('to disperse oneself all over the place/be out of control') was framed negatively, as a complete violation of marriage. These MSP typologies were coherent across sites (Said, 2008), and served as key components of the resulting intervention.

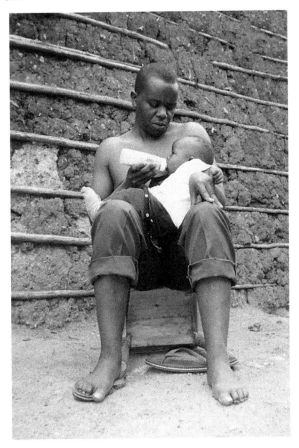

Figure 5. Scripted photo: Man with baby. Source: ©2003 Jones Kilonzo, Courtesy of Photoshare.

Discussion: advantages of projective photo-based elicitation

PTs yielded richer data on sexual norms and attitudes than we believe direct questioning methods would have elicited, generating new findings (described elsewhere [Holman, 2008; Said, 2008; Said & Figueroa, 2008]). We encourage researchers to consider PTs, especially when studying complex or invasive topics, when seeking to avoid circumscribing participants' responses, or when facilitators may have limited qualitative experience.

Feasibility. Facilitators new to PTs mastered the tools rapidly. Group participants quickly grasped the third-personing exercises and their implied relationship to 'real life' issues.

Increased comfort, reduced bias. Participants enjoyed the photos, became emotionally and intellectually engaged, and stayed interested through long discussions. Conversations about fictional characters' sex lives were surprisingly relaxed, suggesting the groups had created a safe setting for participants to discuss topics that could have been awkward with traditional facilitation. Even quieter group members participated, thereby reducing selection bias by including their perspectives, echoing others' findings that photos can bring fuller participation from those with less 'verbal skill' or inclination (Curry, 1986). PT transcripts yielded very few self-disclosures and made any first-person stories seem hypothetical, bolstering participants' confidentiality and protecting against 'overdisclosure of sensitive information' – a potential pitfall of traditional focus groups (Morgan & Krueger, 1993, p. 7).

Order of elicitation. We found it was important to introduce ambiguous photos early in the process, to create space for participants to introduce taboo topics in local vernacular. Thus, the framing later introduced with structured questions still invited the breadth of associations previously brought to unscripted photos.

Rich stories and dialogue. Participants told informative and detailed stories when they 'read' visuals. Stories created a more palpable, intricate depiction of behavioural context than a generalising exercise such as concept mapping, where essential categories of influence are generated but illustrative details are not. Mock dialogues modelled communication within couples and communities. These conversations were useful in designing vignettes, slogans, and other content for communication programmes that resonated with the audience.

Narrative participation. Although researchers selected photos and vignettes, participants appropriated them and imposed their own personal and collective interpretations. In this 'narrative participation,' they could adopt, tincture, or override meanings researchers may have inadvertently embedded. The first mention of 'HIV' in all discussion groups was from a participant, not the facilitator. Compared to a traditional focus group, the facilitator played a much reduced role in terms of summarising and framing the discussion. The ambiguous photos and unfinished vignettes constituted engaging 'puzzles of desire' that participants wanted to solve, 'pav[ing] the way for shared interpretations of intimate encounters' (Groes-Green, 2012, p. 57). These 'problem-solving' opportunities (Wutich et al., 2010) further increased member participation.

Eliciting normative and minority scripts. Participants' multiple interpretations allowed for full expression of marginal views that might have been 'crossed off the list' in a consensus-seeking methodology like participatory appraisal. These alternative viewpoints are essential to health communication interventions, which often engage existing scripts and promote a minority viewpoint as a means to changing behaviour (Do, Kincaid, & Figueroa, 2014; Kincaid, 2004). Photo-elicitation opened a safe space that allowed participants to express thoughts and opinions normally suppressed in the 'spiral of silence' (Noelle-Neumann, 1974) maintained around MSP (Said & Figueroa, 2008). With PTs, they could speak indirectly about normative local practices without implicating their town or neighbours.

Implicit attitudes. Another advantage of PTs was that participants did not have to explicitly articulate their attitudes to convey them. Attitudes are complex, multifaceted, and even contradictory within the individual, and such 'emotional ambiguities' are critical for understanding sexual research informants (Groes-Green, 2009b, p. 657). A participant's beliefs may not be evident even to herself, and can be missed in methods that rely on direct questioning (Calvert, Fulcher, Fulcher, Foster, & Rose, 2014). With PT, participants inevitably shared their sentiments about MSP through the *way* they talked about characters' motivations, actions and consequences, generating attitudinal data that included consciously retrievable opinions as well as below-the-surface feelings and assumptions.

Vernacular phrasing. Instead of directly asking for opinions about 'concurrent partners' or 'extramarital affairs,' we showed photos of couples and asked 'What do you think is happening here?' This enabled participants to articulate a range of MSP behaviours in informal language, allowing forms of MSP to come up in participants' own words without introducing technical phrases that may be referentially unclear or meaningless.[4] These day-to-day expressions and concepts were invaluable when designing the subsequent MSP communication interventions.

Quality of projective data

In terms of the 'dependability' (Lincoln & Guba, 1985) of PTs as a qualitative method, we observed thematic and linguistic repetition across study sites and instruments. Similar ideas, associations, and phrases about MSP emerged across gender groups, urban and rural zones, and provinces (Said, 2008). Key conclusions were compatible with results of direct questioning in the key informant interviews conducted within the same study. Positive evaluations of the resulting communication interventions (discussed below) helped corroborate the 'transferability' (Lincoln & Guba, 1985) of the PT findings to the broader population. Finally, results from other studies in Mozambique were consistent with ours (Jana, Nkambule, & Tumbo, 2008; PSI, 2010).

Limitations of PTs in the formative research study

Photo-elicitation became tiring with too many photos. We eventually downsized from 24 photos per discussion to 10–12, which better suited adult attention spans.

When individually administered, projection exercises could be vulnerable to exaggeration; however in a group setting, fellow participants could correct atypical portrayals.

In terms of renderings, the organisational photos used in our study were inescapably representational. Pauwels (2011) cautions against assuming that photographs' depicted scenarios are unproblematic stand-ins for the real life scenarios to which they are intended to refer (2011). He warns that the 'inevitable difference' between the two 'can seriously influence or even misinform' participants' views on the actual behaviours (2011, p. 11). We found photographic details such as age and facial expression were both a boon and a burden: realistic images prompted a strong emotional engagement with the scenes, but may have suggested demographic profiles that restricted or triggered certain projective associations.

Uniqueness of projective data

Photo-elicitation opened the space for non-normative opinions to be discussed in front of neighbourhood peers. Participants actively critiqued male concurrency vignettes, to the point that *negative* appraisal of these partnerships dominated in some male discussion groups and in most female discussion groups. These new findings offered communication programme designers a 'window of opportunity' to reverse the spiral of silence and rally endorsement of fresh ways of thinking to change HIV risk behaviour (Said, 2008; Said & Figueroa, 2008).

Visual projection brought forth a greater range of MSP metaphors and sub-types than direct qualitative questioning could have elicited. This approach could be especially useful for public health studies seeking to explore the definitional boundaries of social behaviours.

We also found that direct qualitative inquiry has been effective in learning about *drivers* of MSP (Jana et al., 2008; N'weti, 2008; PSI, 2010), while third person photos and vignettes were especially useful in bringing up perceived *consequences* of MSP. Participants were eager to chime in about 'what happens next?' Their responses contributed to our understanding of perceived impacts of MSP – conflict, suffering, and disorganisation within the couple, family, and broader community (Holman, 2008; Said, 2008; Said & Figueroa, 2008).

Fictional third-personing elicited complex descriptions of the internal conflict or shame a man or woman might feel in succumbing to or attempting to resist gendered peer pressure around MSP, which we had not found in previous focus group research.

We believe PTs more readily achieved the sharing of equivocal, conflicted, and minority attitudes towards MSP because the 'proper' or normative opinion was less strongly embedded in the projective instruments, compared to instruments that use direct inquiry. A more comprehensive depiction of the nature of MSP emerged than the study team had anticipated. These rich data were creatively used in developing the communication interventions described below.

Resulting health communication programmes

Based on the PTs formative research findings, two HIV prevention communication interventions were developed to reduce MSP and increase other HIV preventive behaviours. The *Tchova Tchova, Histórias de Vida* (Push forward, life stories) programme used a community-dialogue approach to influence ideational factors such as interpersonal communication, beliefs and values, perceived risks, and other cognitive and affective factors (Kincaid et al., 2012), as well as collective norms associated with HIV prevention behaviours. This approach involved small group discussions and debates that created social dialogue space for participants to confront underlying social and gender norms that encourage MSP and other HIV risk behaviours. The original programme ran from August 2008 to March 2010, and some components were retained in follow-up initiatives. The evaluation showed that the programme positively influenced attitudinal changes in gender roles, partners' communication about HIV, perceived HIV risk of MSP and reported MSP behaviour (Figueroa et al., 2016).

The second intervention consisted of a mass media MSP prevention campaign titled *Andar Fora e Maningue Arriscado* (stepping outside – cheating – is risky business). The campaign was part of a broader collaborative effort among several organisations in Mozambique. The year-long campaign started in December 2009, increasing the visibility of MSP attitudes identified by the PTs formative research and the knowledge that MSP increases HIV risk. The campaign's impact evaluation found a dose–response relationship in the expected direction: those with greater recall of the *Andar Fora* campaign messages were twice as likely to hold unfavourable attitudes towards MSP, more likely to have talked to their partner about MSP risk, and less likely to have engaged in MSP in the last 12 months (Figueroa et al., 2014).

The positive impact of these two programmes signals substantial qualitative validity of the PT findings on which the programmes were based, both internally among participants and externally in the general population. The *Andar Fora* multimedia campaign created television spots that were sympathetic to those who confront peer pressure, and modelled how to avoid succumbing. For example, in one spot a young woman effectively, but diplomatically, resists the pro-MSP advice of female elders; in another a man adeptly encourages his male co-worker to abandon MSP and focus on his marriage, but without undermining the co-worker or himself (JHU-CCP, 2011). The degree to which Mozambicans responded favourably to the programmes' health communication messages indicates attentive processing of the messages, signalling that messages effectively keyed in to individuals' understandings of MSP and underlying norms. These positive impact evaluations of the *Andar Fora* interventions help corroborate the quality of the projective data that informed their development.

Conclusion

We believe this is the first study to use visual PTs to broach challenging topics of multiple and concurrent sexual partnering in sub-Saharan Africa. Projective elicitation was relatively simple to administer and can effectively deepen understanding on multiple ideational communication constructs in one study. They can be useful for exploratory studies, especially of private or stigmatised topics, or when researchers want to maximise the talents of local facilitators without circumscribing participants' responses.

The third-person orientation fostered comfortable group dynamics and reduced pressure to provide socially acceptable answers or withhold information. Talking about a third person provided participants a 'safe space' to offer dissenting views about normative attitudes and practices without fear of criticism, embarrassment, or reprisal. The unstructured nature of photo-elicitation enabled richer discussion, granting participants wide latitude in their comments and the opportunity to work through associations activated by personal and peer experience. Used in a group setting, PTs generated a fertile conversation that gave insight into both mainstream perceptions and underground evaluations, providing an emotional and motivational context for these mental maps – fear, empathy, humiliation, and desire. Such factors are often deep-rooted and difficult to articulate in response to direct inquiry, especially when asking about sexual behaviour.

In the process of interpretation, participants also modelled typical interpersonal communication around sex and gender roles, and shared local terms and phrases used to refer to behavioural categories and relevant social ideals. This combination of constructs and portrayals was uniquely valuable to the development of effective health communication campaigns.

Communication programmes stand to gain from the use of visual-based PTs at appropriate points in their research-to-practice cycle, either at the formative stage, for message and image testing, or as a qualitative sub-study embedded into a larger survey evaluation.

Our conclusions on PTs facilitating open participation, social details, and both conscious and subconscious attitudes squares with the experience of political marketing researchers recently employing qualitative PTs for attitudinal elicitation (Pich & Dean, 2015).

We recommend consideration of photo-elicitation and other visual PTs in qualitative or mixed-method health communication research. We believe PTs, used carefully and thoughtfully, can help elicit and triangulate hard to reach psychosocial constructs and established norms that sustain risky behaviours. It can also improve the quality and use-fulness of exploratory data, and improve participant experience in sexuality research. Verbal projections onto photographs offered a new perspective for understanding how Mozambicans talk and think about MSP. Findings permeated the language and images that went into the communication campaign, and enabled the development of an HIV intervention that spoke to people in familiar terms, addressed ideals that were relevant to their universe of experience, and kept sexual behaviour comfortably at the centre of the conversation.

Acknowledgements

The regional MCP campaign activities were coordinated by the National AIDS Council (CNCS) in Mozambique, with complementary components designed and implemented by JHU-CCP, Funda-ção para o Desenvolvimento da Comunidade (FDC), PSI, and N'weti Health Communication. The contents of this article are the responsibility of the authors and do not necessarily reflect the views of the U.S. Government or above donors or collaborators. We would like to thank Patricia Poppe and Patrick Devos for their skilled assistance in the organisation of the study; Rajiv Rimal for his meth-odological insights during data analysis; the talented facilitators who so capably and effectively con-ducted the PT groups; and the study participants who candidly contributed their time and experiences. Finally, we would like to acknowledge the thoughtful feedback of the anonymous reviewers of this manuscript. E. Holman assisted with pretesting the instruments in Mozambique, conducted data analysis, and drafted the first version of the manuscript. C. Harbour conducted the literature review and selected findings from the overall project report for this manuscript. R. Azevedo Said participated in development of the PT tools, coordinated and led data collection, analysis, and preparation of the overall study report. M.E. Figueroa led design of the overall study and development of the PT tools, and collaborated on data analysis and the overall study report. All co-authors contributed to this manuscript.

Notes

1. More recent 2011 sentinel survey data place national adult HIV prevalence at an estimated 15,8%, rising to 23,6% in the southern provinces (CNCS, 2014).
2. The National AIDS Council still considers multiple partnerships to be a critical concern in the national epidemic (CNCS, 2014).
3. The larger study included key informant interviews with traditional leaders, religious leaders, sexual initiation counselors (*madrinhas* and *padrinhos*), school teachers, and truck drivers.
4. See Groes-Green (2009b) for useful reflection on how introducing sexual health jargon into a research interview can be off-putting to participants, limit their engagement, and yield 'inadequate answers and unproductive' encounters (p. 656).

Disclosure statement

No potential conflict of interest was reported by the authors.

Funding

The formative PTs study was funded by the President's Emergency Plan for AIDS Relief (PEPFAR) through the U.S. Agency for International Development (USAID). It was led by the Johns Hopkins Center for Communication Programs (JHU-CCP) in partnership with World Vision and the

International HIV/AIDS Alliance. The *Tchova Tchova* programme was funded under USAID Leader/Associate Award [# GPH-A-00-00008-00].

References

Aboim, S. (2009). Men between worlds: Changing masculinities in urban Maputo. *Men and Masculinities, 12*(2), 201–224. doi:10.1177/1097184X07313360

Agadjanian, V. (2002). Men doing 'women's work': Masculinity and gender relations among street vendors in Maputo, Mozambique. *Journal of Men's Studies, 10*(3), 329–342. doi:10.3149/jms.1003.329

Agadjanian, V. (2005). Gender, religious involvement, and HIV/AIDS prevention in Mozambique. *Social Science & Medicine, 61,* 1529–1539. doi:10.1016/j.socscimed.2005.03.012

Agha, S., Kusanthan, T., Longfield, K., Klein, M., & Berman, J. (2002). *Reasons for non-use of condoms in eight countries in sub-Saharan Africa.* Retrieved from http://www.aidsmark.org/resources/pdfs/sub-saharanafrica.pdf

Audet, C. M., Burlison, J., Moon, T. D., Sidat, M., Vergara, A. F., & Vermund, S. H. (2010). Sociocultural and epidemiological aspects of HIV/AIDS in Mozambique. *BMC International Health and Human Rights, 10*(15), 1–10. doi:10.1186/1472-698X-10-15

Bagnolle, B., & Chamo, E. (2003). *'Titios' e 'catorzinhas': Pesquisa exploratória sobre 'sugar daddies' na Zambézia (Quelimane e Pebane)* [Exploratory study on 'sugar daddies' in Zambézia]. U.K. Department for International Development/PMG Mozambique.

Baltazar, C. S., Horth, R., Inguane, C., Sathane, I., César, F., Ricardo, H., ... Young, P. W. (2015). HIV prevalence and risk behaviors among Mozambicans working in South African mines. *AIDS and Behavior, 19*(Suppl. 1), S59–S67. doi:10.1007/s10461-014-0941-6

Bandali, S. (2011). Exchange of sex for resources: HIV risk and gender norms in Cabo Delgado, Mozambique. *Culture, Health & Sexuality: An International Journal for Research, Intervention and Care, 13*(5), 575–588. doi:10.1080/13691058.2011.561500

Belk, R. W. (2006). *Handbook of qualitative research methods in marketing.* Cheltenham: Edward Elgar.

Calvert, G., Fulcher, E., Fulcher, G., Foster, P., & Rose, H. (2014). Using implicit methods to develop an objective measure of media brand engagement. *International Journal of Market Research, 56* (1), 15–32. doi:10.2501/ÜMR-2014-004

Catterall, M., & Ibbotson, P. (2000). Using projective techniques in education research. *British Educational Research Journal, 26*(2), 245–256. Retrieved from http://www.jstor.org/stable/1501597

CNCS. (2014). *Global AIDS response progress report (GARPR), country progress report, Mozambique.* Retrieved from http://www.unaids.org/sites/default/files/country/documents/MOZ_narrative_report_2014.pdf

Collier, J. (1967). *Visual anthropology: Photography as a research method.* New York, NY: Holt, Rinehart & Winston.

Conselho Nacional de Combate ao HIV e SIDA [National Council for the Combat of HIV and AIDS]. (2006, June). *Estratégia nacional de comunicação para o combate ao HIV/SIDA* [National communication strategy to combat HIV/AIDS]. Maputo. Retrieved from http://www.ilo.org/wcmsp5/groups/public/—ed_protect/—protrav/—ilo_aids/documents/legaldocument/wcms_172573.pdf

Conselho Nacional de Combate ao HIV e SIDA [National Council for the Combat of HIV and AIDS]. (2014). Global AIDS response progress report (GARPR), country progress report, Mozambique. Retrieved from http://www.unaids.org/sites/default/files/country/documents/MOZ_narrative_report_2014.pdf.

Curry, T. J. (1986). A visual method of studying sports: The photo elicitation interview. *Sociology of Sport Journal, 3,* 204–210.

Do, M., Kincaid, D. L., & Figueroa, M. E. (2014). Impacts of four communication programs on HIV testing behavior in South Africa. *AIDS Care: Psychological and Socio-medical aspects of AIDS/HIV*, *26*(9), 1109–1117. doi:10.1080/09540121.2014.901487

Donoghue, S. (2000). Projective techniques in consumer research. *Journal of Family Ecology and Consumer Sciences*, *28*, 47–53. doi:10.4314/jfecs.v28i1.52784

Figueroa, M. E., & Kincaid, D. L. (2014). *Evaluating the impact of a communication campaign on multiple sex partnerships in Mozambique: Final report*. Baltimore, MD: USAID, Project Search: Research to Prevention. Retrieved from http://www.jhsph.edu/research/centers-and-institutes/research-to-prevention/publications/Mozambique_FinalReport.pdf

Figueroa, M. E., Kincaid, D. L., & Hurley, E. A. (2014). The effect of a joint communication campaign on multiple sex partners in Mozambique: The role of psychosocial/ideational factors. *AIDS Care: Psychosocial and Socio-Medical Aspects of AIDS/HIV*, *26*(Sup1), S50–S55. doi:10.1080/09540121.2014.907386

Figueroa, M. E., Poppe, P., Carrasco, M., Pinho, M. D., Massingue, F., Tanque, M., & Kwizera, A. (2016). Effectiveness of community dialogue in changing gender and sexual norms for HIV prevention: Evaluation of the Tchova Tchova program in Mozambique. *Journal of Health Communication: International Perspectives*. doi:10.1080/17441692.2016.1170870

Groes-Green, C. (2009a). Safe sex pioneers: Class identity, peer education and emerging masculinities among youth in Mozambique. *Sexual Health*, *6*, 233–240. doi:10.1071/SH09021#sthash.bYxxPNKK.dpuf

Groes-Green, C. (2009b). Health discourse, sexual slang and ideological contradictions among Mozambican youth: Implications for method. *Culture, Health & Sexuality*, *11*(6), 655–668. doi:10.1080/13691050903040188

Groes-Green, C. (2010). Orgies of the moment: Bataille's anthropology of transgression and young men's defiance of danger in post-socialist Mozambique. *Anthropological Theory*, *10*(4), 385–407. doi:10.1177/1463499610386662

Groes-Green, C. (2012). Ambivalent participation: Sex, power, and the anthropologist in Mozambique. *Medical Anthropology: Cross-Cultural Studies in Health and Illness*, *31*(1), 44–60. doi:10.1080/01459740.2011.589418

Groes-Green, C. (2013). 'To put men in a bottle': Eroticism, kinship, female power, and transactional sex in Maputo, Mozambique. *American Ethnologist*, *40*(1), 102–117. doi:10.1111/amet.12008

Groes-Green, C., Barrett, B. A., & Izugbara, C. (2011). Introduction: Intimate studies and ethnographic sensitivity. In B. A. Barrett, & C. Groes-Green (Eds.), *Studying intimate matters: Engaging methodological challenges in studies of gender. Sexuality and reproductive health in sub-Saharan Africa* (pp. 1–15). Kampala: Fountain Publishers.

Halperin, D. T., & Epstein, H. (2004). Concurrent sexual partnerships help to explain Africa's high HIV prevalence: Implications for prevention. *The Lancet*, *364*(9428), 4–6. doi:10.1016/S0140-6736(04)16606-3

Harper, D. (2002). Talking about pictures: A case for photo elicitation. *Visual Studies*, *17*(1), 13–26. doi:10.1080/14725860220137345

Hawkins, K., Mussá, F., & Abuxahama, S. (2005). *'Milking the cow'. Young women's constructions of identity, gender, power and risk in transactional and cross-generation sexual relationship: The implications for behavior change interventions*. Maputo: Population Services International. Retrieved from http://www.psi.org/publication/milking-the-cow-young-womens-construction-of-identity-and-risk-in-age-disparate-transactional-sexual-relationships-in-maputo-mozambique/

Holman, E. S. (2008). *Walking around [Andar Fora] in Central Mozambique: Meanings and normative perceptions encasing concurrent sexual partnerships* (thesis). Masters in Health Science, Submitted to Dept. of Health, Behavior and Society, Johns Hopkins University Bloomberg School of Public Health, Baltimore, US, 151 pgs.

James, W. (1909). *A pluralistic universe: Hibbert lectures at Manchester College on the present situation in philosophy*. New York, NY: Longmans, Green. Retrieved from https://books.google.com/books?id=1PiCjgEACAAJ

Jana, M., Nkambule, M., & Tumbo, D. (2008, August 10). *One love: Multiple and concurrent sexual partnerships in Southern Africa*. A ten country research report. The Soul City Institute Regional Program. Retrieved from http://www.comminit.com/africa/content/one-love-multiple-and-concurrent-sexual-partnerships-southern-africa

Johns Hopkins Center for Communication Programs. (2011, February 10). *Mozambique HIV/AIDS: 'Andar Fora e Maningue Arriscado' Campaign (Spot 1)*. Retrieved from https://www.youtube.com/watch?v=aWhXE7lyvO0

Karlyn, A. S. (2005). Intimacy revealed: Sexual experimentation and the construction of risk among young people in Mozambique. *Culture, Health and Sexuality, 7*(3), 279–292. doi:10.1080/13691050412331334362

Kincaid, D. L. (2000). Mass media, ideation & behavior: A longitudinal analysis of contraceptive change in the Philippines. *Communication Research, 27*(6), 723–763. doi:10.1177/009365000027006003

Kincaid, D. L. (2004). From innovation to social norm: Bounded normative influence. *Journal of Health Communication, 9*(Suppl. 1), 37–57. doi:10.1080/10810730490271511

Kincaid, D. L., Delate, R., Storey, J. D., & Figueroa, M. E. (2012). Closing the gaps in practice and in theory: Evaluation of the scrutinize HIV campaign in South Africa. In R. Rice, & C. Atkin (Eds.), *Public communication campaigns* (4th ed., pp. 305–320). Thousand Oaks, CA: Sage.

Korchin, S. (1976). *Modern clinical psychology*. New York, NY: Basic Books.

Kuate-Defo, B. (2004). Young people's relationships with sugar daddies and sugar mummies: What do we know and what do we need to know? *African Journal of Reproductive Health, 8*(2), 13–37. doi:10.2307/3583175

Lapenta, F. (2011). Some theoretical and methodological views on photo-elicitation. In E. Margolis, & L. Pauwels (Eds.), *The SAGE handbook of visual research methods* (pp. 201–213). London: Sage. doi:10.4135/9781446268278.n11

Lilienfeld, S. O., Wood, J. M., & Garb, H. N. (2000). The scientific status of projective techniques. *Psychological Science in the Public Interest, 1*(2), 27–66. Retrieved from http://www.jstor.org/stable/40062280

Lincoln, Y. S., & Guba, E. G. (1985). *Naturalistic inquiry*. Beverly Hills, CA: Sage.

Luke, N., & Kurz, K. (2002). *Cross-generational and transactional sexual relations in Sub-Saharan Africa: Prevalence of behavior and implications for negotiating safer sexual practices*. Population Services International & International Center for Research on Women. Retrieved from http://www.icrw.org/files/publications/

Machel, J. (2001). Unsafe sexual behavior among schoolgirls in Mozambique: A matter of gender and class. *Reproductive Health Matters, 9*(17), 82–90. doi:10.1016/S0968-8080(01)90011-4

MacPhail, C. (2003). Challenging dominant norms of masculinity for HIV prevention. *African Journal of AIDS Research, 2*(2), 141–149. doi:10.2989/16085906.2003.9626568

Manuel, S. (2005). Obstacles to condom use among secondary school students in Maputo city, Mozambique. *Culture, Health and Sexuality, 7*(3), 293–302. doi:10.1080/13691050412331321302

Manuel, S. (2007, July). *Multiple concurrent partners: Revisão de literatura*. Maputo: N'weti Comunicação para a Saúde (Unpublished manuscript). Retrieved from www.nweti.org/publicacoes/download/multiple-concurrent-partnership

Morgan, D. L., & Krueger, R. A. (1993). When to use focus groups and why. In D. L. Morgan (Ed.), *Successful focus groups: Advancing the state of the art* (pp. 3–19). Newbury Park, CA: Sage.

Morris, M., & Kretzschmar, M. (1995). Concurrent partnerships and transmission dynamics in networks. *Social Networks, 17*(3–4), 299–318. doi:10.1016/0378-8733(95)00268-S

Nalá, R., Cummings, B., Horth, R., Inguane, C., Benedetti, M., Chissano, M., … Lane, T. (2015). Men who have sex with men in Mozambique: identifying a population at high-risk for HIV. *AIDS & Behavior, 19*(2), 393–404. doi:10.1007/s10461-014-0895-8

Noelle-Neumann, E. (1974). The spiral of silence: A theory of public opinion. *Journal of Communication, 24*(2), 43–51. doi:10.1111/j.1460-2466.1974.tb00367.x

N'weti Comunicação para a Saúde. (2008, May). *Silêncio, Segredos e Mentiras. MCP – Relatório de Pesquisa de Audiência, Parceiros Múltiplos e Concorrentes (HIV)* [Silence, secrets and lies:

Formative research report, multiple and concurrent partners]. Retrieved from http://www.nweti.org/index.php/publicacoes/2012-02-14-00-20-27

O'Sullivan, G. A., Yonkler, J. A., Morgan, W., & Merritt, A. P. (2003). *A field guide to designing a health communication strategy*. Baltimore, MD: Johns Hopkins Bloomberg School of Public Health/Center for Communication Programs. Retrieved from http://ccp.jhu.edu/documents/AFieldGuidetoDesigningHealthComm Strategy.pdf

Pauwels, L. (2011). An integrated conceptual framework for visual social research. In E. Margolis, & L. Pauwels (Eds.), *The SAGE handbook of visual research methods* (pp. 3–40). London: Sage. doi:10.4135/9781446268278.n1

Pearson, C. R., Cassels, S., Kurth, A. E., Montoya, P., Micek, M. A., & Gloyd, S. S. (2011). Change in sexual activity 12 months after ART initiation among HIV-positive Mozambicans. *AIDS and Behavior, 15*(4), 778–787. doi:10.1007/s10461-010-9852-3

Pearson, C. R., Kurth, A. E., Cassels, S., Martin, D. P., Simoni, J. M., Hoff, P., … Gloyd, S. (2007). Modeling HIV transmission risk among Mozambicans prior to their initiating highly active anti-retroviral therapy. *AIDS Care, 19*(5), 594–604. doi:10.1080/09540120701203337

Pich, C., & Dean, D. (2015). Qualitative projective techniques in political brand image research from the perspective of young adults. *Qualitative Market Research: An International Journal, 18*(1), 115–144. doi:10.1108/QMR-12-2012-0058

Pinto, E. R. (2014). Conceitos fundamentais dos métodos projetivos [Fundamental concepts of projective methods]. *Ágora: Estudos em Teoria Psicanalítica, 17*(1), 135–153. Retrieved from: http://ref.scielo.org/7tcrps

Piotrowski, C. (2015). Clinical instruction on projective techniques in the USA: A review of academic training settings 1995–2014. *Journal of Projective Psychology and Mental Health, 22*(2), 83–92.

Population Services International. (2010, July). *Understanding drivers of concurrent partnerships in Mozambique*. Poster session for the 2010 International AIDS Conference, Vienna. Retrieved from http://www.psi.org/publication/iac-2010-mozambique-understanding-drivers-of-concurrent-partnerships/

Prata, N., Morris, L., Mazive, E., Vahidnia, F., & Stehr, M. (2006). Relationship between HIV risk perception and condom use: Evidence from a population-based survey in Mozambique. *International Family Planning Perspectives, 32*(4), 192–200.

Prosser, J. (2006, July). *Researching with visual images: Some guidance notes and a glossary for beginners* (Real Life Methods working paper series). Manchester: University of Leeds. Retrieved from http://www.socialsciences.manchester.ac.uk/medialibrary/morgancentre/research/wps/3-2006-07-rlm-prosser.pdf

Regan, M., & Liaschenko, J. (2008). In the margins of the mind: Development of a projective research methodology for the study of nursing practice. *Research and Theory for Nursing Practice, 22*(1), 10–23. doi:10.1891/0889-7182.22.1.10

Rimal, R. N., & Lapinski, M. K. (2009). Why health communication is important in public health. *Bulletin of the World Health Organization, 87*(4), 247–247.

Said, R. (2008, April). *Pesquisa formativa: Normas sociais, dinâmicas familiares e de género que impulsionam a epidemia do HIV em Moçambique* [Formative research: Social norms and family and gender dynamics driving the HIV epidemic in Mozambique]. Maputo: Johns Hopkins University Center for Communication Programs. 185p.

Said, R., & Figueroa, M. E. (2008). *New gender dynamics for HIV prevention: Windows of opportunity in Mozambique*. Maputo: Johns Hopkins University Center for Communication Programs. Retrieved from http://ccp.jhu.edu/documents/NewGenderDynamicsforHIVPrevention-WindowsofOpportunityinMozambique.pdf

da Silva, B., Nhalivilo, B., Nobela, C., Osório, C., Machungo, F., da Silva Carrilho, L., … da Silva, T. (2006). *Para além das desigualdades 2005: A mulher em Moçambique* [Beyond inequalities 2005: The woman in Mozambique]. Maputo: Fórum Mulher, SARDC WIDSAA. Retrieved from http://www.sardc.net/books/moz2005port/moz2005port.pdf

Soley, L. C. (2006). Measuring responses to commercials: A projective-elicitation approach. *Journal of Current Issues and Research in Advertising, 28*(2), 55–64. doi:10.1080/10641734.2006.10505198

Soley, L. C. (2010). Projective techniques in US marketing and management research: The influence of 'The Achievement Motive'. *Qualitative Market Research: An International Journal, 13*(4), 334–353. doi:10.1108/13522751011078782

South African Development Community. (2006, July). *Expert think tank meeting on HIV prevention in high-prevalence countries in southern Africa.* Maseru: Author. Retrieved from http://data.unaids.org/pub/Report/2006/20060601_sadc_meeting_report_en.pdf

Timberg, C., & Halperin, D. (2012, March 9). A smarter way to fight AIDS in Africa. *The Washington Post.* Retrieved from http://www.washingtonpost.com/opinions/a-smarter-way-to-fight-aids-in-africa/2012/02/17/gIQAEpkd1R_story.html

UNAIDS. (2008). *UNAIDS Mozambique 2008.* Progress Report for the UNGASS on HIV/AIDS. Retrieved from data.unaids.org/pub/Report/2008

United Nations Joint Programme on HIV/AIDS. (2007). *UNAIDS expert consultation on behaviour change in the prevention of sexual transmission of HIV: Highlights and recommendations.* Geneva: Author. Retrieved from http://data.unaids.org/pub/Report/2007/20070430unaidsexpertconsultationonbehaviourchangereport_en.pdf

Vera Cruz, G., & Maússe, L. (2014). Multiple and concurrent sexual partnerships among Mozambican women from high socio-economic status and with high education degrees: Involvement motives. *Psychology, 5,* 1260–1267. doi:10.4236/psych.2014.510138

Ward, V. M., Bertrand, J., & Brown, L. F. (1991). The comparability of focus group and survey results: Three case studies. *Evaluation Review, 15*(2), 266–283. doi:10.1177/0193841X9101500207

Wiehagen, T., Caito, N. M., Sanders Thompson, V., Casey, C. M., Weaver, N. L., Jupka, K., & Kreuter, M. W. (2007). Applying projective techniques to formative research in health communication development. *Health Promotion Practice, 8,* 164–172. doi:10.1177/1524839906289818

Wutich, A., Lant, T., White, D. D., Larson, K. L., & Gartin, M. (2010). Comparing focus group and individual responses on sensitive topics: A study of water decision makers in a desert city. *Field Methods, 22*(1), 88–110. doi:10.1177/1525822X09349918

Visual methodologies and participatory action research: Performing women's community-based health promotion in post-Katrina New Orleans

M. Brinton Lykes[a] and Holly Scheib[b]

[a]Department of Counseling, Developmental and Educational Psychology, Center for Human Rights & International Justice, Boston College, Chestnut Hill, MA, USA; [b]Disaster Resilience Leadership Academy, School of Social Work, Tulane University, New Orleans, LA, USA

ABSTRACT

Recovery from disaster and displacement involves multiple challenges including accompanying survivors, documenting effects, and rethreading community. This paper demonstrates how African-American and Latina community health promoters and white university-based researchers engaged visual methodologies and participatory action research (photoPAR) as resources in cross-community praxis in the wake of Hurricane Katrina and the flooding of New Orleans. Visual techniques, including but not limited to photonarratives, facilitated the health promoters': (1) care for themselves and each other as survivors of and responders to the post-disaster context; (2) critical interrogation of New Orleans' entrenched pre- and post-Katrina structural racism as contributing to the racialised effects of and responses to Katrina; and (3) meaning-making and performances of women's community-based, cross-community health promotion within this post-disaster context. This feminist antiracist participatory action research project demonstrates how visual methodologies contributed to the co-researchers' cross-community self- and other caring, critical bifocality, and collaborative construction of a contextually and culturally responsive model for women's community-based health promotion post 'unnatural disaster'. Selected limitations as well as the potential for future cross-community antiracist feminist photoPAR in post-disaster contexts are discussed.

Disaster response and intervention has moved beyond a one-dimensional, stage-oriented, and linear approach towards acknowledging variability, inequality, diversity, and social disparities that precede a disaster and contribute to its wake. Central to this reframing is an understanding that local, national, and global systems shape not only populations' differential risks in disasters, but also how they recover from them (SPHERE, 2011). For example, underlying historical tensions (e.g. institutionalised racism) and global and national systems of aid generate differential vulnerabilities where those marginalised

222

from access to resources and power before a disaster are most likely to suffer the greatest impacts and remain on the margins of recovery processes and resources. In August 2005, Hurricane Katrina and the US government's responses to it revealed the global situated-ness of New Orleans and the US as well as the former's pre-existing racial and economic inequalities and the limits of the local, state, and federal governments' responses to the city's majority populations of colour.

Structural inequalities and disaster in New Orleans

Racial and economic inequalities in New Orleans had increased in the decades prior to Katrina. Demographics in Orleans Parish (equivalent to a county) between 1960 and 2000 had shifted from 62.6% white and 37.2% black, to 28.1% white and 67.3% black (U.S. Bureau of Census Data, cited by Frailing & Harper, 2007, p. 57). Black unemploy-ment rates were consistently double those of whites in the 1960s, rising to six times higher in 1990 (Frailing & Harper, 2007, p. 57). In 2004, 22% of the population earned less than $10,000/year and 84% of New Orleans residents living in poverty were black (Masozera, Bailey, & Kerchner, 2007). High unemployment rates and poverty within the black community compounded with limited resources to address adequate housing and health care, food insecurity, and systemic violence contributed to the racialised stra-tification of goods and services delivery and structured inequality.

Violent crime focused in the black community contributed to New Orleans' reputation as the 'murder capital of America', a 1994 moniker (Brown, 1997) that continued to describe high rates of violence in the city's poorer sections in the twenty-first century. For example, in 2004, the year before Katrina, the murder rate was 56 per 100,000 resi-dents, more than 4 times the rate for a US city of similar size (Gelinas, 2007). Crime was and remains highly associated with poverty. Thus, prior to the storm, New Orleans was characterised by high crime rates, low-wage jobs, and a poverty rate that was more than twice the national average and deeply racialised (Center for Progressive Reform, 2005; Gault, Hartmenn, DeWeever, Werschkul, & Williams, 2005). A white-black binary of haves and have nots that characterised pre-Katrina New Orleans played out in the storm's aftermath. Specifically, while there was little difference in flooding and immediate displacement between high- and low-income neighbourhoods (Masozera et al., 2007), a higher percentage of poor people lived in areas that sustained higher levels of damage due to Katrina and post-Katrina flooding (Logan, 2006) and longer-term effects (Plyer, 2011).

Interestingly, 'issues of structured inequality and stratification have long been under-studied within the disaster context' (Barnshaw & Trainor, 2007, p. 91). Rather, the disaster literature and disaster responsivity have focused on disaster as a 'disruptive event', contri-buting to event-driven individual responses to what are frequently identified as 'natural disasters' rather than to systemic responses to situations generated by, among other things, longstanding structural injustices. 'Disaster relief' that ignores structural inequities and related barriers to recovery resources fails to address immediate post-disaster needs, further exacerbates inequalities, and sets into motion processes with long-term deleterious effects. These tendencies framed initial responses to Katrina that both failed to recognise how diverse groups within New Orleans differentially experienced the storm and its wake and how structural inequalities constrained government and non-governmental agencies' actions. In short, most of the population suffered in the wake of Katrina but those with the fewest resources prior to Katrina suffered disproportionately in its aftermath (Plyer, 2011).

Survivors' culturally and contextually relevant responses to disaster

As argued above, disaster response requires a structural analysis and differentiated responses that recognise diverse needs. As importantly, these responses must be intersectional, that is, designed in response to the particular cultural, linguistic, racial, and gendered realities of the survivors. For example, many long-term African-American residents within the post-Katrina context were unable to return home post-disaster as the barriers for recovery and the scramble for resources proved too challenging. Those returning to rebuild their lives faced immediate losses that ensued from the above-mentioned structural inequalities. Moreover, the population of the city was changing. Perhaps most notably, lower-income jobs in rebuilding efforts attracted a high number of undocumented labourers, arriving from Northern states or crossing Southern borders and needing housing. Official estimates, which are acknowledged as greatly underestimated, show a doubling of the Latino population in New Orleans between 2000 and 2010, from approximately 3% to nearly 6%, with adjacent Jefferson Parish increasing to 14% (The Data Center, 2014). This population change was racialised by local media who represented these realities as competition and conflict between African-American and Latino workers over scarce housing and job opportunities (Keyes, 2010).

In the first few years after the storms, neighbourhoods – particularly those of the city's non-white and low-income residents – lacked basic services including hospitals, schools, housing, public transportation, gas, and electricity. The absence of rebuilding initiatives in these areas echoed a historic lack of opportunities for African-American New Orleanians. Displaced New Orleanians and newly arrived immigrants faced particular socio-emotional challenges that involved not only their own and their family's recovery, but the collective healing of an increasingly diverse city in a context of longstanding unanswered demands for social redress of historic and contemporary inequities. The absence of basic services contributed to an increased reliance on community-based health workers. The latter were challenged to provide sustainable socially and culturally relevant material and psychosocial responses. Moreover, the destruction of all levels of the city's functioning dissolved traditional distinctions between service providers and clients as everyone remaining in or returning to the city was challenged to participate in both personal and professional recovery endeavours.

PAR and visual methodologies as one post-disaster response

University-based white researchers (one a native New Orleanian, the other a long-time resident) joined Latinas and African-American women who sought to document local women's community-based health promotion in New Orleans through collaboratively designing a photoPAR process (Scheib & Lykes, 2013). Photo documentation and elicitation strategies complemented other creative techniques developed in prior work in contexts of war and post-conflict recovery (Lykes, 1994, 2001) and were engaged in this work. The first author drew from the psychologically grounded photo-elicitation strategy of Giuseppe Costantino's TEMAS (Costantino, Malgady, & Flanagam, 2001) and Ximena

Bunster's 'talking pictures' (Bunster & Chaney, 1989) whereby photographs developed with Peruvian market women were used to elicit narratives from other women in similar contexts. Finally, the participatory photography methodology developed by Caroline Wang and her associates in China, photovoice (Wang, Burris, & Ping, 1996), was critical to the development of *photoPAR*, a methodology deployed in rural Guatemala (Lykes, 2001) and then in this research (Scheib & Lykes, 2013). In contrast to many PAR and photovoice processes, the photoPAR process described herein emphasises participation and engagement of co-researchers at all levels of the research process as well as transformative actions (Lykes, 2013).

PhotoPAR begins with individual storytelling in which the photographer narrates what she has learned from taking a picture – both through observation and/or from interviewing those who are in her photograph. She then pairs that story and photograph, creating a phototext (photograph + story). Multiple phototexts are individually developed and then iteratively organised and re-organised. Higher level concepts are constructively generated through co-researchers' interpretations and critical analyses of the combined phototexts. The co-researchers collectively elaborate a third iteration, that is, a photonarrative reflecting a 'mini-theory' (a la Charmaz, 2014). The authors argue below that the collective photonarratives included herein re-present several of the shared understandings and performances of women's community-based health praxis (multiple individual phototexts + critical bifocality (see below) + constructivist interpretations → a collective photonarrative).

The first author developed these processes in earlier work with community-based women's groups. With that as an antecedent, she initiated a series of meetings with local non-profit health organisations in New Orleans to explore her tentative vision for a project that would use the above participatory action research and visual methodologies in a proposed collaboration. She noted multiple reports on post-Katrina recovery that had neglected women's contributions, expressing interest in redressing those erasures through partnering with local women of colour responders. She approached the directors of two New Orleans-based community health organisations who had previously facilitated meetings between their respective African-American and Latina staff. They reported that their organisations' outreach work responded to unique and shared needs articulated within African-American and Latino communities in New Orleans. The second author was, at that time, a public health PhD student with a history of volunteer translation work with one of these programmes, background in photography, and academic training in photovoice, all of which were recognised as important resources for the project. Subsequent group meetings included discussions of possible project foci, potential benefits and challenges for organizations and their staff, estimated time for the collaboration and its anticipated effects on participants' work time, proposed compensation for participant co-researchers, and space for workshops.

Once all agreed to undertake the photoPAR project, they finalised a proposal, secured approval from the Institutional Review Board of the sponsoring university, and funding from a private foundation. The collaborating organisations supported the work through paying community co-researchers for one day per month to work with the project – and provided space for meetings and resources for some aspects of the fieldwork. The external funding supplemented this, supporting all other costs of the fieldwork and offering the co-researchers a small honorarium each month. Initial team-building workshops focused on getting to know each other, creating a safe space, practicing 'listening' and 'being heard', and the multiple ethical procedures and practices of participatory action research. Trust-building participatory processes laid the groundwork for the first phase of this inquiry process: the development of a shared research focus.

That focus emerged from a brainstorming exercise through which health promoters enumerated what they perceived to be community issues and concerns. Their list included: the [lack of] health insurance, financial burdens, literacy and communication challenges, violent communities, flood-remediated housing, transportation, confronting pride of needy families who resist help, knowing what services had returned to the city, if and where records may have been saved, and finding ways to coordinate available services. The promoters' consensus was to focus the project on their roles and actions as women community health workers in greater New Orleans post-Katrina, seeking to explore how they were resources for both their own and their communities' recovery. They titled the project: 'Voices and Photographs of Community Health Work and Workers in Post-Katrina New Orleans' and developed what they called a project 'tag line': 'Two Communities/One Photovoice'.

This overall photoPAR process lasted from 2006 through 2009 and documented local women's community-based health promotion in the New Orleans post-Katrina context. It sought to enhance women's understanding and valuing of health promotion that crosses racial, ethnic, and linguistic barriers to forge collaborative responses to health-related needs within a deeply racialised and fractured post-Katrina context. It was designed as a reflection-action process through which co-researchers would educate themselves and the wider New Orleans community about the nature and significance of such work.

Collaborators included the white university-based researchers, authors of this article, two health promotion programme coordinators – one a Caribbean migrant and the other from Latin America, both with masters' degrees in pubic health – four African-American health promoters, self-described as 'walkers-talkers', a name reflecting their home visiting and community-based delivery processes, and three Latinas who called themselves *promotoras,* Spanish for *promoter* of community health. The seven health promoter participants, referred to as co-researchers in this article, took photographs and generated stories about them to document and generate knowledge about how they and other historically marginalised groups were surviving and responding to multiple personal and community-based post-disaster realities that directly affected their health and wellbeing and that of their communities.

This paper focuses on the processes through which these health promoters developed as co-researchers and post-disaster health responders with a particular emphasis on developing, representing, and performing 'critical bifocality' (Weis & Fine, 2012). The latter refers to the capacity to name and interpret the relationships of power circulating within and between micro and macro systems in which one lives and works. The authors facilitated processes through which critical bifocality was developed as a core element in women's post-disaster cross-community-based health promotion. They designed and facilitated workshops drawing on visual resources, including individual and collective drawings, as well as a range of photography-based techniques (i.e. photo elicitation, photovoice, and photonarratives) and oral and performance-based resources (i.e. creative storytelling and embodied image generation and analysis) (Lykes, 2001). They documented co-researchers' storying of a selection of the hundreds of photographs that they had taken as well as their analyses of their stories about or in-depth interviews with the people in the photograph.

Co-researchers thereby developed and operationalised critical bifocality through documentation, critical analysis, and re-presentation. They enhanced their skills through participatory teaching-learning processes that facilitated individual and collective meaning-making about health promotion and advocacy in a post-disaster context. One example, discussed in greater detail below, is reflected in the co-researchers' documentation and analyses of ethnically diverse health needs post-Katrina. Through photoPAR they reframed post-Katrina health disparities as rooted in, and a consequence of, racialised and gendered inequalities in New Orleans. They took collective actions as health promoters discussing the products of their analyses with those whose pictures and stories they had re-presented as well as with a range of community groups.

The two phototexts and two photonarratives discussed in this paper reflect co-researchers' self-recognition as survivors and agents of change. The research summarised below focuses on these processes and on the 'outcome' or actions, that is, the sections from the co-researchers' community presentations that exemplify a particular cross-community women's health praxis in response to disaster in a context of ongoing gendered and racialised inequalities post-disaster. The authors conclude by discussing some of the limitations of this work as well as the importance of visual strategies and PAR as resources in post-disaster praxis wherein those responding are themselves direct survivors of the disaster.

Feminist antiracist photoPAR

Enhancing personal and cross-community communication through photo storytelling

Visual methods facilitated participation across a diverse range of linguistic skills and formal educational experiences. These methods facilitated participants' deployment of non-verbal communication and embodied self-expression, enhancing their self-understanding as co-researchers and the emergence of a cross-community research team. The following activity exemplifies these processes.

Early on in the project, co-researchers and organizational directors were invited to bring in photographs of personal importance to them. The strategy was designed to provide a context for deeper personal sharing among co-researchers as well as to generate a teaching-learning photo-elicitation experience. Women brought family photographs and images representing important life events or meaningful contexts. Each participant shared her photograph, explained its significance, and then exchanged it, inviting another group member to story the photograph, that is, to develop a story based on what they learned about the person whose photograph they now had from the previous sharing. Each participant experienced having an 'other' tell a story about the image she had brought to the workshop. Stories included particular preparations of food by Latina promoters that were compared to and contrasted with experiences of African-American cuisine. Participants spoke of their shared experiences of the significance of food as generative of community, despite particular differences in the choices of what was eaten and its preparation. A home in rural Colombia revealed professional class privilege that was contrasted with urban cramped housing revealed in an African-American walker-talker's photograph and story. As these stories were exchanged and discussed, participants were encouraged to document what in the narrative represented the experience that had been shared by the person who brought the photograph and initially shared it and what the multiple other storytellers had added. They were also encouraged to think about what underlying assumptions might have led the storytellers to generate the stories they had shared.

Co-researchers thus developed skills in telling their own and each other's stories and in listening to variations of their own stories as others were telling them. In reflecting upon themselves and their emotions, and in coming together to think through the connections and disjunctures between their known or lived experiences and these experiences re-storied by someone else, this within-gender, cross-ethnic and cross-racial exercise and subsequent discussion elicited sharing about ethnic, linguistic, class, and national differences. It also facilitated the introduction of an intersectional framework as a resource for analysing one's own and another's life experiences.

Creative exercises deploying visual resources were repeated throughout the length of the project. As facilitators the authors sought to encourage co-researchers' expression of personal feelings and thoughts in the service of the photoPAR process, and, more specifically, to negotiate meaning-making through the construction of photonarratives. Visual techniques facilitated engagement with what co-researchers brought into the research process and contributed to their developing use of reflexivity as a research tool as well as to their engaged dialogue with each other and with the authors, that is, a listening process through which they valued each other's diverse ethnic, linguistic, and economic positionalities as well as their own and each other's lived experiences. These initial exercises contributed to the co-researchers acknowledgement and analysis of how they personally had been directly impacted by New Orleans's racialised inequality and differentially affected by Katrina.

The photo-sharing and storying exercise contributed to building co-researchers' self- and other-awareness and to generating a shared language and enhanced communication skills among Latina and African-American co-researchers. These were complemented by embodied practices including dramatic play, dramatic multiplication (Pavlovsky, 1990) and image theatre techniques (Boal, 1992). For example, co-researchers were invited to choose another's photo-based story, discuss it within a small group, and represent it or an imagined 'next step' through dramatic play and/or Boal's image theatre. Co-researchers' trust and comfort levels with each other were supported and stimulated through these embodied practices. Significant time, coordination, and training using these resources occurred prior to engaging together in a more formal community-based data-gathering process. In addition to enhancing co-researchers' skills, these processes contributed to developing 'just enough trust' (Maguire, 1987) within and across communities that were frequently re-presented through public media in New Orleans and beyond as competing with each other for scarce resources and/or engaging in discriminatory and stereotyping behaviours. Moreover, these collaborative activities were critical to enhancing the participants' wellbeing, allowing this group of survivors to value their coming together to support each other and to visualise their often unrecognised or undervalued knowledge as community-based health promoters.

As university-based researchers who designed and facilitated processes through which co-researchers documented and built on their own and others' ongoing recovery in a post-disaster context, the authors sought to support the insiders' personal journeys. They recognised that taking time to honour the unique experiences of displacement and loss that each co-researcher had endured was an important step towards individual resilience. Personal sharing of experiences, engaged listening, and empathetic representations reflecting understanding facilitated participants' self-knowledge and valuing of each other, towards a strength-based focus on those beyond their group. These processes facilitated their communication within and between ethnic-racial groups and organisations as well as their engagement with broader collective responses to organisational and citywide upheavals and health disparities in disaster's wake.

Critically interrogating Katrina through phototexts and collective storytelling

As discussed above, photoPAR integrates community-based PAR principles, participants' documentary photography as visual elicitation resources, their individual and small group analyses, and narrative interview methods. The steps in this process were designed to support co-researchers' self-appraisal as survivors and as cross-community responders and their development of critical bifocality as well as its extension through actions (Lykes & Scheib, 2015). With these bifocal lenses, co-researchers visualised and storied relationships among power structures, social and cultural practices, and historical and socio-political formations, and both named their praxis as women community-based health promoters and generated a particular framework for engaging women's health advocacy and actions.

The four African-American and three Latina promoters shared personal experiences and achievements, noting barriers to health and wellness in their individual communities through these documentation and analytic processes. They took more than a thousand photographs over a two-year period, recorded over a hundred individual stories and interviews, and wrote and re-wrote dozens of collective stories, thereby crafting phototexts and then photonarratives of Katrina's effects and the communities' challenges and resilience in responding. One of the early themes they selected to explore was public safety, a topic they photographed and analysed in relation to health, inequalities, racism, and recovery. Photographs included crime scenes, anti-violence posters, victim memorials, and locations of accidents, robberies, and gun violence familiar to the photographer. Some photographs were intensely personal, including a photograph of the site where a member of a co-researcher's immediate family had been murdered. Individual stories highlighted the strain on families who sought to live healthy lives, the losses communities experienced, and the fear of not being supported by local authorities. Participants documented how their community health outreach was restricted in some areas of need due to ongoing community violence, including restrictions in neighbourhoods where some lived or had grown up.

Figure 1 depicts 'everyday life' post-Katrina. The photographer's story about this image is below it, in italics. She aptly captured the dichotomy between the billboard and its context, illuminating the way in which a phototext (photograph + story) is generated to describe and illuminate a lived experience and then re-used to elicit a critical analysis of incongruities and/or contradictions co-researchers experience each day.

While going through the streets of New Orleans, I spotted this sign from the NOPD [New Orleans Police Department]. It is showing a happy family. The reality is that if you look

229

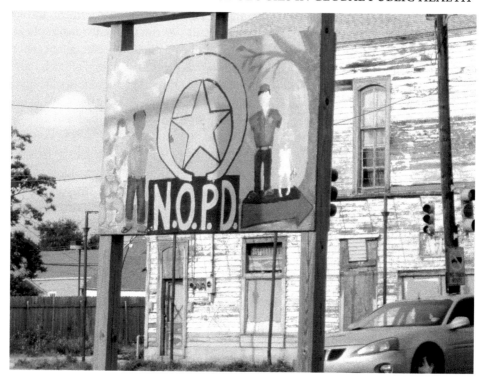

Figure 1. 'The New Orleans police department's vision, our realities'. Used with permission of co-researchers.

at the background, it paints a different story. The reality of the residents of New Orleans now as we were just named 'The Murder Capital of the USA' is one of frustration, sadness. And with very little faith in the Criminal Justice System. The city leaders need to have a reality check and do something to stop the violence on the streets of New Orleans and then you may see happy families again.

This New Orleans Police Department's (NOPD) 'self-image' or 'self-presentation' and the co-researcher's understanding of the community's self-understanding, that is, their 'frustration, sadness, little faith in the ... system' are storied in the phototext. The latter is informed by the storyteller's knowledge of media representations of her city, as the 'murder capital of the USA' and concludes with a challenge to city leaders to 'stop violence on the streets'. By inviting the photographer to story her image and then to present it to her co-researchers, photoPAR encourages processes of close observation, critical engagement with contradictory knowledge that may have been constructed in the phototext and identification of possible actions or responses. The photographer-storyteller's dialogue with co-researchers whose observations and interpretations sometimes differ from her own challenge her to clarify her perspective and to dialogue with their understandings. The next iteration of this action-reflection process draws heavily on this latter step.

Underemployed men emerged repeatedly in the co-researchers' photographs. Many were clients they encountered during community outreach. Latinos were photographed in public spaces where they awaited day-labour opportunities. African-Americans were photographed outside a neighbour's home or in a community centre. Co-researchers' individual stories of the photographs they took included their descriptions of the context and stories shared by the men they had photographed and interviewed. Through their photographs, stories, and discussions about their individual phototexts, co-researchers recognised similarities across the 'different' groups of men, first categorising them as 'under-utilised' and 'under-appreciated', and then recognising that the experiences they were photographing reflected systemic factors that rendered these members of their own and each other's communities as 'highly vulnerable to exploitation', and as they were often in public spaces, 'visible symbols of inequality and racism'.

A second iteration of the photoPAR process invited co-researchers to look across their individually developed photographs and stories, clustering the first level phototexts thematically, and then analysing the cluster. The goal was to generate a shared understanding of multiple phototexts, exploring similarities and differences in order to thicken the description and analysis, thereby facilitating a critical bifocal analysis of the previously more descriptive phototexts. Figure 2 represents a clustering of photographs, that is, a group of three phototexts that were combined into a single unit and restoried. The clustered phototext reflects the second iteration of the constructivist and critical analyses within the photoPAR process.

Exploitation can take different forms in the community; exploitation is a major cause of problems yet it's not very obvious to the people who are being affected. Most workers, Latinos and African Americans, are being exploited. They are being taken advantage of because they are undocumented or desperate. Their faces reflect the worry and uncertainly of not being able to find reliable work, of not knowing if they will have the luck to find someone who

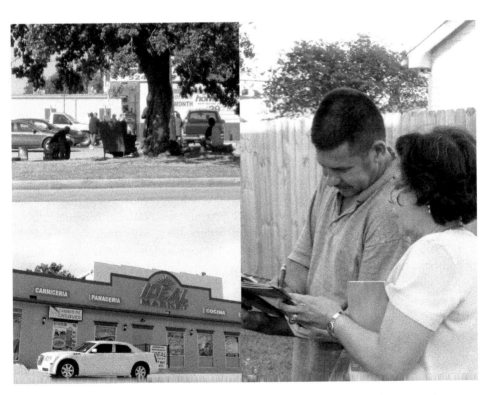

Figure 2. 'Living exploitation in English and Spanish'. Used with permission of co-researchers.

will give them work even for a couple of hours a day. When they don't find a job, they hang out all day and purchase alcohol from local corner stores and have nothing productive to do. Local check cashing businesses ... [are] convenient for people who do not have access to a bank. They don't realize that they are being exploited with the high fees that they are being charged to cash the money they earned. ...

As community health workers [it] is part of our responsibility to educate these individuals who don't have the basic knowledge in the areas they work for. Providing them with resources will help them to be less vulnerable to exploitation.

Earlier experiences of intercultural sharing – and an exercise through which health promoters 'shadowed' each other at their respective work sites (Scheib & Lykes, 2013) – enabled Latinas and African-Americans to look within and across linguistic and cultural differences and recognise cross-community similarities. Although the three images that are clustered represent sites of Latino unemployment and poverty, the particularities of African-American unemployment were reported by co-researchers from their communities who juxtaposed their 'desperation' to the images and story of Latino undocumented status, noting that these are 'different forms of exploitation'. Both communities are characterised as vulnerable to exploitation and each lacks reliable employment. The unemployed are 'worried and uncertain', and some turn to alcohol in response to the confluence of systemic oppression and self-doubt, irrespective of ethnicity or race. Lack of access to banking services represents another constraint imposed on undocumented Latino 'poor'. Through juxtaposing diverse images of Latino undocumented men and crafting a story that represents the men within and across their respective communities, the co-researchers identify a shared underlying causal factor, that is, racialised exploitation. This is an example of how participants began honing comparative skills that were deployed in the third iterative step of photoPAR, that is, the construction of a collective photonarrative (see Figure 3). The latter exemplifies their critical bifocality, reflecting their empathy with individual suffering within and across communities, while situating the causes of these men's pain within structures of marginalisation and exploitation which they named as generating health disparities and a public health crisis within pre- and post-Katrina New Orleans. Although the identified solution proposed by the co-researchers in the second iteration of clustered phototexts – educating these men about their rights – does not attack the underlying exploitation, it reflects their cross-community knowledge as well as an engaged empathy for and understanding of the men's lived experiences. This may be a realistic strategy for their taking action within what they understood to be their roles as community-based health promoters which include providing educational resources through which men themselves can take action 'to be less vulnerable to exploitation'. The next iteration or collective photonarrative is the process through which co-researchers reflect on and construct their most explicit re-presentation of circulations of power and experiences of marginalisation and oppression within their communities.

The representations of the third iteration of the photoPAR process evolved in response to the co-researchers action goals. As participants in this photoPAR process the co-researchers engaged in structured conversations about how to share their understandings of themselves as health advocates in cross-community health promotion (ideas represented in their photoPAR analyses and actions) with members of the wider New Orleans communities. They were challenged to put the various pieces of the process

CHALLENGES FACING AFRICAN AMERICAN FAMILIES

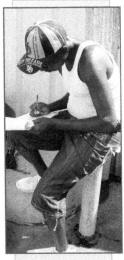

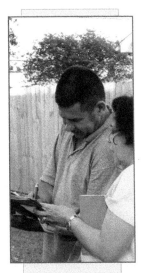

LATINOS AND LATINAS MOVE TO NEW ORLEANS

Pre-Katrina there were housing developments up and running for low-income families. Post-Katrina, only three of the housing developments remain open, with limited housing available. The rest were demolished when there were hundreds of families with homeless children, living under bridges in tents. Instead of opening these housing units, the government stated that they were unsafe and people had to live in tents that were neither safe nor sanitary.

The St. Bernard Housing Development is an example. It housed over 200 families and had a Community Center and Offices. When families came back after Katrina to live here because they were not damaged, they were arrested for trespassing in their own homes.

Discrimination and exploitation take different forms in the community and are a major cause of health problems yet its not very obvious to the people who are being affected. Most Latino and African American workers are taken advantage of because they are either undocumented or desperate. Their faces reflect the worry and uncertainty of not being able to find reliable work, of not knowing if they will have the luck to find someone who will give them work even for a couple of hours a day. When they don't find a job, they hang out all day and purchase alcohol from local corner stores and have nothing productive to do.

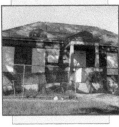

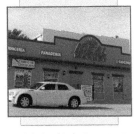

Mr. Helms's unemployment benefits were ending earlier than he had expected. He stated that the government talks about black men not wanting to work but that he is a black man who wants to work and needs to work but can't find a job.

Local check cashing businesses are more convenient for most people who do not have access to bank accounts. They don't realize that they are being exploited with the high fees that they are being charged to cash the check and get the money that they have earned.

These are examples of how, post-Katrina, the system is not working for the people. These people could have helped themselves if they had a little help from the government. YES WE CAN!

As community health workers, part of our responsibility is to educate these individuals, providing them with resources that will help them to be less vulnerable to exploitation.

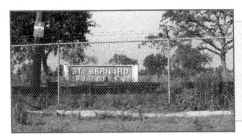

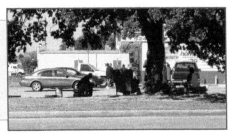

Figure 3. 'African American and Latino families and communities'. Used with permission of co-researchers.

into a larger, integrated whole. In order to share their collaborative work with organisational leaders, friends and families, clients (i.e. those featured in the photonarratives), and the community-at-large, they would have to move their work from one site to another. The idea of 'movable banners' displaying the collectively generated photographs and stories, that is, the collective photonarratives, was a feasible solution given these multiple goals.

Performing women's community-based health promotion through photonarratives

Co-researchers generated five photonarratives and printed them on banners where images and stories were threaded to report the higher level themes through which they storied their co-construction of meanings made and actions taken as women's community-based health promoters in a post-Katrina context. To create these banners they re-analysed and sometimes re-interpreted individual (e.g. Figure 1) and collective (e.g. Figure 2) phototexts that they regrouped and restoried to create a collective photonarrative. They preceded the five collective photonarratives with a banner that described the photoPAR methodology and book-ended them with a banner that included a photograph of all co-researchers, programme coordinators, and the authors. Two of these seven photonarratives are discussed herein: 'Challenges facing post-Katrina African American and Latino communities' (see Figure 3) and 'Analyzing Systemic Oppression and Racism' (see Figure 4).

The first banner (see Figure 3) is divided in two, with one side focusing on experiences of African-Americans and the other, those of Latinos, the two ethnic-racial-linguistic communities in which the co-researchers lived and worked. Featured on the banner are photographs of the St. Bernard Housing Development, where African-Americans who lived there prior to the storm had been arrested when they returned to homes that, despite reports of liveability, the federal government had decided to tear down. This was interpreted by most as an explicitly racist response to the African-Americans' Katrina-driven displacement and as contributing to the inability of many African-Americans to return to New Orleans. The Latino experience storied in this banner reflects challenges confronting undocumented migrants and the photographs were storied in the clustered phototext in Figure 2 and are now reorganised and directly contrasted with 'similar' experiences in the African-American community. While including the particularities of each community, the underlying cause for each exemplar of social suffering is clearly identified as exploitation. The co-researchers included the government's failure to generate work and housing for New Orleanians of colour as one explanation of this exploitation. As importantly, the texts and the photographs are organised to create a rethreaded whole, one that both embodies the co-researchers' critical bifocality and affirms through representation the project's tagline, 'two communities, one photovoice'.

The second collective photonarrative included herein extends earlier analyses and reflects the health promoters' developing critical bifocality through their juxtaposition of the individual-level experiences and systemic circulations of power they documented and co-analysed. The banner explicitly contrasts the ways in which the government – in this case the New Orleans Police Department (NOPD) – presents itself and the New Orleans community via the billboard described previously in Figure 1 and the co-researchers' images and analyses of New Orleanians post-Katrina.

In this re-presentation of the original phototext, the co-researchers are more explicit about implicating the NOPD as intentionally misrepresenting the lived experiences of many in New Orleans. They named the causes of community members' 'depression and sadness', to be lack of housing, closed businesses, graffiti on buildings, and a failure of the police to protect them. Significantly, they spoke about the entire community, not only the African-American and Latino communities, acknowledging the social suffering of all New Orleanians. The transitional story implicates government labour policies as

ANALYZING SYSTEMIC RACISM AND OPPRESSION

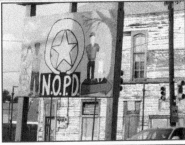

Paint a Perfect Picture

The city of New Orleans has been trying to paint a perfect picture with billboards depicting happy families being supported by NOPD post-Katrina. In reality, people are suffering from depression and sadness due to the lack of housing, closed businesses with graffiti on the buildings, and lack of visible police patrols and protection in their neighborhoods.

These pictures show how government policies impact people, leaving them to fight on their own. In the long run people lose hope and become products of a failed system.

This is a call to government to change some policies in order to be able to work with people who are unemployed, to protect immigrants who have come to help rebuild the city and work in the United States, and to provide affordable housing for low-income families.

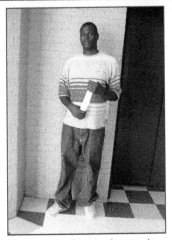

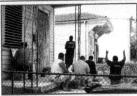

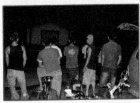

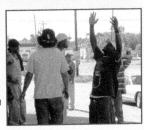

We have a group of Latino men who are currently unemployed. They sometimes get daily work, but never with a steady employer. They are scared to leave their homes because when they do, they are being assaulted because people think that they have cash in their pockets. Because these men are undocumented, they are unable to receive a paycheck from their employer or open up a bank account because the employer would be in trouble for hiring undocumented workers. So instead they just hang out at home. Who is responsible for helping these people?

Another Latino man is unemployed and uncertain about finding work because many employers are tricking Latinos into working for them but do not want to pay when the work is done. Mr. Suazo compares his hard times with the good times just after Katrina when there was great demand for workers and helpers of any kind, as opposed to now where he can't really trust others when it comes to getting paid. Through his time of need, he remains patient because he feels that some work will come. He is always hopeful through his belief that God will look after him and his people to protect them.

Mr. Anthony is an African-American man who has spent his best years in jail. He has been on the street for six months but he is still trapped in the system due to his background. He is a convicted felon who wants to do better but doors are steadily closing in his face. Mr. Anthony is trapped in the system. What can we do so that he can put himself back into society so that he can be a productive citizen?

HOLD ON . . . just a little while longer . . .

Figure 4. 'Analysing systemic racism and oppression'. Used with permission of co-researchers.

the source of people's 'losing hope' and becoming products of a failed system. The examples of African-American and Latino men describe in detail their efforts to find work, not handouts, as well as the systemic barriers preventing each from success. In Louisiana, a criminal record is costly to expunge, and carries lengthy qualifying time periods, which severely limit opportunities for employment (Burris, 2011). Federal law requires citizenship or employment papers for migrants. Just as the men were limited by these policies, the community health workers felt frustrated that they could not better support this population. The walker-talkers and *promotoras* often encountered men in their communities who were looking for support in securing employment who visibly represented the racialised systemic unemployment and poverty in New Orleans. These men approached community health workers walking in their neighbourhoods as 'first responders', expecting them to 'solve' the challenges they faced as they struggled to support themselves and their families. The community-based health workers resituated male unemployment and/or the lack of documents as structural injustices that limited the men's abilities to support their families and sustain their communities. Ironically, perhaps, they did not include a gendered analysis that might have, for example, illuminated differential rates of education and employment within the African-American communities and contributed a more intersectional analysis.

The photonarrative banners displayed multiple themes which told stories of the two communities and how they, African-American and Latina community-based health promoters, were responding to some of Katrina's effects and documenting and analysing broader social disparities that contributed to and ensued from the disaster. The banners were translated into Spanish, and two sets (a Spanish and an English) were designed and printed for exhibition. Visitors were invited to walk around the exhibit and experience it in both languages. Co-researchers accompanied the exhibit, introducing the work to the public and then conversing with visitors as they circulated. Analysis of post-presentation interviews that the authors conducted with co-researchers (Scheib & Lykes, 2013) suggest that these presentations challenged co-researchers to interpret their creative, participatory, and action research work in conversation with deeply familiar dialogic partners (e.g. family, co-workers) and those whom they had never met (e.g. other New Orleanians, community health promotion colleagues, conference attendees in Boston). They performed some of the skills that they had developed through the photoPAR processes and recognised the significance of what they had done: that they indeed were researchers who had documented and critically interpreted the lived experiences of many in their communities, including themselves, and their work as women community-based health promoters. The photoPAR process facilitated this documentation and exhibition of an emergent model of women's post-disaster response, where health promotion is community-based, centres in self-help and cross-community support, provides interracial empathy, and draws on and re-presents critically bifocal analyses from which future, more systemic, actions can be derived.

Challenges, limitations, and lessons learned

This participatory action research process was infused – and transformed – by the visual and dramatic performances of local African-American and Latina community-based health promoters in collaboration with their work-based supervisors and white antiracist feminist university-based researchers. In contexts in which individuals, families, employers and employees, and systems of service provision have been shattered, participatory action-reflection research processes, infused by visual techniques and informed by empathetic listening and critical bifocality, facilitated local protagonists' documentation and critical analyses of their lived experiences in the wake of a humanitarian disaster. They also enhanced their self-confidence in negotiating with and responding to Katrina's individual and collective health-related effects through their ongoing participation in these iterative processes. The co-researchers in this project were, themselves, in recovery processes. When they joined the collaboration some were living in temporary housing, some were rebuilding homes, and all sought to support parents and children as well as extended families and communities while working full-time as community-based health promoters. Through protagonism, evidenced in their ongoing performances as co-researchers and in the banners they produced, they embodied 'wounded healers' (Nouwen, 1972). They cared for themselves and each other as survivors of and responders to this post-disaster context. The process also offered them professional and personal opportunities to rethread their communities, make meaning of and perform their work as ethnically, racially, and linguistically diverse women community-based health promoters, and recover from some of the personal and social psychological losses experienced post-disaster.

Secondly, photoPAR facilitated co-researchers' critical bifocality and created new audiences whom they could educate about the potential contributions of cross-community Latinas and African-Americans engaged in health promotion. Their analyses of the racialised inequities underlying the pre- and post-Katrina environment exposed racist assumptions that African-Americans were a drain on the New Orleans system, a group to be flushed out, while the recent influx of Latino labourers were described as the 'salt of the earth'. They exposed and challenged these assumptions, explaining underlying systems of exploitation and exclusion shared by both communities in photonarratives accessible to multiple linguistic and differently educated communities. They challenged media images by narrating through word and image the lived experiences of African-American men and Latinos, advocating for them as under-used and inaccurately represented in post-disaster planning and rebuilding systems. Their work challenges dominant media images and government and NGO practices of racialised disaster and recovery responses. Cultural sharing contributed to strengthening the co-researchers' cross-community empathy and to developing workplace solidarity and resilience that they extended to each other and to each other's communities.

Thirdly, this research report documents women's cross-community-based health promotion as embodied by two groups of promoters who were themselves directly affected by Katrina and crossed racial-ethnic-linguistic barriers to perform women's health advocacy and praxis. These walkers-talkers and *promotoras* collaborated in generating opportunities for their own and each other's recovery at a time of public conflict between African-Americans and Latinos. The work strengthened the women's personal resilience as well as their recognition of their own roles as health promoters, their positionalities within and across their diverse communities, and the importance of their performances as community-based health promoters in a post-disaster context. Each of these contributes importantly to their work as health advocates and deliverers in this vulnerable context of recovery.

The authors argue that the photonarratives reflect post-disaster women's health promotion and can serve as critical resources for other global health promoters who have survived and are responding to disaster(s). PhotoPAR processes facilitated and documented the promoters' developing critical bifocality and restorying of Katrina as an 'unnatural disaster'. Their knowledge production and actions suggest the need to rethink post-disaster health promotion along lines proposed by SPHERE (2011), and a strategy for extending them. Thus this research is about both the PAR processes the women engaged as Katrina survivors and the ways in which these processes constituted their self-help and health advocacy within their own and each other's communities. The outcomes or actions, that is, the situating of Katrina and its effects and recovery processes in the context of structural injustices generated by circulations of power and systemic racialised inequities, constitute a critical and bifocal understanding of disaster. Moreover, they constitute a potential public health model for disaster relief, wherein women working in community health promotion take leadership roles in outreach, informational resources, and cross-community organisation in post-disaster contexts.

Despite these multiple strengths, there were a number of limitations to this work. Organisational realities and subsequent disasters in the Gulf of Mexico (Norse & Adams, 2010) limited the project's reach despite earlier desires to replicate it with members of each of the co-researchers' communities who would themselves be co-researchers. Local co-researchers were enthusiastic about the processes and deeply engaged in many aspects of the project. Yet the project consumed considerably more of co-researchers' time and energy than they had anticipated at its outset. Thus low-income women with limited resources, who were themselves survivors of the disaster, were volunteering time and resources on top of the multiple professional and personal challenges facing them. Their recognition and celebration of their enhanced personal and professional skills and resources – and their enthusiasm for taking pictures and story-ing them – were often punctuated by stories of exhaustion and over-extension. Similar challenges faced the NGOs in which they were working and their supervisory staff who collaborated in some of these processes. University-based researchers are challenged to rethink some of the expectations surrounding participation at all levels of a photoPAR process while also ensuring that community-based co-researchers are enhancing long-term skills and opportunities through the photoPAR process.

Secondly, those in and from vulnerable and marginalised communities may view visual techniques, particularly those reliant on photography, with suspicion despite the cameras ubiquitous presence in contemporary US life. Although most community members invited to participate in the photoPAR process were willing, sometimes eager, to share their stories and allow themselves to be photographed, undocumented migrants were par-ticularly cautious, and co-researchers took extra care to protect identities, photographing people from behind, or taking photos without human figures. Others have written about the camera as an instrument of surveillance in contexts of state-sponsored violence or war (Prins, 2010). Disaster and post-disaster contexts are, arguably, similar particularly in con-texts of racialised and gendered inequities where law enforcement is frequently seen as inadequate or outright hostile to majority minoritised communities.

Finally, as antiracist and feminist university-based white researchers, the authors con-fronted contradictions and challenges throughout this photoPAR. Their underlying assumptions and critical antiracist and feminist epistemologies sometimes contrasted with the cultural diversities and more traditional personal-community values that infused the co-researchers lives and narratives. The repeated almost exclusive selection of pictures of men to include in multiple phototexts and narratives about discrimination, unemployment, and institutional racism reflect their disproportionate presence among the unemployed and their overrepresentation among first returnees and undocumented migrants, as well as more traditional or stereotypical gender assumptions of many of the co-researchers. The authors engaged in ongoing discussions among themselves to deconstruct the co-researchers' representations and to identify some of the complex circulations of power within and across the 'two communities' as well as the representations of gender reflected in many of the photonarratives. Project supervisors served as critical colleagues in many of these analyses. Yet, the co-authors deferred to the co-researchers' meaning-making, cognizant of their own university-based power and racialised white privilege and of cautions from others in the feminist development community who work in the global South. Andrea Cornwall, for example, (Cornwall & Anyidoho, 2010) cautions those in such positions to honestly engage the challenges – and limitations – of enhancing critical skills and actions among women when structural patriarchal realities in which they live and work often limit their exercise of this newly identified power.

Additionally, the authors self-consciously positioned themselves as antiracist feminist activist scholars, drawing on Aronson, Yonas, Jones, Coad, and Eng (2008) examination of the corrosive and limiting effects of white privilege on community-based participatory research, wherein they urge outsider researchers to problematise and engage racism prior to and throughout a cross-race or interracial collaborative partnership and on the first author's experiences with the New Orleans-based People's Institute for Survival and Beyond (www.pisab.org) to situate the project. Yet neither the authors nor the co-researchers analysed or de-constructed the co-authors' white privilege as it may have influenced the photoPAR processes or subsequent benefits to them through presentations and publications. Despite this, the co-researchers' election of the project tagline, 'two communities, one photovoice', referring explicitly to the African-American and Latino communities, may reflect a racialised sense of 'self and other' implicit in the co-researcher team and their erasure of whiteness. The failure to more intentionally interrogate these more local and immediate circulations of power is a yet to be addressed challenge in this process – and a critical agenda for our future antiracist feminist photoPAR processes. Despite these limitations and cautions vis-à-vis the use of visual methodologies, the authors advocate their inclusion in cross-community collaborative and participatory processes that utilize feminist antiracist approaches to research that is guided by and invests in communities shattered by disaster and defined by long standing racism and inequalities.

Acknowledgements

Thanks, first and foremost, to the Latino and African-American communities in New Orleans for sharing their experiences and stories with the community health promoters who serve their neighbourhoods. Thanks also to the health promoters, programme coordinators, and executive directors of the New Orleans collaborating organisations for their confidence in the project – and for sharing its results with their constituencies. Finally, thanks to Verena Niederhoefer, MA, Boston College, who served as a research assistant throughout this process and to the two anonymous reviewers, for their thoughtful reflections and feedback.

Disclosure statement

No potential conflict of interest was reported by the authors.

Funding

Health Care for All, Kingsley House, and the Latino Health Access Network of Catholic Charities provided in-kind support for this project and collaborated through the contribution of one day's labour for each participating health promoter. Institutional support from the Center for Human Rights and International Justice and Media Technology Services at Boston College was critical to the production of the banners while a grant from the K and S Fund of the Community Foundation of Greater Birmingham supported project expenses.

References

Aronson, R. E., Yonas, M. A., Jones, N., Coad, N., & Eng, E. (2008). Undoing racism training as a foundation for team building in CBPR. In M. Minkler & N. Wallerstein (Eds.), *Community-based participatory research for health: From process to outcomes* (2nd ed., pp. 447–452, Appendix I). San Francisco, CA: Jossey-Bass.

Barnshaw, J., & Trainor, J. (2007). Race, class, and capital amidst the Hurricane Katrina diaspora. In D. L. Brunsma, D. Overflet, & J. S. Picou (Eds.), *The sociology of Katrina: Perspectives on a modern catastrophe* (pp. 91–105). New York, NY: Rowman & Littlefield.

Boal, A. (1992). *Games for actors and non-actors*. London: Routledge.

Brown, E. (1997, November 6). New Orleans murder rate for year will set record. *The Guardian.* Retrieved from http://www.theguardian.com/world/2007/nov/06/usa

Bunster, X., & Chaney, E. M. (1989). Epilogue. In X. Bunster & E. M. Chaney (Eds.), *Sellers & servants: Working women in Lima, Peru* (pp. 217–233). Granby, MA: Bergin and Garvey.

Burris, A. (2014, September 30). Getting a second chance after a criminal record. *The Shreveport Times.* Retrieved from http://www.shreveporttimes.com

Center for Progressive Reform. (2005). *An unnatural disaster: The aftermath of Hurricane Katrina.* Report. CPR Publication, vol. 512.

Charmaz, K. (2014). *Constructing grounded theory* (2nd ed.). Thousand Oaks, CA: Sage.

Cornwall, A., & Anyidoho, N. A. (2010). Women's empowerment: Contentions and contestations. *Development, 53*(2), 144–149. doi:10.1057/dev.2010.32

Costantino, G., Malgady, R. G., & Flanagam, R. M. (2001). Narrative assessment: TAT, CAT and TEMAS. In L. A. Suziki, J. G. Ponterotto, & P. J. Meller (Eds.), *Handbook of multicultural assessment* (2nd ed., pp. 217–237). San Francisco, CA: Jossey-Bass.

Frailing, K., & Harper, D. W. (2007). Crime and hurricanes in New Orleans. In D. L. Brunsma, D. Overflet, & J. S. Picou, (Eds.), *The sociology of Katrina: Perspectives on a modern catastrophe* (pp. 51–68). New York, NY: Rowman & Littlefield.

Gault, B., Hartmenn, H., DeWeever, A. J., Werschkul, M., & Williams, E. (2005). *The women of New Orleans and the Gulf coast: Multiple disadvantages and key assets for recovery. Part I. Poverty, race, gender and class.* Washington, DC: Institute for Women's Policy Research.

Gelinas, N. (2007, May 13). New Orleans still drowning in crime. *The Dallas Morning News.* Retrieved from http://www.dallasnews.org/

Keyes, A. (2010, August 10). Racial tensions linger in Post-Katrina New Orleans. *National Public Radio.* Retrieved from http://www.npr.org/

Logan, J. R. (2006). *The impact of Katrina: Race and class in storm damaged neighborhoods.* Providence: Brown University. Retrieved from http://www.s4.brown.edu/Katrina/report.pdf

Lykes, M. B. (1994). Terror, silencing, and children: International multidisciplinary collaboration with Guatemalan Maya communities. *Social Science and Medicine, 38*(4), 543–552. doi:10.1016/02779536(94)90250-X

Lykes, M. B. (2001). Creative arts and photography in participatory action research in Guatemala. In P. Reason & H. Bradbury (Eds.), *Handbook of action research* (pp. 363–371). Thousand Oaks, CA: Sage.

Lykes, M. B. (2013). Participatory and action research as a transformative praxis: Responding to humanitarian crises from the margins. *American Psychologist, 68*(8), 772–783. doi:10.1037/a0034360

Lykes, M. B., & Scheib, H. (2015). The artistry of emancipatory practice: Photovoice, creative techniques, and feminist anti-racist participatory action research. In H. Bradbury-Huang (Ed.), *Handbook of action research III* (pp. 131–142). Thousand Oaks, CA: Sage.

Maguire, P. (1987). *Doing participatory research: A feminist approach*. Amherst, MA: UMass Center for International Education.

Masozera, M., Bailey, M., & Kercher, C. (2007). Distribution of impacts of natural disasters across income groups: A case study of New Orleans. *Ecological Economics, 63*, 299–306. doi:10.1016/j.ecolecon.2006.06.013

Norse, E. A., & Adams, J. (2010). *Impacts, perceptions, and policy implications of the deepwater horizon oil and gas disasters*. Washington, DC: Environmental Law Institute.

Nouwen, H. J. M. (1972). *The wounded healer: Ministry in contemporary society*. New York, NY: Doubleday.

Pavlovsky, E. (1990). Psícodrama analítico: Su historia. Reflexiónes sobre los movimientos rances y Argentino [Analytic psychodrama: Its history. Reflections on the French and Argentine Movements]. *Clínica y análisis grupal [Clinical and Group Analysis], 12*(1), 9–45.

Plyer, A., (Ed.). (2011). *Resilience and opportunity: Lessons from the U.S. Gulf coast after Katrina and Rita*. Washington, DC: Brookings Institution Press.

Prins, E. (2010). Participatory photography: A tool for empowerment or surveillance? *Action Research, 8*, 426–443. doi:10.1177/1476750310374502

Scheib, H., & Lykes, M. B. (2013). African American and Latina community health workers engage *PhotoPAR* as a resource in a post-disaster context: Katrina at 5 years. *Journal of Health Psychology, 18*(8), 1069–1084. doi:10.1177/1359105312470127

SPHERE. (2011). The sphere handbook: Humanitarian charter and minimum standards in humanitarian response. Retrieved from http://www.spherehandbook.org/

The Data Center. (2014). The Data Center analysis of U.S. Census Bureau data from Census 2000 and Population Estimates 2014. Retrieved from http://www.datacenterresearch.org/data-resources/who-lives-in-new-orleans-now/

Wang, C., Burris, M. A., & Ping, X. Y. (1996). Chinese village women as visual anthropologists: A participatory approach to reaching policymakers. *Social Science & Medicine, 42*(10), 1391–1400. doi:0277-9536(95)00287-1

Weis, L., & Fine, M. (2012). Critical bifocality and circuits of privilege: Expanding critical ethnographic theory and design. *Harvard Educational Review, 82*(2), 173–201.

The heroines of their own stories: Insights from the use of life history drawings in research with a transnational migrant community

Jennifer S. Hirsch[a] and Morgan M. Philbin[b]

[a]Department of Sociomedical Sciences, Mailman School of Public Health, Columbia University, New York, NY, USA; [b]HIV Center for Clinical and Behavioral Studies, New York State Psychiatric Institute and Columbia University, New York, NY, USA

ABSTRACT

In this paper, we discuss how life history drawings can serve as a valuable method for global health research. The introduction discusses qualitative approaches to concepts such as reliability, validity and triangulation, and situates the use of participatory visual methods within the broader field of participatory research. The paper reports on an experience using life history drawings as part of extended ethnographic research in rural Mexico and among Mexican migrants living in Atlanta. The primary method for that parent project was comparative ethnographic research, which included life histories collected from 13 pairs of women over 15 months of participant observation. Early in the research, the drawings contributed to a major reorientation in the direction of the research project. The insights generated through analysis of the life history drawings exemplify how this participatory research technique can direct attention to social processes that feel salient to community members. In this case, they called attention to the enormity of social change in this community over one generation, reorienting the study from one focused on change causes by migration to one that focused on two trajectories of change: generational and migration-related.

Introduction

This paper discusses how a participatory research method, life history drawings, can contribute to global health research by increasing the reliability and validity of qualitative research through the targeted elicitation of insider perspectives on social change. It does so by describing their application within a multi-sited ethnographic exploration of gender, sexuality and reproductive health among Mexican women (Hirsch, 2003). The study initially employed the life history drawing method to generate information on study participants' most significant life experiences, with a goal of ensuring that the subsequent life history interview field guides included questions on culturally significant life course events. The participatory drawings served this purpose, but they also generated compelling representations of women's dreams, losses, goals and values. These representations provided an unusual source of data on the enormity of generational changes in family dynamics and structure in this Mexican community over the past 30 years and on the social context of reproductive health. Data from the drawings contributed to a substantial reorientation of the research, including a rethinking of the sampling plan so that it included diversity in generation as well as in relation to migration status.

We argue that life history drawings show promise as a means to enhance qualitative health research and in particular how the drawings can capture themes that reflect the experiences of the wider community of which the participants are members. We first describe how life history drawings fit into the broader field of participatory research and how the use of participatory methods for triangulation might strengthen the policy-relevance of qualitative research. We use the term qualitative methods to refer to the collection of textual, visual and narrative data via methods that include interviews, participant observation, participatory methods and focus groups. As such, both ethnographic research (which frequently relies in particular on participant observation and in-depth interviews) and participatory methods overlap with the broad category 'qualitative methods.' But they are distinct from it in a number of ways, including the fact that both ethnography and participatory methods can include quantitative data collection. We then describe the research project within which the life history drawings were used and explain how the exercise was conducted and how the drawings were subsequently interpreted. This drawing method, which is uncomplicated, inexpensive and easily replicated, can help global health researchers – particularly those who do not have the luxury of extended periods of fieldwork – to produce more robust, reliable and valid data.

Triangulating qualitative methods to enhance validity and reliability

The production of reliable and valid data is a critical element in policy-relevant research, since researchers are ultimately suggesting that their findings should be the basis for policy formation and the allocation of public resources. Over the past decade health researchers have increasingly used qualitative methods to reach hidden populations and to understand the social processes that undergird strongly quantified but poorly understood correlations (NIH, 2000). Despite the power of personal stories in shaping policy, qualitative data are still frequently regarded as less generalisable (and thus potentially less useful in shaping policy) than population-level surveys. Such assumptions reflect misunderstandings about the ways qualitative findings may be generalised. The paper draws on Popay's (Popay, Rogers, & Williams, 1998) definition: ' ... the aim is to make logical generalizations to a theoretical understanding of a similar class of phenomena rather than probabilistic generalizations to a population.' We employ the terms reliability and validity based on their standard definitions for qualitative research: validity refers to the degree to which findings correspond with participants' realities (or construction of realities) whereas reliability ensures that the findings are dependable and that the methods are described with enough detail for a future researcher to repeat the work. It is in this way, as discussed below, that participatory drawing exercises can enhance the reliability and validity, and thus generalisability of qualitative research – even short term fieldwork – by pointing to key forms of social difference, or meaningful social phenomena, within a community.

Understanding what generalisability means in qualitative research is a critical first step in considering how visual participatory methods can help produce research on social processes in one place that is useful in thinking about social context in other places. Mauss, in his classic work *The Gift* (1954/1990), called our attention to the uses and complexities of gifting relationships, providing an excellent example of what qualitative generalisability means. Gifting practices vary, but their importance in constructing society is of universal relevance. What is 'generalisable' from these works is the questions and concepts they generate and the ways in which they help build conceptual frameworks useful for exploring similar phenomena in other contexts. One would not, for example, expect to find a ceremonial exchange of pigs or yams connecting elites in Boston, but researchers might draw on the broad ideas described in Mauss' work, or the very specific descriptions of gift-giving as productive of social bonds in other classic ethnographic monographs (Malinowski, 2002/1932), to look at how ceremonial gift-giving creates social connections and marks social inequalities.

Participatory research and methods

Participatory research methods, which are increasingly recognised as valuable by public health researchers, involve sequential reflection and action conducted with and by communities versus the more traditional linear research model that conducts research 'on' communities (Cornwall & Jewkes, 1995; Khanlou & Peter, 2005). Participatory research emerged to address concerns that most research is conducted by relatively powerful and privileged people with subjects who are less so (Cornwall & Jewkes, 1995). Proponents of participatory approaches seek to ameliorate socially organised power differences by including participants in a way that is substantial enough to affect the outcome of the research (De Koning & Martin, 1996; Gatenby & Humphries, 2000). De Koning and Martin write that the 'researcher and participants develop a critical awareness of circumstances influencing their lives, reflect on what this means in their individual and communal situation and decide what action would be most important and feasible to take' (1996, p. 5).

Participatory research has been used with increasing frequency in social science research as a way to include grassroots-level perspectives on public health problems and on their solutions (e.g. arts-based, visual methodologies; Theron, Mitchell, Smith, & Stuart, 2011). Starting in the early 1970s geographers and psychologists had participants draw 'mental maps' to represent their local environments (Cornwall & Jewkes, 1995). Methods then expanded through the early 2000s to include social maps that describe households and families, drawings that depict social hierarchies and stratifications, and participatory maps of the body (Theron et al., 2011). When drawings are used in research it is important to engage participants in talking about and making meaning of their own drawing, as participants are sometimes willing to use drawings to depict challenges they would not otherwise verbalise (Theron et al., 2011). This also ensures the researcher correctly interprets the drawing, and also allows for a collaborative research process (Guillemin, 2004).

It is important to distinguish between participatory research as a *process*, the goal of which is to ensure that the community has more control over research, and participatory research *methods*, the goal of which is to involve members of the community collaboratively in data collection. Participatory research as a process necessarily involves methods of organizing a research project or collecting data that are participatory, but the use of participatory methods alone does not necessarily imply ceding (or even sharing) control of the research topic. Furthermore, as noted, the extent to which the research process is participatory does not necessarily correspond to a qualitative or ethnographic approach; it is possible to include an element of community participation in large scale surveys by working with the community to select the research topics, define the specific questions and share the results of data collection.

There are three general categories of visual participatory research methods that create opportunities for community-level participation in research: (1) video and photography; (2) music and theatre; and (3) drawings and pictures. Video and photography has been used to help asthma patients explore their perceptions of illness aetiology and coping strategies (Rich, Patashnick, & Chalfen, 2002) and as a strategy for the development of health education materials. Music and theatre co-produced or led by community participants, sometimes drawing on indigenous theatrical traditions, has featured music and performances that address health and social issues in their communities (Elkind, Pitts, & Ybarra, 2002; Ghosh, Patil, Tiwari, & Dash, 2006). Pictorial approaches include body mapping (Cornwall, 2002), community mapping (Lynn et al., 2000), sexuality life lines (McConville, 1997), sunburst diagrams, pictorial bar charts, time lines and calendars (Kesby, 2000; Howson & Smith, 2000) and reproductive life lines (Stewart, 2000). If culture is the 'taken for granted' background that shapes everyday life, then analysing what people choose to draw and how they choose to draw it can be one way to see culture. In the following section, we discuss how life history drawings were used to understand goals and dimensions of value structures among rural Mexican women and female Mexican migrants in the US.

Using participatory research to study gender, sexuality and reproductive health

Sampling framework

These data were generated as part of a comparative ethnographic study with two primary objectives: (1) to explore differences in social constructions of gender and sexuality among women and men in rural Southwestern Mexico and among Mexican migrants in Atlanta, GA and (2) to see how these differences might contribute to variations in reproductive health practices in these two different locations of a transnational community. The drawings were collected in 1999 and 2000 as part of the first author's dissertation fieldwork; work with the community has been on-going since that time, with new work attesting to the continued or even intensified pace of generational change first identified through the life history drawings (Hirsch, 2003; Hirsch, 1999).

The core sample from the parent study included 13 pair of women who were either sisters, sisters-in-law or, in one case, best friends. In each pair, one of the women lived in Atlanta, GA, and the other was interviewed in her hometown in rural western Mexico. The initial plan for purposive sampling sought diversity based on marital status, parity, age, education, migration experience and work experience; the women were systematically selected to represent the social and economic diversity of the larger community (Hirsch, 2003). Of the migrant women, some had driver's licences, working papers, and spoke English, while others spoke no English had no kin in Atlanta, and were thus far more dependent on their husbands than if they had remained in Mexico (Hirsch, 1999; Hirsch, 2003). Women who participated in the drawings ($n = 32$) came from the first round of women recruited in rural Mexico. These women were all non-indigenous; the overwhelming majority of people in that part of the Mexico are Mestizo.

The primary data collection methods used during the 15 months of fieldwork were participant observation and 6 life history interviews with each of the 26 women in the core sample, exploring (1) childhood and family life, (2) gender and differences between life in the US and in Mexico, (3) the organisation of productive and reproductive work in their families, (4) pregnancy, menstruation and reproduction, (5) fertility control and sexually transmitted diseases, and (6) sexuality in the context of courtship and marriage. The initial goal of the life history drawings was to ensure that the life history interview instruments included locally significant life cycle events. Given the project's reliance on life history narratives, the drawings were also useful as a technique for triangulation, since they provided women in the community an opportunity to represent their own vision of what a 'life history' was.

Subsequent reorientation

The life history drawings pointed to specific life cycle moments to include in the interviews, but they also contributed more generally to a reorientation of the study, which was initially focused entirely on examining migration-related change in gender, sexuality and reproductive health, to examine generational changes. Reflecting that new interest in change over time, some life history informants over the age of 40 were recruited into the core sample (adding diversity in addition to reproductive experience, social class and location of residence), and eight of the life history informants' mothers were recruited for key informant interviews, with a new field guide written expressly to explore their perspectives on how gender, sexuality and marriage had changed over their lifetime.

These drawings helped build iterativity into the research design, ensuring that the data collection on women's life histories would include women's ideas about key moments in a life history. The initial life history interview field guide, for example, asked about women's memories of their childhood birthdays but this was dropped when pictures of quinceañera celebrations and migration-relation gifts suggested that these were more important markers of life transition and moments of socially significant gift exchange. Seeing the drawings and talking with women as they produced them generated questions about first communions, graduation from primary school, quinceañeras, opportunities to work in the careers for which they had studied (for the few who had post-secondary education), and whether the tortillas they heated for their families were made from nixtamal they had taken to the mill to grind, or purchased at the corner store.

Experiences using life history drawings participatory method

Early on in the research in both Atlanta and Mexico fieldsites, the first author met with women – sometimes individually, but usually in groups – to explain that she was interested in learning about women's lives in their community and wanted to ensure that she was asking about things that were important to them. These women were asked to draw after they had been recruited into the study and completed a qualitative interview. This allowed for a sense of rapport that facilitated the drawing process. She asked that women draw pictures of the most important moments in their past, present and future; there were no explicit instructions regarding what to draw. The women were provided with large sheets of blank newsprint and magic markers.

The researchers acknowledge that this process can be challenging if participants feel that their drawing skills make them appear unsophisticated in the way they represent their lives. However, these participants were also able to express their experiences verbally (and thus in more sophisticated ways) through the in-depth interviews and the conversation that accompanied the drawing process. The researcher also addressed power dynamics by working closely with the women to create a space where they could express their opinions through drawing (i.e. a 'reassuring invitation to draw') (Theron et al., 2011, p. 23), regardless of their drawing ability (e.g. by being reassured that it did not matter what the drawing itself looked like – the researcher frequently noted that she also used stick figures when asked to draw humans).

The analysis employed a method of similar to the critical visual methodology framework outlined in Rose (2001), which focuses on the drawing itself (i.e. the technological, compositional and social), as well as having the women describe what they drew and what it means to them (Guillemin, 2004; Mair & Kierans, 2007). Women were asked if they wanted to codify the issues, themes or theories that arose from their drawings; the drawings also served as prompts to ask why they had included a specific aspect of their drawing. After the subjects completed these drawings, they discussed them as a group, which allowed participants to talk about the meaning in their drawings (Rose, 2001); this shared analysis also facilitates the production of valid and reliable knowledge (Guillemin, 2004). These drawings were referred to during subsequent individual interviews as a way to clarify specific aspects of the drawing, or verify whether emerging themes related to other participants' drawings resonated with the women.

The analysis began by the researcher asking specific questions regarding what the drawing depicted and what it meant, its spatial organisation and why people were (or were not) present (Cahill, 2007; Guillemin, 2004). Given the project's specific goal of using the drawings to validate the substantive content of the life history interview guides, another part of the analysis was to look specifically for milestone events depicted in the drawings to make sure they were included in the subsequent interviews. The drawings also served as means to ensure that the a priori selected axes of diversity around which the sample was built actually represented the most critical forms of stratification within the community; as noted above, the drawings also led to the inclusion of a fourth axis of diversity in the sampling. The analytic approach was framed using different axes of diversity to compare the women (e.g. age, profession, residence, education levels, etc.), which helped the first author to uncover themes related to generational differences in how women portray themselves as individuals and represent their own life history and future life course. This framework included examining which drawings were similar, and then assessing other similarities among the women who drew them. In addition, the broader themes of generational differences described by the women were discussed with men in the village in order to assess its relevance.

The goal of these drawings was to learn about how people see their world and what was important to them by examining differences in how people in the community represent themselves to an outsider. As such, these drawings should not be taken as transparent representations of truths about the community any more than interview data should be assumed to represent the 'truth' about an interviewee. Rather, the drawings should be seen as strategic representations, or visual portrayals of what each participant wanted the researcher to know about her life. These drawings were a process of self-crafting that revealed underlying value structures related to what a woman might want somebody to know about her and social position (e.g. whether to focus on her current life or future aspirations). Though rich in meaning, the interpretation and analysis of these drawings would not have been as nuanced in the absence of other data or contextual knowledge about the community (derived from the first author living there for 15 months). These drawings would remain useful, however, even without such 'insider' knowledge; they still paint the central themes in women's lives.

Generational differences in life history drawings

The most important finding from the drawing exercise – the finding that led to a substantial shift in direction for the research project – was that the younger women had an entirely different sense than the older women of what it meant have a life history. (In both this analysis and the subsequent research, 'younger women' refers to women born in the 1960s and after, while 'older women' refers to women born before that.) In spite of the fact that women were provided with the same instructions, and that the drawing groups were often mixed in age, the older women almost unanimously represented themselves by drawing pictures of their houses. There were differences in the ways younger and older women presented themselves and contrasted their former and current lives; these differences are discussed in more detail in the sections, below.

Figure 1, by a woman who lives in an agricultural community, shows a well-kept traditional rancho house. The drawing depicts the quiet of dawn, with the moon hanging low and the sun just rising. Most women in the rancho rise early for their morning chores, and in the drawing we see how this woman, when asked what is important about her life, draws our attention to the products of her round-the-clock labour – the chickens, the clean yard and the flower pots.

In Figure 2, by an older woman who grew up in a rural village but now lives in town, we see the gendered division of labour that characterised life in rural Mexico, with men planting and hoeing (the cowboy hats and large shoes indicate that they are men) while the women draw water and kneel to make tortillas on the comal. The drawing shows a number of physical features – the ox, the prickly pear cactus, the dry stone wall, the rows of corn plants – that characterise rural life in Mexico, indicating both the challenges of a life of subsistence agriculture and a sense of place to which Mexicans who move to town, or to the US, feel intense nostalgia.

The strikingly different drawings of the younger women illustrate the vast social, economic and demographic changes that have occurred in Mexico in the past several decades. Rising rates of female education have transformed the lives of girls in rural Mexico. In 1960, census reports suggest that 32% of the population in this region of Mexico was illiterate, by 1990 that had dropped to 11% (Hirsch, 2003, p. 166). While many young women in rural Mexico do not continue their studies beyond secondary school, it would be very unusual for a girl not to attend primary school. In many of these drawings, people sketched version of their younger selves, proudly going off to school. In the third frame of Figure 3, for example, a young girl marches into a modern cement school building

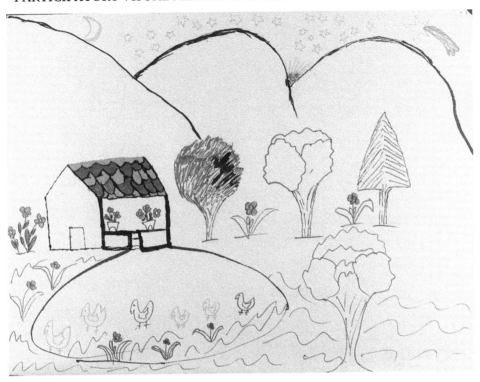

Figure 1. Drawing 1.

with a metal window frame. In the first frame of Figure 4, a girl depicts herself studying, with the following caption: 'it was in the year 1976 in my childhood, I went to school with my companions and I was very happy'. The third frames of Figures 5 and 6 depict an even higher level of educational attainment, with girls proudly displaying their high-school diplomas.

The material conditions of everyday life in rural Mexico have changed radically over the past generation, even if most people in this community are still far from wealthy. The percentage of homes with running water in the county in which the research was conducted grew from 12% in 1960 to 92% in 1990; similarly, in 1960 only 4% of homes had electricity, while in 1990 this figure was 97% (Hirsch, 2003, p. 166). The second frame of Figure 5, completed by a young woman from a relatively well-off family, depicts an elaborate quinceañera celebration, complete with a mariachi serenade and a bus trip for a group of friends to a mountain lake. In Figure 7, a young woman from the rancho illustrates her past by showing her own splendid quinceañera celebration (for which her sisters who were migrants in Atlanta all contributed to the cost of her huge pink dress), followed by her pride at her family's current access to electricity, and her bold dreams of car-ownership in the future.

The way social and economic change has remade the routine of daily life is also evident in the younger women's inclusion of leisure time, toys and play. While their mothers surely also played, it was unlikely they did so with toys such as the elaborate doll carriage shown in frame 1 of Figure 8, in which the young girl's arms seem overflowing with toys,

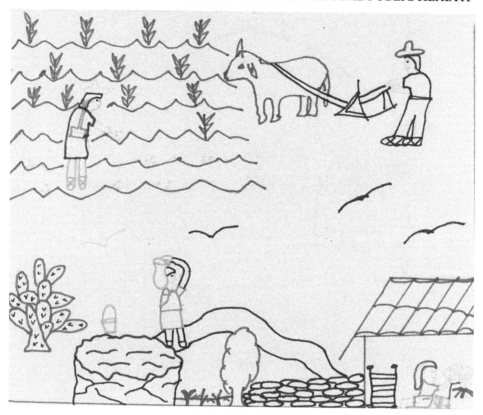

Figure 2. Drawing 2.

or the balloons and balls deliberately referred to in the caption that accompanies the second frame of Figure 3 ('playing with balloons, balls, etc.'). The material transformation of everyday life is perhaps most obvious in Figure 9, in which a well-to-do woman in Mexico contrasts her rural past (water from a pump, one-room adobe house with tiled roof, farm animals) with her current prosperity, as indicated by a car and a cement house with two well-furnished rooms featuring a refrigerator, a sink, a stove, furniture, a television and art on the walls.

'Now my husband is in the United States so we can finish building our house'

Migration and social status

The drawings of many women, both young and old, call attention to the omnipresence of migration as a source of social stratification and a strategy for social mobility. Figure 10 shows a one-room house with a neat yard and tiled roof (much like the drawings done by older women), but is distinguished by the antenna topping the roof. These antennas – supplanted in the 1990s by *antennas parabolicas* (satellite dishes) and now replaced by cable TV – were a luxury that was only accessible to those with a family member working in the US. They represent the economic success and continued commitment of

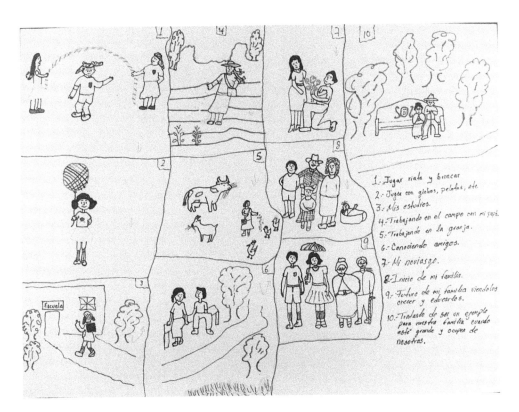

Figure 3. Drawing 3.

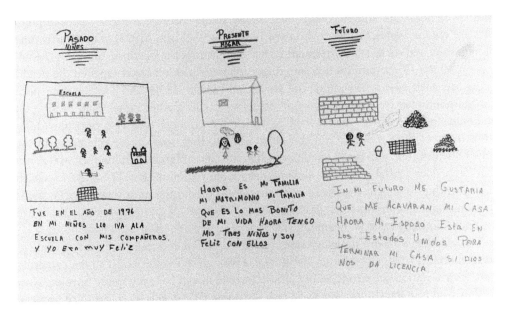

Figure 4. Drawing 4.

251

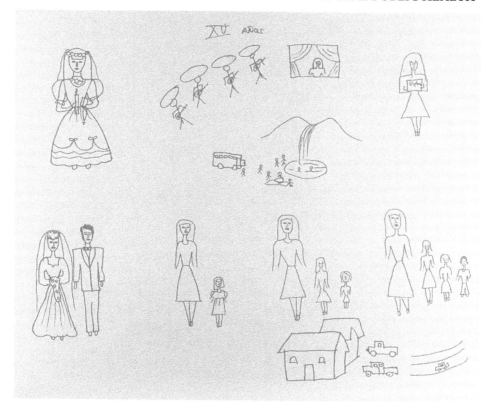

Figure 5. Drawing 5.

this migrant to his (or her) home town and family, but they also indicate what Luin Goldring has referred to as 'transnational systems of social status', in which families in rural Mexico demonstrate and negotiate their social status through forms of consumption that are only available to those who earn in dollars (Goldring, 1998). The intertwining of migration and social status-oriented forms of consumption, of course, predates the television. In the 1970s, families tied into migration networks may have ensured the neighbours saw their new refrigerators and stoves, and in the 1950s and 1960s conspicuous consumption may have meant showing off store-bought clothes rather than those spun at home. In spite of the many ways in which the younger women's drawings differ from those of their mothers and the older women, they share these references to the way in which the purchases made possible through migrant remittances are a key marker of local social status in these transnational communities. The ways in which these drawings highlight the use of consumption to mark migration-related social status in transnational communities illustrate how this type of participatory method can produce knowledge that is meaningful outside of its specific time and place.

The younger women's drawings suggest that migration continues to be a key route to social mobility. In the third frame of Figure 4, a woman shows her house under construction, with a caption she wrote: 'in my future, I would like to have my house finished. Now my husband is in the United States to finish the house if God wills it'. In the third frame of Figure 8, another young woman demonstrates a similar dream for her future – a finished

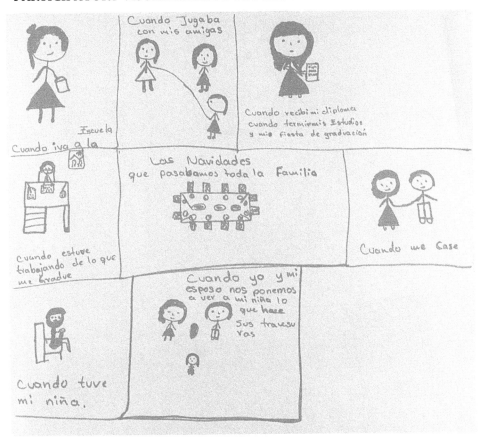

Figure 6. Drawing 6.

(and furnished) house, and the chance to provide an education for her children – neither of which would be easily accessible to her without her husband's earnings as a plumber in Atlanta. The cars featured in Drawings 5 and 7 are relatively common possessions for migrant Mexican women in the US; for women who stay behind in rural Mexico, the social and physical mobility a car would offer is a distant dream.

The women's drawings also frequently included features of life common in a transnational community. The gifts that return migrants bring are evident in the father's suitcase in Figure 11, as is the envy of those who do not have access to these gifts, which comes through in the caption to Figure 12: 'when my cousin went to California, I saw all of her clothes and everything that she put on, which was so nice, and I dreamed about coming to the US.' That same woman, who currently lives in Atlanta, shows the hard work that migrants put into staying in touch in Figure 13, which depicts talking on the phone with her mother in Mexico as one of the most important aspects of her 'present'.

Heroines of their own stories

While all the drawings represented signifiers of consumption (e.g. a car or TV antenna), the differences between the younger and older women's drawings focus attention on historical time, highlighting the many ways that life in rural Mexico has changed over the past

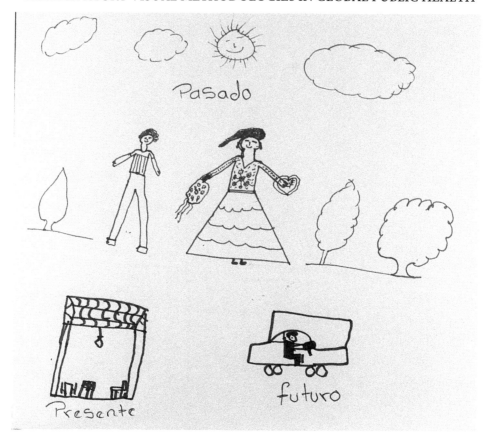

Figure 7. Drawing 7.

generation – changes which have accelerated to a breath-taking pace since initial data collection (Hirsch & Vasquez, 2012). The younger women's drawings, however, also direct our attention to individual chronological time and the trajectories of women's lives; they seem to demonstrate a different idea than the older women's drawings about what it means to have a life history. Many of the older women's drawings present a house in one frame; when compared with the graphic novel orientation used by younger women, the older women's drawings suggest that being part of a family and a homeowner is the one thing they most wish to communicate about themselves. The older women's drawings seem to say 'I am my house', whereas the younger women's drawings communicate both that being a member of a family was the crucial aspect of identities and that younger women wish to represent themselves as individuals, with individually variable life stories. The younger women's drawings tell us much more about the particularities of their achievements and relationships, hinting at the emergence of affective individualism in a way that resonates with the substantial social science literature on the phenomenon (Stone, 1979). With a narrative style that seems to draw on the Mexican popular tradition of fotonovelas (for example, in Figure 3 small arrows on the top right hand corner of each frame instruct the naïve viewer of the order in which to read the story), the younger women are the heroines of their narratives; frame by frame, the drawings depict the

254

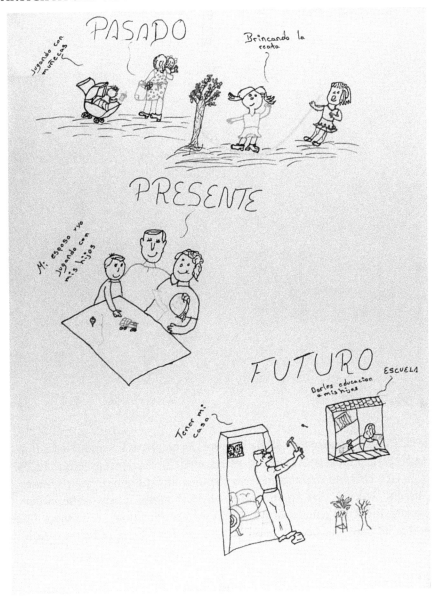

Figure 8. Drawing 8.

highlights of these women's childhoods, courtships and marriages, as well as their hopes for a prosperous and loving future. The sense of the passage of time over the life course is palpable from these drawings. They create an expectation of change, of development, implying that the choices women make matter, that they can shape their own lives, and that these women have clear hopes for what the future holds, both in terms of the affective quality of their marriages and their styles of consumption.

As is discussed at great length elsewhere (Hirsch, 2003) – and as is clear from the smiling, hand-holding couples in drawings three, six, seven and eight – the way that younger women depict their marriages in these drawings provides yet more evidence

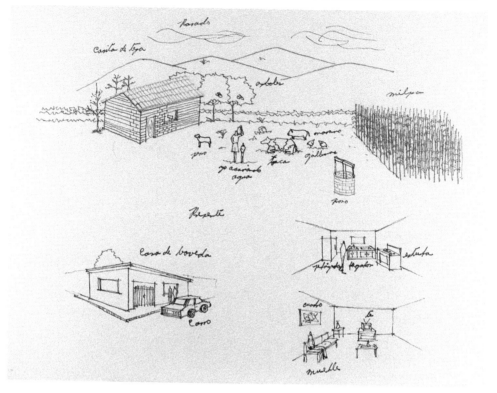

Figure 9. Drawing 9.

that marital ideals in Mexico have shifted towards an emphasis on emotional intimacy and cooperation as key criteria for the successful modern relationship. None of the older women, in fact, chose to draw themselves standing anywhere near their spouses. While this is hardly evidence that emotional or physical intimacy was unimportant to the older women, the stark generational different in representations of intimacy underlines the way that intimacy has become more prominent as a feature of marital ideals.

Discussion

This shift in the research design and questions for this project was also, ultimately, key to the intellectual significance of the project – that is, its ability to answer the questions it purported to and to present the women's realities. This use of visual participatory methods to facilitate triangulation (i.e. validity) can be extended to other populations (e.g. racial and sexual minorities, rural populations and children), as noted in Popay's (Popay et al., 1998) definition of qualitative generalisability that focuses on understanding similar classes of phenomena rather than making statements about the likelihood it will occur across a population. Specifically, this research demonstrates how integrating participatory methods into qualitative research can generate questions and conceptual frameworks useful for exploring related phenomena in other contexts. A concrete example would be that these drawings remind us that other work on gender and sexuality, whether in migration-related contexts or not, should attend to change over time rather

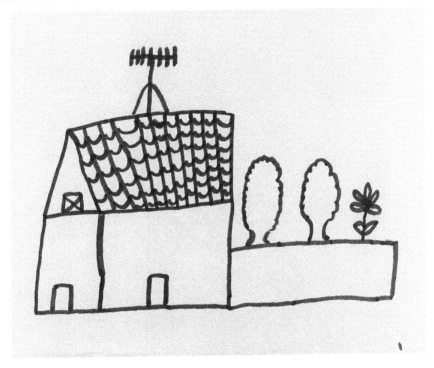

Figure 10. Drawing 10.

than assuming that the social organisation of gender or notions of personhood are unchanging.

Finally, in addition to the role the drawings played in shaping the overall project, they are compelling in and of themselves as representations of women's dreams, losses, goals and values. They provide an unusual source of data on changing notions of individuality, on how women have experienced the vast social and economic changes that have taken place in this Mexican community over the past 30 years and, ultimately, on the social context of reproductive health.

Guillemin (2004) notes that this type of drawing method works best to increase trustworthiness when incorporated into an ethnographic or interview project similar to that presented here. In addition to enhancing the validity and reliability of this life history research, the drawings generated compelling evidence of two critical forms of internal stratification within the community – generation and migration – and indeed these were ultimately the two axes of diversity around which the sampling was organised (Hirsch, 2003, pp. 1–56). They served, then, to increase the significance of the data collected by pushing the research questions towards topics that were of great significance locally but that had not been included in the initial research design.

These methods are particularly useful for researchers who lack extended time in the field as they can be conducted quickly, at low cost, and in a group setting; analysis can also begin without transcription. Multiple studies have applied these methods in short periods of time with excellent results (Theron et al., 2011). An advantage of life history drawings is that they allow for iterativity because they produce immediately analysable

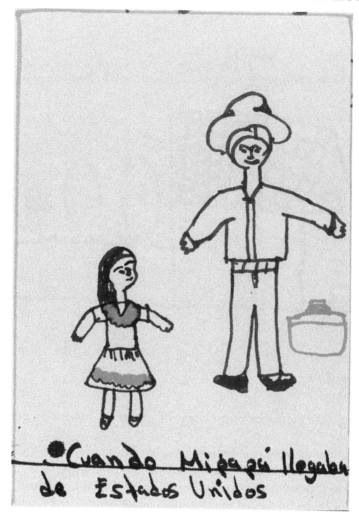

Figure 11. Drawing 11.

data available to team members not based in the field; for team-based projects, in which the bulk of data comprises taped interviews, which must be transcribed and coded prior to analysis, this level of iterativity is rarely achieved.

It is important to note that what was produced through the drawings was likely affected by the positionality of the American researcher who, to many, represented modernity and consumption. For example, the participants often described inter-generational differences in stark and broad-brush strokes. Though these themes may have been emphasised more because of the researcher, this does not mean that such themes are not valid. Positionality is discussed in more detail elsewhere (Hirsch, 2003).

The limitations inherent in participatory research methods, particularly life drawings, also existed in this project. We addressed these limitations by working with the participants to have them explain the meaning in their drawing and why they chose to represent what that they did. However, as MacEntee and Mitchell (2011) note, it is also important for researchers to understand the community context and thus be able to critically explore

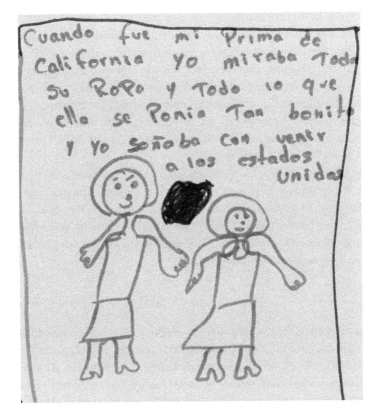

Figure 12. Drawing 12.

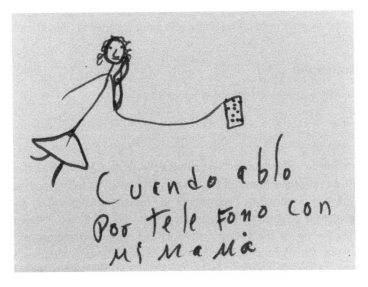

Figure 13. Drawing 13.

any potential limits of a particular participant or the group's perspective to avoid a positivist framework. The issue of validity is a common critique of visual methodologies, with claims that the interpretation of images is subjective and ambiguous (Guillemin, 2004). However, qualitative research acknowledges the existence of multiple truths, and that the images are strategic representations of what somebody wants to portray, not always a singular truth. To address this critique the study analysed the drawings and the participants' interpretations of the drawings in conjunction with interviews and participant observation. The triangulation of these data increased validity by allowing participants multiple ways to express their experiences.

This research used ethnographic methods, with objectives developed by the researcher rather than by the community. As basic social science research, the goal was not to inform behavioral change or impact community-level health directly. However, data generated from this study have been cited in Ministry of Health reports to argue for an increased focus on migration as a risk factor for HIV infection (Magis-Rodríguez, Bravo García, Gayet-Serrano, Rivera-Reyes, & De Luca, 2008).

Conclusions

These findings demonstrate how participatory research methods such as life history drawings can be a valuable tool in global public health research. By uncovering local phenomenon, and connecting them to broader social forces (which in the data presented here include consumption, changing notions of individuality and reproductive health) participatory research methods can increase the reliability and validity of qualitative research, with an ultimate goal of developing policy that takes into account both those critical social forces and the way people experience them.

Acknowledgements

Jennifer S. Hirsch gratefully acknowledges research assistance from Laurie Helzer, who conducted a literature review for an early draft of this paper, and from Caroline M. Parker.

Disclosure statement

No potential conflict of interest was reported by the authors.

Funding

The data collection for this research was supported by the Andrew Mellon Foundation through a grant to the Department of Population Dynamics at Johns Hopkins University, the National Science Foundation Programme in Cultural Anthropology (SBR-9510069) and the International Migration Programme at the Social Science Research Council. Jennifer S. Hirsch receives institutional support from the Department of Sociomedical Sciences and from the Columbia Population Research Center, which is supported by the Eunice Kennedy Shriver National Institute of Child Health and Human Development (R24HD058486). Morgan Philbin is supported by an NIMH postdoctoral training grant (T32 MH019139, Principal Investigator, Theodorus Sandfort, Ph.D.) at the HIV Center for Clinical and Behavioral Studies at the New York State Psychiatric Institute and Columbia University (P30-MH43520; Principal Investigator: Robert H. Remien, Ph.D.). The content is solely the responsibility of the authors and does not represent the official views of the National Institutes of Health.

References

Cahill, C. (2007). Participatory data analysis. In S. Kindon, R. Pain, & M. Kesby (Eds.), *Participatory action research approaches and methods: Connecting people, participation and place* (pp. 181–187). Abingdon: Routledge.

Cornwall, A. (2002). Body mapping: Bridging the gap between biomedical messages, popular knowledge and lived experiences. In A. Cornwall & A. Welbourne (Eds.), *Realizing rights: Transforming approaches to sexual and reproductive wellbeing* (pp. 219–234). New York, NY: Zed Books.

Cornwall, A., & Jewkes, R. (1995). What is participatory research? *Social Science & Medicine, 41* (12), 1667–1676.

De Koning, K., & Martin, M. (1996). *Participatory research in health: Issues and Experiences.* New York, NY: Zed Books.

Elkind, P. D., Pitts, K., & Ybarra, S. L. (2002). Theater as a mechanism for increasing farm health and safety knowledge. *American Journal of Industrial Medicine, 42*(S2), 28–35. doi:10.1002/ajim.10053

Gatenby, B., & Humphries, M. (2000). Feminist participatory action research: Methodological and ethical issues. *Women's Studies International Forum, 23*(1), 89–105. doi:10.1016/S0277-5395(99)00095-3

Ghosh, S. K., Patil, R. R., Tiwari, S., & Dash, A. P. (2006). A community-based health education programme for bio-environmental control of malaria through folk theatre (Kalajatha) in rural India. *Malaria Journal, 5*(1), 123. doi:10.1186/1475-2875-5-123

Goldring, L. (1998). The power of status in transnational social fields. *Comparative Urban and Community Research, 6,* 165–195.

Guillemin, M. (2004). Understanding illness: Using drawings as a research method. *Qualitative Health Research, 14*(2), 272–289. doi:10.1177/1049732303260445.

Hirsch, J. S. (1999). 'En El Norte La Mujer Manda' Gender, generation, and geography in a Mexican transnational community. *American Behavioral Scientist, 42*(9), 1332–1349.

Hirsch, J. S. (2003). *A Courtship after marriage: Sexuality and love in Mexican transnational families.* Berkeley: University of California Press.

Hirsch, J. S., & Vasquez, E. E. (2012). Mexico-US migration, social exclusion and HIV risk: Multisectoral approaches to understanding and preventing infection. In K. Organista (Ed.), *HIV prevention with Latinos: Theory, research and practice* (pp. 103–120). London: Oxford University Press.

Howson, J., & Smith, A. (2000). 'Safely through the night': A review of behaviour change in the context of HIV/AIDS. *PLA Notes, 37,* 92–99.

Kesby, M. (2000). Participatory diagramming as a means to improve communication about sex in rural Zimbabwe: A pilot study. *Social Science & Medicine, 50*(12), 1723–1741. doi:10.1016/S0277-9536(99)00413-X

Khanlou, N., & Peter, E. (2005). Participatory action research: Considerations for ethical review. *Social Science & Medicine, 60*(10), 2333–2340. doi:10.1016/j.socscimed.2004.10.004

Lynn, H., Ward, D., Nugent, C., Potts, L., Skan, L., & Conway, N. (2000). Putting breast cancer on the map. *PLA Notes, 37,* 106–112.

MacEntee, K., & Mitchell, C. (2011). Lost and found in translation: Participatory analysis and working with collections of drawings. In L. Theron, C. Mitchell, & J. Stuart (Eds.), *Picturing research: Drawing as visual methodology* (pp. 89–104). Rotterdam: Sense.

Magis-Rodríguez, C., Bravo García, E., Gayet-Serrano, C., Rivera-Reyes, P., & De Luca, M. (2008). *El VIH y El SIDA en México al 2008: Hallazgos, tendencias y reflexiones.* Mexico, DF: CENSIDA.

Mair, M., & Kierans, C. (2007). Descriptions as data: Developing techniques to elicit descriptive materials in social research. *Visual Studies*, *22*(2), 120–136. doi:10.1080/14725860701507057

Malinowski, B. (2002). *Argonauts of the Western Pacific: An account of native enterprise and adventure in the archipelagoes of Melanesian New Guinea*. London: Routledge. (Original work published 1932).

Mauss, M. (1990). *The gift: The form and reason for exchange in archaic societies*. New York, NY: Norton. (Original work published 1950).

McConville, F. (1997). Sexuality lifelines: Participatory assessment of reproductive health. *Participatory Learning and Action*, *1*, 90–91.

NIH. (2000). Qualitative methods in health research: Opportunities and considerations in application and review. *Office of Behavioral and Social Sciences Research*. Retrieved from http://obssr.od.nih.gov/pdf/Qualitative.pdf.

Popay, J., Rogers, A., & Williams, G. (1998). Rationale and standards for the systematic review of qualitative literature in health services research. *Qualitative Health Research*, *8*(3), 341–351. doi:10.1177/104973239800800305

Rich, M., Patashnick, J., & Chalfen, R. (2002). Visual illness narratives of asthma: Explanatory models and health-related behavior. *American Journal of Health Behavior*, *26*(6), 442–453.

Rose, G. (2001). *Visual methodologies: An introduction to the interpretation of visual materials*. London: Sage.

Stewart, K. A. (2000). Toward a historical perspective on sexuality in Uganda: The reproductive lifeline technique for grandmothers and their daughters. *Africa Today*, *47*(3), 122–148. doi:10.1353/at.2000.0075

Stone, L. (1979). *The family sex and marriage: In England 1500–1800*. New York, NY: Harper & Row.

Theron, L., Mitchell, C., Smith, A. L., & Stuart, J. (Eds). (2011). *Picturing research: Drawing as visual methodology*. Rotterdam: Sense.

Community health workers as cultural producers in addressing gender-based violence in rural South Africa

Naydene de Lange[a] and Claudia Mitchell[b]

[a]Faculty of Education, Nelson Mandela Metropolitan University, Port Elizabeth, South Africa; [b]Department of Integrated Studies in Education, McGill University, Montreal, Canada

ABSTRACT

South Africa has been experiencing an epidemic of gender-based violence (GBV) for a long time and in some rural communities health workers, who are trained to care for those infected with HIV, are positioned at the forefront of addressing this problem, often without the necessary support. In this article, we pose the question: How might cultural production through media making with community health workers (CHWs) contribute to taking action to address GBV and contribute to social change in a rural community? This qualitative participatory arts-based study with five female CHWs working from a clinic in a rural district of South Africa is positioned as critical research, using photographs in the production of media posters. We offer a close reading of the data and its production and discuss three data moments: CHWs drawing on insider cultural knowledge; CHWs constructing messages; and CHWs taking action. In our discussion, we take up the issue of cultural production and then offer concluding thoughts on 'beyond engagement' when the researchers leave the community.

and we go from house to house … and place to place … (Community health worker, *Our photos, our videos, our stories*; Mitchell, Mak, & Stuart, 2005)

Introduction

The national news media in South Africa highlighted the actions of a group of community health workers (CHWs) in the Free State who silently protested against the sliding quality of public health care in the province with a sit-in ('Free State health workers arrested over sit-in', 2014). In doing so, they positioned themselves as concerned health workers acting on what they perceived to be poor service delivery by the provincial health department. Their silent protest signalled the type of action CHWs can take around issues of importance to them and their communities (in spite of the fact that they are at the low end of the earning scale and have little status and power). This feeds into a critical debate in South Africa: '[Are CHWs] to be viewed as agents of community empowerment or

263

narrow functionaries of the health system?' (Schneider, Hlophe, & Van Rensburg, 2008, p. 180). As Schneider et al. point out, the concept of CHWs as 'community/lay workers in the health sector' (p. 180) was introduced in South Africa at a time when addressing HIV and AIDS was a priority, and consequently, community health work focused on providing home care to patients dying of AIDS.[1] CHWs are community members typically selected by the local community, through their local clinic, to be trained in basic health services and to provide these services to members of their communities (Berman, Gwatkin, & Burger, 1987); in effect decentralising the clinic approach to health care (Storer, 2013). Indeed, CHWs are at the forefront of rural health, particularly in the context of HIV and AIDS and observe, close-up, the drivers of the infection, namely poverty (Nelson Mandela Foundation, 2005) and gender-based violence (GBV) (Garcia-Moreno & Watts, 2000; Maman, Campbell, Sweat, & Gielen, 2000), in the everyday lives of their clients.[2] The rural context in which work opportunities are scarce not only deepens poverty but contributes to people's material deprivation, which affects relationships and fuel GBV.

In this article, we explore the engagement of a group of five female CHWs from a clinic in rural KwaZulu-Natal, South Africa, and focus on their frontline action, through a lens of cultural production, to address GBV. It has been widely documented that violence profoundly affects every aspect of life in South Africa (Dartnell & Gevers, 2015), and that the country has one of the highest rates of sexual assault in the world (Abrahams et al., 2009). In spite of the difficulties of measuring the extent of the problem, it is estimated that only 1 in 25 women who are raped report it to the police (Machisa, Jewkes, Lowe-Morna, & Rama, 2011). As Mullick, Teffo-Menziwa, Williams, and Jina (2010) highlight, such violence is gender-based and embedded in pre-existing social, cultural, and economic inequalities between men and boys and women and girls, and according to Jewkes, Flood, and Lang (2014, p. 2) is linked to 'the social values, roles, behaviours, and attributes thought to be appropriate and expected for men and women'. We concur with Jewkes et al. (2014) that addressing the different types of GBV and their contexts, as well as same-sex GBV (Dunkle, Jewkes, Murdock, Sikweyiya, & Morrell, 2013; Posel, 2005), entails 'transforming relations, norms, and systems that sustain gender inequality and violence' (Jewkes et al., 2014, p. 1). It is therefore necessary to consider context and culture as starting point in addressing GBV, engaging with the power that shapes social relations (silencing or empowering) and working from where people are and what they think they can do. This is necessary particularly in rural contexts (see e.g. Amnesty International, 2008) and for us, is at the centre of our work with CHWs in addressing GBV because CHW are right there and go from 'house to house' in the community. There is still not enough known about the intimate reality of the family and local community and, concomitantly, about the place of local engagement and local solutions, particularly in rural contexts. We thus focus on local engagement and the idea of local solutions in this article. We ask ourselves what role CHWs, a group typically marginalised in relation to health and social policies, can play in addressing GBV and contributing to social change in a rural community. How might they participate as cultural producers in media making to address GBV? How can this work inform the everyday work of addressing GBV in rural South Africa? To what extent can CHWs become 'action oriented' in addressing GBV?

We first contextualise the study in participatory arts-based research and its relationship to taking action to address critical social issues at the community level, and then link to cultural production, media making, and social change, in a conceptual framework to shape the study but also to make meaning of the work produced by the CHWs. We explain the methodology of the study and how the health workers produced the media posters and then offer a close reading of the data around the process and products. Finally, we offer a discussion of CHWs as cultural producers in addressing GBV in a rural community. In so doing, we return to what the role of CHWs could be in South Africa.

Participatory arts-based research and cultural production

The idea of using local participatory arts-based and other media productions to address critical health and social issues is part of a burgeoning body of work that draws on tools and methods such as photovoice, participatory video, and digital storytelling (De Lange & Geldenhuys, 2012; Gubrium & Harper, 2013; Milne, Mitchell, & De Lange, 2012; Mitchell, 2011; Vaughan, 2014). Such work facilitates the process of gaining greater insider knowledge on how participants themselves view issues, and at the same time allows for raising participant and community awareness of the issues under investigation through, for example, local photo exhibitions and screenings of the videos. The work referred to in the article adds to other community-based projects in South Africa, which investigate the ways in which media making and arts-based approaches can help to confront GBV (see e.g. the 2007 'Clothesline Project' in Cape Town). While these projects draw on the perspectives of local participants, all in the service of challenging dominant images of girls and women in subordinate positions, we would argue that there is a need for a more nuanced understanding of what it means for local community members – in this instance CHWs – to disrupt the automatic transmission of cultural norms which underpin GBV across generations through media making as cultural production.

At the same time, however, as Vaughan (2014) points out in her work with youth, and especially in relation to the idea of developing a critical consciousness through participation, that there may be limitations to what this work can accomplish. On the one hand, she argues, Freire's theory of critical consciousness 'underpins participatory research projects where collective action for social change is a desired outcome' (p. 185), and 'the development of critical consciousness through reflection is inextricably linked with the critical capacity to make choices to transform reality through critical action' (p. 185). On the other hand, her work with youth shows that being engaged in a participatory project, which encourages critical thinking and raises awareness, does not naturally lead to taking action for positive social change. This may be particularly so in adult-driven projects. In the case of our work with CHWs, which extends over several years, it was the women themselves who wanted to create media productions which are locally relevant and could be used in their day-to-day work, and in this respect they were the ones seeking to take action in the community to bring about positive social change.

Cultural production, media making, and change

Our participatory study with CHWs to address GBV in their community is informed by the work of various media theorists on cultural production, media making, and taking action. Fiske's (1987) work has been particularly important in understanding various forms of text in cultural production: primary texts, or what is produced (a film, photo exhibition, collage, media poster); producer text (the perspectives of the participants engaged in producing media texts); and audience texts (the critical reception by viewers of what is produced). We link Fiske's forms of texts in cultural production to media making, and draw on the work of Buckingham and Sefton-Greene (1994) which has contributed to shifting the idea of engagement with media from a passive reception of media messages to an active engagement of producing media messages. A particular genre of media making that characterised Buckingham and Sefton-Green's (1994) work with youth, and which we use, is the production of media posters as a familiar form in the everyday lives of the youth (they produced media posters using photographs with short accompanying texts to address youth identity). Turning to GBV, Walton (1995), in her work with Grade 6 girls in the UK, also used the genre of media poster as a type of political poster. The girls, tired of being sexually harassed by boys in their school, produced media posters using photographs, drawings, and slogans, targeting the boys as audience and taking action to stop the harassment. Using the work of these researchers, conceptually organised around the idea of disruption through media posters, we were interested in how cultural production through making media posters might contribute to CHWs taking action to address GBV in their everyday work in the community.

The project: community health workers making media to address gender-based violence

Who are the producers?

The women were all isiZulu first-language speakers based at and employed as CHWs at a clinic in a rural KwaZulu-Natal district. Each attended to 60 homes, and received a monthly stipend of R1000 (€65 or $95). In total, the 5 health workers with whom we worked were reaching 300 homes in the rural community. The backstory to this media-making project with the five CHWs, all between the ages of 50 and 62 years, started several years earlier when they were participants in a project on the role of communities in addressing GBV (Hamon, 2011). In the project organised by Hamon (2011), the women participated in a series of arts-based workshops to consider both the issues and actions that could be taken to combat the high levels of GBV, which they were witnessing in their community. A GBV guide, '*Vimba ukuhlukumeza* [Stop abuse]' (Hamon, 2011), was produced as part of the project in both isiZulu and English, for use when they were out doing their work in the community. What also came out of the study was a commitment on the part of this small group of CHWs to keep going with GBV work even after the project was over (De Lange et al., 2010; and the follow-up, Moletsane et al., 2010), and it was indeed possible to keep going. We discovered this in a follow-up workshop session a few months after the completion of the 'Stop abuse' guide (2011) when the group requested additional visual material to support their work on addressing GBV as they went from house to house. One woman pointed out:

> I would compile a file of such pictures, will show them [the community] those [photographs] which could affect her [a woman living with HIV] badly and those which will make her want to go on.

The setting

Building on what the CHWs requested (visual material which they could use in their day-to-day work), we organised an overnight residential workshop at a guest lodge. We have long been interested in the importance of participants, especially women, getting away from the challenges of their double and triple shifts as mothers, community members, and workers (see Khau, 2009 and Masinga's 2012 study), in order to fully participate in research. The guest lodge close to the community was familiar to the women because they had visited it for previous workshops but it was sufficiently far away from their regular world to truly make it a getaway. The sessions in the participatory workshop were videotaped and transcribed for further analysis.

Producing the media poster texts

Part one: the steps in production of the primary texts

Here we map out the series of steps we followed in the media-making workshop which took place over two days.

Step 1 – initial engagement. We screened 'Our Stories' (Mitchell, De Lange, Moletsane, & Stuart, 2006); a composite video made up of short participatory videos produced several years earlier by secondary school youth from the community telling their stories about GBV. The CHWs confirmed that GBV was still an ongoing issue and that there was abuse happening even at primary school level.

Step 2 – identifying key themes. The women then brainstormed key issues underpinning GBV which they thought needed to be addressed and which they felt could be addressed in the community. The issues they identified included the following: children not respecting older people, grandmothers being raped, domestic violence where the woman is beaten by a man, the danger of having multiple sex partners, the effects of alcohol abuse, and keeping silent when it is the bread winner who is the abuser. We noted these down on a flip chart. The women discussed, in isiZulu, whether these were indeed the most important issues to be addressed and if so what relevant media posters could be produced to enable them to engage with the community around the issues.

Step 3 – taking the photographs. The women carefully planned the construction and framing of the photographs for each issue identified. Using digital cameras to take the photographs; some with objects symbolic of an issue and others involving the staging or acting out of an issue, they also ensured that visual ethical issues such as anonymity were adhered to so that their work would do no harm to anyone when it was used in the community (Figure 1).

When considering how to show that GBV affects the family, the women realised it would be difficult to take a photograph of a family because there were not whole families nearby to photograph, and if they did they might have been constrained by visual ethics from taking a photograph. In such cases, we suggested that they draw a picture to use with community members when talking about how GBV affects the family (See below four of the drawings created by the CHWs.) (Figure 2).

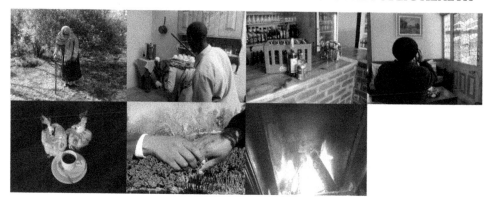

Figure 1. Photographs depicting the different issues identified.

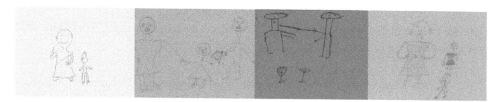

Figure 2. Drawings made to depict the effects of gender violence.

Step 4 – creating captions or messages. Once printed, the photographs were mounted on construction paper and the women created captions, in this case slogans, for each image. They discussed these at length because they wanted the messages to be simple but clear, and wanted to use appropriate isiZulu words. They also agreed that the captions should be both in isiZulu and English and with the assistance of the co-facilitator,[3] the captions were translated and written in English.

Step 5 – producing the package of media posters. A total of 10 media posters were produced. These 10 posters in draft format were then transformed into digital format for reproduction by our research assistant. Multiple sets of media posters were reproduced so that each community health worker could own a set. The sets were laminated and a copy of the 'Stop Abuse' guide (2011) was included to complement the set of media posters. The sets were neatly packaged in plastic envelopes and handed over to the CHWs (Figure 3). We documented the handover by taking photographs that could be displayed in their clinic.

Part two: data moments
In this section, we offer an analysis of both the process and the products created in relation to cultural production. Using a close-reading approach (Tobin, 2000), we analysed the transcripts from the workshop, the media posters, and our field notes, and offer what we call 'data moments'.

Data moment 1 – CHWs with insider cultural knowledge. The insider cultural knowledge revealed by the women as they discussed their images and messages highlighted what they

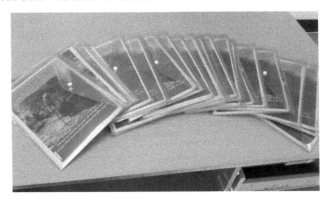

Figure 3. The sets of media posters.

saw to be critical issues related to sexual violence. In this regard, Vaughan (2014, p. 184) reminds us that when we explore the health-related knowledge of our participants 'that [such] knowledge is an expression of historically, socially and psychologically situated lived experience'. While, as noted below, these are not necessarily new issues, the ways in which the women expressed the issues and how they saw them as interrelated, are important. As the five women brainstormed and discussed what they saw as key areas to address, they began to comment on what they were seeing, from the inside, in relation to GBV. First they related the work to their own positions in the family, namely that of grandmothers. They spoke about how GBV against grandmothers relates to the myth of curing AIDS in males who sleep with a virgin and how *gogos* (grandmothers) have now become victims of this violence:

> They [males] saw that when sleeping with a virgin nothing happened. If you have virus you still have HIV, now they have changed to the old women. You know, they started from the very young children and they saw that the virus didn't be cured. They proceeded to the virgin and so the HIV is still there and now they are with older womans, old *gogos*.

Another woman added: 'The elderly women, they are no longer interested in these sexual activities so it's very annoying to her.' They also spoke up on the pervasive silences around certain forms of violence and the difficulty of naming violence: 'As you hear there is that woman, if that one asks "Did he hit you?" she said, "It's not violence, it's just his way." It means she have accepted everything what her husband does to her.' Another woman commented: 'The problem is with us women because we always accept everything because we don't know [what rules] our husbands.' Moletsane (2011) drew attention in her work on culture, memory, and sexuality, to the ways in which culture is often seen to be static, and synonymous with what the dominant group defines as culture, and how it contributes to the normalisation of GBV.

Intergenerational sexual violence in the family (see e.g. Andersson, Ho-Foster, Mitchell, Scheepers, & Goldstein, 2007; Jewkes, Levin, & Penn-Kekana, 2002; Madu & Peltzer, 2000) featured in their discussion, as can be seen in comments about incest:

> You know ... to speak out is a very [big] message because even the mother at home knows that her child is being raped by her father, she just keeps silent. As we are working at the community we can't work because the mother you ... you mustn't talk about that because the dad is going to be arrested and he's a bread winner and what are you going to eat?

They also spoke about fear of their own grandsons: ' ... our grandsons beat us'. Whether they referred to their own experiences or to the community in general, this points to both sexism and ageism. In this regard, Jewkes and Morrell (2010) argue that because of patriarchy still being dominant in South Africa and possibly more so in rural areas, the superiority of men is accepted as the norm and the subservence of both young and old women increases their vulnerability. Russell et al. (2014) also argue that patriarchal culture combined with a legacy of violence creates a society of boys who believe that they may control girls and women, and that they are entitled to use force to do so. Jewkes (2002) makes the point that poverty increases the risk for women; when men do not have economic power and are materially impoverished, they may make up for it by exerting power over women.

Finally, the women commented on other behaviours, which they also regarded as acts of sexual violence even though these might not typically figure in the 'official literature' of sexual violence. It included swearing: 'We can teach the boys you mustn't call your sisters names like "bitch", all that names. Yes. We too we must tell the boys [what] they must do to girls'; the fact that children often witness their parents fighting: 'Yes, it's true because while the mother and father are fighting the children are scared'; and shouting: 'Even shouting to you is a violence.' In the discussions, the women talked about the relationship between young people taking drugs and abuse: 'Children are taking drugs then they are doing their own things, then I'm saying "What is the message in that?" They abuse the community.'

Data moment 2 – constructing the messages. Creating social messages whether for media posters, public service announcements for a video, or slogans to appear on shirts, involves thinking about the target audience and who needs to see or hear the message, the type of image to be presented to the audience, and the words of the slogan. In total, the women created eight messages: 'Violence affects everyone in the family', 'Teach your children to respect people', 'Being beaten by your husband, brother, son or grandson is violence, SPEAK OUT!'; 'Any abuse in the family must be reported even if it is the breadwinner'; 'Think before you do things, your choices have consequences'; 'A real man has only one partner'; 'Having sex with elderly women (*gogos*) does not cure AIDS and it affects the *gogos*' health'; and 'Alcohol and drug abuse contributes to violence and destroys the community. DO NOT DRINK TOO MUCH!' The images and slogans are interesting because they do not simply repeat the many billboard messages in government and NGO-led campaigns about GBV. Rather, they represent what could be regarded as 'fresh eyes' from a group of women who draw on their lived experiences and who have seen a great deal of pain and suffering in the course of their travels from house to house. While it is not possible here to go into depth on the production of all the messages, we offer a verbatim account below of a discussion between Naydene as the researcher and workshop facilitator, and several of the women on the topic of violence against *gogos* (elderly women or grandmothers) as an example of the process of cultural production (Figure 4).

Naydene:	So what would the first message be? *(Starts jotting their ideas on the flipchart)*
Jabu:	Stop violence against old women.
Naydene:	Why?

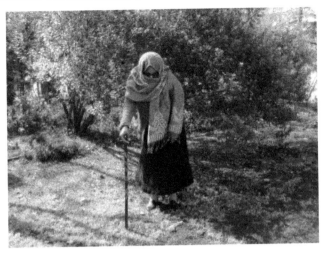

Figure 4. The photograph taken to show the vulnerability of gogos.

Jabu:	So if you say stop violence against the *gogos*, it's right, violence against everybody must stop, but ...
Busi:	People have sex and they get infected.
Naydene:	The *gogos*?
Busi:	Yes.
Naydene:	But why do the men go to the *gogos*? Because they think ... ?
Jabu:	They think the HIV and AIDS can be cured.
Naydene:	OK, so what is the message? Having sex with *gogos* does not cure AIDS?
Thandiwe:	Yes.
Naydene:	You see the point?
Thandiwe:	Yes.
Naydene:	We want to say stop violence against the *gogos*.
Thandiwe:	Yes.
Naydene:	But that's not helping people who think that they are going to be cured? OK is that a good message?
Fikele:	Yes.
Naydene:	So we can also translate that into Zulu later.
Jabu:	If we can say that having sex with elder women affects their health.
Naydene:	OK, and does not cure AIDS?
Jabu:	Because the main point why they do this to old *gogos*.
Naydene:	And affects their health, the *gogos'* health? Is that it?
Jabu:	Yes.
Naydene:	Now let's imagine ... how would you show, what picture would you now take to add this text to. You are not going to take a picture of a *gogo* being raped, no? So what would you use to make the people have empathy and to care about the *gogo*? What kind of picture would that be?
Jabu:	What if you take a picture of a *gogo* that is ill?
Naydene:	Hmmm ... What does a *gogo* look like? What does a *gogo* do in your community?

271

Jabu: Gogo who is being raped. You are asking about *gogo* who ...
Naydene: I'm just asking about *gogos*. What makes a *gogo* in your community?
Thandiwe: Holding a stick and going like this (*hunching forward*).
Jabu: Yes.
Naydene: So you can take a picture of a *gogo* with a walking stick. It can be one of you, and we put the *doek* [head covering] over the head so that we don't see who the *gogo* is?

Data moment 3 – taking action and the significance of audience texts. In a follow-up meeting sometime after the residential workshop, we discussed the use of the media posters with the women. Each was equipped with a set of posters contained in a plastic envelope and showed a feeling of importance and what appeared to be an enhanced sense of their own selves in doing the job that they love. In a sense, they were the first audience of their own work and appreciated what the package of posters would allow them to do. At this point, however, they indicated that to extend the value of their work it would make sense for all of the 30 or so CHWs working out of the same clinic to each own a set of the media posters. This in itself was taking action as they realised that 30 CHWs could do far more than 5. We had 30 more sets of the media posters produced and made a point of officially handing the sets over to the clinic head, who requested a picture taken of the handover so that the head of the district could see and value the work that the women (and the clinic) had done. Some of the women themselves offered comments on why this handover was important:

Jabu: I am quite interested about what we were doing today and hope that even the community will see that gender-based violence is not acceptable.
Thandiwe: We had a wonderful day and hope that we will continue passing the message to the community so that the gender-based violence will be minimal.
Gethwana: We had a wonderful day and this all what is happening today is very encouraging and we are going to show the community the impact of this gender-based violence.
Fikile: I enjoyed to be here today, but what is very interesting is that it's about these visual aids that we are going to use them to the community and the other thing which is very annoying and irritating to me is that ... most of current affairs issues based on gender-based violence pertaining to elderly people who are being raped.

While it is beyond the scope of the work presented here to offer further examples of follow-up in terms of the use of the media posters in the community or the ways that different audiences (especially the community members) might receive the messages of the posters, the fact that the women themselves saw the value of having the head of the clinic involved in the handover speaks to a certain political savvy on their part, and an awareness of how things are, from the inside, in terms of bringing about change. Akintola (2010) writes that there is very little research on the rewards that volunteer caregivers of people living with HIV (also CHWs) in South Africa experience. We deduce from our example that producing the media posters for use in the community, which the clinic serves, was rewarding to the CHWs as it seemed to have enabled capacity development which added to their status in the clinic and the district. This is not something we as out-siders would necessarily have thought to do, and indeed, we might even have thought that just the women possessing the materials would give them some added cultural currency in the community.

Discussion

We believe that this work around the data moments helped to deepen an understanding of the meaning of cultural production in relation to GBV and positive social change in the community. In doing this work, we drew on the critical practice-based work of Bucking-ham and Sefton-Greene (1994), and would like to return here to the question of insider cultural knowledge and generational knowledge as key aspects to understanding and addressing GBV. This is critical in relation to thinking about how change can take place in rural areas where certain aspects of patriarchal culture dominate. As noted above, the generational knowledge of the women about the vulnerability of *gogos*, about abusive grandsons, about forced sex, and about the role of alcohol in abuse which was pro-duced during the workshop brings forward knowledge that is neither typically addressed in GBV campaigns, nor in a format that is both local and relevant to the rural context.[4] At the same time, the messages produced by the women bring in a generational component with additional layers of concern. For example, the women produced a poster with the slogan 'Teach your children to respect people'. As Moletsane (2011) argues in her work on culture and nostalgia in rural South Africa, there is a need to contest certain discourses. While we are not arguing against the value of respect, the respect that is entirely attached to age (elders) and sex (male power) can be problematic in addressing GBV.

Although the idea of the media poster is not new to social research we want to draw attention in this research, to the particular social space occupied by a group of lay health workers whose status as cultural producers or knowledge producers is quite differ-ent from what is typically seen in the pedagogical space found in school or university class-rooms. CHWs only have a Grade 12 education and occupy a status of para-professionals, and as we found in a previous study involving teachers and CHWs (De Lange, Mitchell, & Stuart, 2011), their status is typically lower in the community than that of teachers. Although they see media posters and billboards every day even in deeply rural areas (especially posters linked to HIV and AIDS), they are not typical agents in the production process. In the instance of this research, they were instrumental in suggesting the pro-duction of visual material for use in the community and what the focus of the each media poster should be. They created the images and the slogans, worked together on the translation into isiZulu, and requested more copies for all other CHWs. In this way, they initiated and owned the idea of the media posters, and with each possessing a set of media posters, we believe they were able to take action and in a small way sustain the 'intervention' in their community.

Building on this work with the five CHWs, we also want to draw attention to possibilities of using media or policy posters in social research. We use the terms *media poster* and *policy poster* interchangeably here with the idea that in the type of social research that sets out to address such issues as GBV and HIV stigma, participants are typically engaged in the process of creating messages and images that are meant to influence or transform social or policy contexts through the use of media. We see the process of producing the posters as a fascinating pedagogical space for engaging in addressing a possible 'So what?' question. The idea that one's images and ideas can reach real audiences is potentially very empowering. While we have in the past drawn on the idea of the narrative poster in photovoice projects, its role was more about process and about participants working with their own images in an analytical way to present them and report to other participants (De Lange, Mitchell, Moletsane, Stuart, & Buthelezi, 2006). The policy poster process by comparison is a carefully crafted multimodal text meant to convey a very specific message to a very specific audience – such as 'wearing our cause' through the social message T-shirt in South Africa (see e.g. Moletsane & Lolwana, 2012). Clearly the media poster genre, which offers media messages through slogans along with single images (photos or drawings), is a mode which has cultural currency, and is useful in low-tech contexts. While the initial production was low-tech in this instance, the final production of the complete set of posters was high tech (see step 5). More than anything we want to highlight that it is within the realm of possibilities for a group of women who walk 'from house to house … through the fields, past cattle … ' to create locally relevant insider messages for bringing about positive social change. Returning to Vaughan's (2014) point that participatory research in and of itself is not sufficient to ensure that participants will take action to bring about change, we believe that the CHWs' own agency to take action was enabled through their own cultural production and the media-making process.

While it is clear that the CHW enjoyed producing their own media posters, we realise that exploring GBV with them might have unearthed memories, both long ago and recent, of own lived experiences of GBV, and that the examples of GBV they wanted to address might have been from their own experiences. This compels us to consider Sikweyiya and Jewkes's (2011, p. 1091) question about whether research on GBV 'pose[s] a greater than minimal risk to researchers and participants'? Would the participants in addressing GBV in their work in their community be at risk? Were they adequately equipped to deal with challenges that might arise? This indeed requires careful rethinking on our part as researchers on how we might build into the project what we have come to see as essential care and support for the researchers (Sexual Violence Research Initiative, 2015) and the participants (Jewkes, Dartnall, & Sikweyiya, 2012) who will be using their cultural productions in the community.

Conclusion

The CHWs drew on their insider cultural knowledge of GBV in a rural community to produce culturally relevant knowledge as represented in their media poster productions, but beyond this produced material which could be used in their daily routines of visiting their allocated households. This work with the CHWs has therefore shifted from what might typically be described as engagement to what we here term 'beyond engagement'.

While Hamon, in her 2011 study, concluded that CHWs have very little input into community efforts aimed at addressing sexual violence even though they are expected to be agents of change in the community, we found that the constraints such as low status in the community, lack of support, and lack of formal recognition in the field (Hamon, 2011), did not hold the women back from articulating what they wanted from our project. Similarly, in our previous work with CHWs attached to a different clinic in KwaZulu-Natal, we noted their enthusiasm to be involved in participatory visual research in projects with teachers in the same rural district aimed at deepening understanding of the critical issues of HIV and AIDS which young people face (De Lange et al., 2004; Mitchell, De Lange, Moletsane, Stuart, & Buthelezi, 2005). We also saw this enthusiasm and commitment in follow-up work where CHWs engaged in participatory analysis of visual images produced in a 'Learning Together' project (De Lange et al., 2011). Given the limitations of a small scale initiative in our current study, we are not in a position to say unequivocally that it would be easy to overturn the situation for CHWs so that they can be positioned more directly as 'agents of community empowerment' (Schneider et al., 2008, p. 108). It is clear, however, from the sit-ins referred to at the beginning of this article and from the cultural production in the media-making project described here, that CHWs have the capacity to raise awareness and act on critical issues in relation to the health and wellbeing of their communities.

Disclosure statement

No potential conflict of interest was reported by the authors.

Funding

This work was supported by the South African National Research Foundation [grant number 78783].

Notes

1. In 2004 there were an estimated 40,000 lay health workers working in South Africa National Department of Health (NDoH) contributing to primary health care (Schneider et al., 2008). Schneider and Lehmann (2010) indicated that the NDoH estimated that the number of CHWs had risen to more than 65,000 in 2008. A new framework, *Primary Healthcare Re-engineering Framework in South Africa* proposes that each CHW would take responsibility for 250 households (Hospice Palliative Care Association of South Africa, 2012) – clearly a considerable workload.
2. Along with the rollout of antiretroviral (ARV) drugs in most segments of the country, new legislation and the *Primary Healthcare Re-engineering Framework in South Africa* (Paulus, 2013) have shifted CHWs' work from offering palliative care to patients dying from AIDS to delivering frontline treatment (Storer, 2013).
3. A local teacher, a woman who had participated in our projects over several years, co-facilitated and translated the English for the CHWs, and the isiZulu for us.
4. We highlight this because of the types of criticisms that have been levelled against loveLife's HIV and AIDS messages (Robbins, 2010) as being too urban and slick and often irrelevant to rural audiences.

References

Abrahams, N., Jewkes, R., Martin, L. J., Mathews, S., Vetten, L., & Lombard, C. (2009). Mortality of women from intimate partner violence in South Africa: A national epidemiological study. *Violence and Victims, 24*, 546–556. doi:10.1891/0886-6708.24.4.546

Akintola, O. (2010). Perceptions of rewards among volunteer caregivers of people living with AIDS working in faith-based organizations in South Africa: A qualitative study. *Journal of the International AIDS Society, 13*(22), 1–10. doi:10.1186/1758-2652-13-22

Amnesty International. (2008). *I am at the lowest end of all. Rural women living with HIV face human rights abuses in South Africa.* London: Amnesty International.

Andersson, N., Ho-Foster, A., Mitchell, S., Scheepers, E., & Goldstein, S. (2007). Risk factors for domestic physical violence: National cross-sectional household surveys in eight southern African countries. *BMC Women's Health, 7*(1), 11. doi:10.1186/1472-6874-7-11

Berman, P. A., Gwatkin, D. R., & Burger, S. E. (1987). Community-based health workers: Head start or false start towards health for all? *Social Science & Medicine, 25*, 443–459. doi:10.1016/0277-9536(87)90168-7

Buckingham, D., & Sefton-Greene, J. (1994). *Cultural studies goes to school.* New York, NY: Routledge.

Clothesline Project. (2007). Saartjie Baartman Centre. Retrieved from http://www.saartjiebaartmancentre.org.za/index.php/our-voices/our-campaigns/76-clothesline-project

Dartnell, E., & Gevers, A. (2015). Editorial: Violence can be prevented. *South African Crime Quarterly, 51*, 3–4. doi:10.4314/sacq.v51i0

De Lange, N., & Geldenhuys, M. (2012). Youth envisioning safe schools: A participatory video approach. *South African Journal of Education, 32*, 494–511.

De Lange, N., Mitchell, C., Moletsane, R., Balfour, R., Wedekind, V., Pillay, G., & Buthelezi, T. (2010). Every voice counts: Towards a new agenda for teachers and schools in rural communities in addressing children's vulnerabilities in the age of AIDS. *Education as Change, 14*(3), S45–S55. doi:10.1080/16823206.2010.517916

De Lange, N., Mitchell, C., Moletsane, R., Buthelezi, T., Mazibuko, F., Stuart, J., & Taylor, M. (2004). *Learning together: Towards an integrated participatory approach to youth, gender and HIV/AIDS interventions in rural KwaZulu-Natal schools* (Unpublished Research Proposal). Pretoria, RSA: National Research Foundation.

De Lange, N., Mitchell, C., Moletsane, R., Stuart, J., & Buthelezi, T. (2006). Seeing with the body: Educators' representations of HIV and AIDS. *Journal of Education, 38*(1), 45–66.

De Lange, N., Mitchell, C., & Stuart, J. (2011). Learning together: Teachers and community health care workers draw each other. In L. Theron, C. Mitchell, A. Smith, & J. Stuart (Eds.), *Picturing research: Drawings as visual methodology* (pp. 177–189). Rotterdam: Sense.

Dunkle, K. L., Jewkes, R. K., Murdock, D. W., Sikweyiya, Y., & Morrell, R. (2013). Prevalence of consensual male–male sex and sexual violence, and associations with HIV in South Africa: A population-based cross-sectional study. *PLoS Medicine, 10*(6), e1001472. doi:10.1371/journal.pmed.1001472

Fiske, J. (1987). *British cultural studies television.* London: Methuen.

Free State health workers arrested over sit-in. (2014, July 10). *News24.* Retrieved from http://www.news24.com/SouthAfrica/News/Free-State-health-workers-arrested-over-sit-in-20140710

Garcia-Moreno, C., & Watts, C. (2000). Violence against women: Its importance for HIV/AIDS. *AIDS, 14*(3), S253–S265.

Gubrium, A., & Harper, K. (2013). *Participatory visual and digital methods.* Walnut Creek, CA: Left Coast Press.

Hamon, J. (2011). Understanding the service delivery of rural community health workers: The example of addressing violence against women and girls in Vulindlela, South Africa (Unpublished master's dissertation). McGill University, Montreal, Canada.

Hospice Palliative Care Association of South Africa. (2012). *The legal aspects of palliative care.* Pinelands, RSA: Author.

Jewkes, R. (2002). Intimate partner violence: Causes and prevention. *The Lancet, 359*, 1423–1429. doi:10.1016/S0140-6736(02)08357-5

Jewkes, R., Dartnall, L., & Sikweyiya, Y. (2012). *Ethical and safety recommendations for research on perpetration of sexual violence*. Pretoria, RSA: Sexual Violence Research Initiative, Medical Research Council.

Jewkes, R., Flood, M., & Lang, J. (2014). From work with men and boys to changes of social norms and reduction of inequities in gender relations: A conceptual shift in prevention of violence against women and girls. *The Lancet, 385*, 1580–1589. doi:10.1016/S0140-6736(14)61683-4

Jewkes, R., Levin, J., & Penn-Kekana, L. (2002). Risk factors for domestic violence: Findings from a South African cross-sectional study. *Social Science & Medicine, 55*, 1603–1617. doi:10.1016/S0277-9536(01)00294-5

Jewkes, R., & Morrell, R. (2010). Gender and sexuality: Emerging perspectives from the heterosexual epidemic in South Africa and implications for HIV risk and prevention. *Journal of the International AIDS Society, 13*(1), 6. doi:10.1186/1758-2652-13-6

Khau, M. (2009). Journeys into the hidden self: Reflections on a collaborative inquiry into women teachers' memories of adolescent sexuality. In K. Pithouse, C. Mitchell, & R. Moletsane (Eds.), *Making connections: Self-study & social action* (pp. 59–75). New York, NY: Peter Lang.

Machisa, M., Jewkes, R., Lowe-Morna, C., & Rama, K. (2011). *The war at home*. Johannesburg, RSA: GenderLinks, and Gender and Health Research Unit.

Madu, S. N., & Peltzer, K. (2000). Risk factors and child sexual abuse among secondary school students in the Northern Province (South Africa). *Child Abuse & Neglect, 24*, 259–268. doi:10.1016/S0145-2134(99)00128-3

Maman, S., Campbell, J., Sweat, M. D., & Gielen, A. C. (2000). The intersections of HIV and violence: Directions for future research and interventions. *Social Science & Medicine, 50*, 459–478. doi:10.1016/S0277-9536(99)00270-1

Masinga, L. (2012). Journeys to self-knowledge: Methodological reflections on using memory-work in a participatory study of teachers as sexuality educators. *Journal of Education, 54*, 121–137.

Milne, E.-J., Mitchell, C., & De Lange, N. (Eds.). (2012). *Handbook on participatory video*. Lanham, MD: AltaMira Press.

Mitchell, C. (2011). *Doing visual research*. London: Sage.

Mitchell, C., De Lange, N., Moletsane, R., & Stuart, J. (2006). *Izindaba Yethu. Our stories* [Video documentary]. Durban: Centre for Visual Methodologies for Social Change.

Mitchell, C., De Lange, N., Moletsane, R., Stuart, J., & Buthelezi, T. (2005). Giving a face to HIV and AIDS: On the uses of photo-voice by teachers and community health care workers working with youth in rural South Africa. *Qualitative Research in Psychology, 2*, 257–270. doi:10.1191/1478088705qp042oa

Mitchell, C., Mak, M., & Stuart, J. (2005). *Our photos, our videos, our stories* [Video Documentary]. Montreal: Taffeta Productions.

Moletsane, R. (2011). Culture, nostalgia and sexuality education in the age of AIDS in South Africa. In C. Mitchell, T. Strong-Wilson, K. Pithouse, & S. Allnutt (Eds.), *Memory and pedagogy* (pp. 193–208). New York, NY: Routledge.

Moletsane, R., De Lange, N., Mitchell, C., Balfour, R., Wedekind, V., Pillay, D., & Chikoko, V. (2010). *Nothing about us without us: Participatory approaches to teacher development and community wellness to enhance teaching and learning in rural schools* (Unpublished Research Proposal). Pretoria, RSA: National Research Foundation.

Moletsane, R., & Lolwana, P. (2012). Wearing our hearts on our sleeves: The T-shirt and the South African activist agenda. In R. Moletsane, C. Mitchell, & A. Smith (Eds.), *Was it something she wore? Dress, identity, materiality* (pp. 277–287). Cape Town, RSA: Human Sciences Research Council Press.

Mullick, S., Teffo-Menziwa, M., Williams, E., & Jina, R. (2010). Women and sexual violence. In S. Fonn & A. Padarath (Eds.), *South African Health Review 2010*. Durban, RSA: Health Systems Trust. Retrieved from http://www.hst.org.za/publications/south-african-health-review-2010

Nelson Mandela Foundation. (2005). *Emerging voices. A report on education in rural South Africa.* Cape Town, RSA: Human Sciences Research Council Press.

Paulus, E. (2013). *Re-engineering public health care in Gauteng. Re-engineering primary health care: A national perspective.* Retrieved from http://www.anovahealth.co.za/images/uploads/Paulus_NDoH_Anova_Conference_28022012.pdf

Posel, D. (2005). The scandal of manhood: 'Baby rape' and the politicization of sexual violence in post-apartheid South Africa. *Culture, Health & Sexuality, 7,* 239–252. doi:10.1080/13691050412331293467

Robbins, D. (2010). *Beyond the billboards: The loveLife story.* Johannesburg, RSA: Porcupine Press.

Russell, M., Cupp, P. K., Jewkes, R. K., Gevers, A., Mathews, C., LeFleur-Bellerose, C., & Small, J. (2014). Intimate partner violence among adolescents in Cape Town, South Africa. *Prevention Science, 15,* 283–295. doi:10.1007/s11121-013-0405-7

Schneider, H., Hlophe, H., & Van Rensburg, D. (2008). Community health workers and the response to HIV/AIDS in South Africa: Tensions and prospects. *Health Policy and Planning, 23,* 179–187. doi:10.1093/heapol/czn006

Schneider, H., & Lehmann, U. (2010). Lay health workers and HIV programmes: Implications for health systems. *AIDS CARE, 22*(1), 60–67. doi:10.1080/09540120903483042

Sexual Violence Research Initiative. (2015). *Guidelines for the prevention and management of vicarious trauma among researchers of sexual and intimate partner violence.* Pretoria, RSA: Author.

Sikweyiya, Y., & Jewkes, R. (2011). Perceptions about safety and risks in gender-based violence research: Implications for the ethics review process. *Culture, Health & Sexuality, 13,* 1091–1102.

Storer, E. (2013). *Nursing a nation: Community health workers in South Africa.* Retrieved from http://thinkafricapress.com/south-africa/role-community-health-workers-against-hivaids

Tobin, J. (2000). *Good guys don't wear hats: Children's talk about the media paperback.* New York, NY: Teachers College Press.

Vaughan, C. (2014). Participatory research with youth: Idealising safe social spaces or building transformative links in difficult environments? *Journal of Health Psychology, 19*(1), 184–192. doi:10.1177/1359105313500258

Walton, K. (1995). Creating positive images: Working with primary school girls. In J. Spence & J. Solomon (Eds.), *What can a woman do with a camera?* (pp. 153–158). London: Scarlet Press.

Champions for social change: Photovoice ethics in practice and 'false hopes' for policy and social change

Gloria Johnston

Department of Sociology, University of New Brunswick, Fredericton, Canada

ABSTRACT
Photovoice methodology is growing in popularity in the health, education and social sciences as a research tool based on the core values of community-based participatory research. Most photovoice projects state a claim to the third goal of photovoice: to reach policy-makers or effect policy change. This paper examines the concerns of raising false hopes or unrealistic expectations amongst the participants of photovoice projects as they are positioned to be the champions for social change in their communities. The impetus for social change seems to lie in the hands of those most affected by the issue. This drive behind collective social action forms, what could be termed, a micro-social movement or comparative interest group. Looking to the potential use of social movement theory and resource mobilisation concepts, this paper poses a series of unanswered questions about the ethics of photovoice projects. The ethical concern centres on the focus of policy change as a key initiative; yet, most projects remain vague about the implementation and outcomes of this focus.

Introduction

In response to the enduring 'crisis of representation', many researchers have sought out research projects collaborative in design to share knowledge and shift traditional researcher–subject relationships. Photovoice, developed by Wang and Burris (1994), offers a research design that requires a positive and engaged audience to affect this desired change. Within the aims of photovoice to elicit social change, critical consciousness and social action mobilisation will be ineffective if the study is negatively received by the wider public or those in positions to commit to actual social change. There are a handful of insightful researchers who have commented that photovoice also has the potential to raise false hopes as when efforts to rally public concern or efforts to inform public policy are unsuccessful (Mitchell, 2011; Tanjasiri, Lew, Kuratani, Wong & Fu, 2011; Wallerstein & Bernstein, 1988). Mitchell has asked 'Why is finding the solution to a social issue always the responsibility of those most affected by the issue?' (2011, p. 14). Wallerstein and Bernstein (1988) argue that people cannot assume the sole responsibility for creating a healthier environment, arguing that individuals alone are not responsible for enacting and changing complex multiple categories and issues. I will begin with a brief overview of photovoice as a methodology and discuss a few key points on this unclear aspect of the photovoice research design. This aspect may imply an imbedded pressure for the participants to be the champions of social change. I propose that photovoice researchers could benefit from reviewing the literature on social movements theory, especially in terms of resource mobilisation, to facilitate social change outcomes.

Methodology

In the course of a thorough reading of the literature, a feature emerged that remains as an unanswered question as to how photovoice is discussed with regard to effecting social change and changing policy. These insights emerged in reviewing photovoice literature for my doctoral research. I am not the first to point out the ethical issues of photovoice as a social change project, but I state that these researchers stand out as the few rather than the many. I performed a scoping review (Armstrong, Hall, Doyle, & Waters, 2011) of 53 published articles that have informed this review. This scoping review began by using a variety of search engines including EBSCO, Sociological Abstracts, SocINDEX, HealthSource, ProQuest, JSTOR and WorldCat accessed through the University of New Brunswick Harriet Irving Library between March 2012 and September 2012. I searched for articles using a variety of keywords: photovoice, community based participatory research, participatory action research (PAR), community photography, reflexive photography, photo narrative and visual self-elicitation. I gathered literature that fit the goals of photovoice and CBPR/PAR with a focus on community involvement and collaboration as part of the research design. As a scoping review, I anticipate that this literature will inform an updated systematic review at a later date (Armstrong et al., 2011). The emergent parameters from this scoping review and the research gap it addresses demonstrate that there is great potential for the development of understanding the ethics of photovoice, false hopes, social and policy change.

Photovoice

Photovoice is an increasingly popular technique also termed 'native image production' (Wagner, 1979), 'cultural self-portrayal' (Pauwels, 2010), 'photo self-elicitation' (Banks, 2001) 'photo novellas' and 'visual narratives' (Guillemin & Drew, 2010). Images in these practices are produced within a research context, although not by the researchers, but rather by the participant. In most projects, the researcher and participant work collaboratively in the selection and analysis of the images. The researcher's control over the production of these images as a process is limited, as the viewpoint of the participant is the focus to provide a unique insider perspective (Pauwels, 2010). It asserts that people and their experience as they see it from their viewpoint are a legitimate and important source of expertise. Photovoice is a community-based participatory action research (CBPR) method (Strack, Magill, & McDonagh, 2004) that expresses the idea that 'power is held by those who have voice, set language, make history, and participate in decisions' (Schneider, 2010, p. 47). Photovoice aims to bring new or seldom-heard ideas, images, conversations and voices into the public forum (Wang, 2001) by creating images from the viewpoint of the participant rather than the images being subjected to the selection of the visual researcher.

Photovoice and community-based participatory research

The 'photovoice' method, a branch of CBPR, has received a growing interest and is practised mainly in health, education and the social sciences. In photovoice projects, participants are invited to express their viewpoint, by exploring community issues and daily-lived experience by taking photographs, discussing the photographs, developing narratives of the photos and participating in social action to enact social or policy change (Wang & Burris, 1994). This commitment to social action may take the form of new expressions of unheard knowledge, social awareness-raising (Wang, 1999; Wilson et al., 2007) or opening dialogue with policy-makers (Wang, 1999; Wang & Burris, 1994). With these aims, photovoice has three main goals: (1) to enable people to record and reflect their community's strengths and concerns, (2) to promote critical dialogue and knowledge about personal and community issues through large and small group discussion of their photographs and (3) to reach policy-makers (Wang, 1999, p. 185). Photovoice is consistent with the core principles of CBPR, also known as PAR. When artistic methods are incorporated, it is called participatory arts-based research and shares similar goals. All participatory methods aim to have researchers and members of a specific community work together as equal partners in the development, implementation and dissemination of research that is relevant to the community. The research approach of CBPR abandons the dominant research tradition of control over the process and the products of research. Participatory research stresses empowerment, education and social action claiming that there is a political nature to all research, and that all research has implications for the distribution of power in society (Schneider, 2010).

Issues of power are central to CBPR/PAR research. Baum, MacDougall, and Smith (2006) state that the general goal of empowerment is a shift in the modes of power and to establish new relationships to reduce inequalities and power differences in access to resources (Baum et al., 2006). When community members are central in the maintenance of research agendas, and are active in research, empowerment emerges as they are established as 'more powerful agents' (Baum et al., 2006, p. 855). Given this framework, in traditional or non-CBPR research settings, people are rarely considered knowledgeable or capable of knowing about their own reality and are accordingly subjected to research projects as objects (Jaggar, 2008, p. 421). In this aim, participatory research expresses that all people, provided with tools and opportunities, are capable of critical reflection and analysis (Castleden, Garvin, & First Nation, 2008). The aim of CBPR is not to position one type of knowledge over one another but to incorporate ignored and subjugated voices into the conversation. It is to reject traditional models of power and knowledge production within the research relationship (Harrison, 2002, p. 862). In this approach, CBPR seeks to equalise the influence and knowledge of community members, organisation representatives and researchers to be equal in authority, responsibility and knowledge. CBPR offers a dialogue approach to research where everyone should participate as equals and co-learners to express social knowledge from various perspectives (Wallerstein & Bernstein, 1988, p. 382). This dialogue approach, as practised in photovoice and similar methods implies a co-action component also consistent with the principles of CBPR.

How is photovoice practised?

The foundational work by Wang and Burris (1994) focused on rural women in China's Yunnan province (Wand, 1999; Wang & Burris, 1994, 1997; Wang, Yi, Tao, & Carovano, 1998) has inspired a wide range of photovoice projects addressing a variety of public health and social concerns ranging from HIV/AIDS (Gosselink & Myllykangas, 2007), cancer survivorship (López, Eng, Randall-David, & Robinson, 2005; Poudrier & Mac-Lean, 2009), women's health (LeClerc, Wells, Craig, & Wilson, 2002; Moffitt & Vollman, 2004; Wang & Burris, 1997), economically disadvantaged youth (Foster-Fishman, Nowell, Deacon, Nievar, & McCann, 2005; Stevens, 2006; Strack et al., 2004; Wang & Redwood-Jones, 2001). older adult communities (Baker & Wang, 2006; LeClerc et al., 2002), youth (Wang et al., 2006), mental illness (Erdner, Andersson, Magnusson, & Lützén, 2009; Sitvast, Abma, & Widdershoven, 2010; Thompson et al., 2008), Aboriginal women's health (Moffitt & Vollman, 2004; Poudrier & Mac-Lean, 2009), lone mothers (Duffy, 2010) and the homeless (Wang, Cash, & Powers, 2000). The photovoice methodology offers many advantages to sociological inquiry. Photovoice situates expert knowledge within the daily-lived experience of the participant because their vision and voice are recognised as equal and valid (Killion & Wang, 2000; Wang & Burris, 1994). The participants of photovoice are often from economically, politically, or socially disadvantaged social groups and the design of photovoice 'reduces the distinction between those seen as experts and non-experts' (Chio & Fandt, 2007, p. 486). The extensive opportunities of access to various groups and personal narrative situate the photovoice methodology as a creative and innovative PAR strategy. The advantages could be seen as a two-stage process: the focus is first on individual development through empowerment and then on hopes of community development and change (Wang & Burris, 1994).

Policy change: what do we DO about it?

Photovoice is, as termed by Wang (1999), Wang and Burris (1994, 1997) and Wang et al. (1998), a combination of several theoretical perspectives that emphasise community participation for social action, including empowerment education and documentary photography. These theoretical perspectives appreciate the value of participants defining and determining the subjects that are documented, with the emphasis on uncovering underlying root causes and identifying policy-oriented actions to address injustices. During analysis of the pictures taken by photovoice participants, many studies state the use of SHOWeD, an acronym developed by Wang and Burris (1994) to explore concepts and meaning representing: What do you See here? What's really Happening here? How does this relate to Our lives? Why does this problem or strength exists? What can we Do about this? (Catalani & Minkler, 2010). SHOWeD is used to identify the root cause of the problem or asset, discuss the image critically and focused mainly to develop strategies for change. The question is a focus on this '*do*' component. It is a built-in to almost every photovoice project, the implied social or policy change spearheaded by the newly empowered participants to engage in their communities and effect real change by reaching policy-makers. This emphasis on involving policy-makers and other community leaders in photovoice projects has been a part of Wang and similar researcher's ongoing work and recommendations for best practices (Catalani & Minkler, 2010; Wang, 1999; Wang &

Redwood-Jones, 2001). It has been stated that this component of effective social change reaffirms community identity and involvement as the narrative comes from within stimulating social action as people become their own advocates (Wang & Burris, 1994, p. 173). Most photovoice projects have a built-in 'research as social change' orientation (Reason & Bradbury, 2001) that normally manifests as a 'research action plan' to be mobilised towards social action.

Social action and photovoice

Social action is an integral part of the conceptual framework of photovoice. Yet, despite the central focus on social action and policy change, there is a vagueness in addressing how to enact social action plans. There are also concerns for the noticeable lack of documented follow-through actions of attempts at social change and project outcomes. The concern of this vagueness is that the inspiration for change, as a participant, a co-leaner, is that the participants are responsible for this change and that a photovoice study will achieve necessary social and policy change. What does this mean for the participants? With such a focus on social and policy change, what if nothing comes about? Why is hardly anyone discussing this issue save a handful of researchers? With the growing popularity of photovoice, this is an important and critical concern.

Wang and Burris (1994) themselves have stated that photovoice projects often require a positive and engaged audience effect. The audiences, of the public or of influential policy leaders, must be open to unconventional ideas and capable of processing criticism (Wang & Burris, 1994, p. 184). Adding that critical conscious raising and social action mobilisation will be ineffective if the study is negatively received by the wider public or those in positions to commit to change (Wang & Burris, 1994). With the acknowledgement of external factors for social and policy change, why is the focus on empowerment leading to policy change initiated by the participants themselves?

False hopes and expectations

There are a few researchers (Catalani & Minkler, 2010; Mitchell, 2011; Tanjasiri et al., 2011), who have commented that photovoice has the potential to raise false hopes when efforts to rally public concern or attempts to change public policy fail (Tanjasiri et al., 2011). Some studies offer few details about the method itself leaving a somewhat romanticised view of participatory photography and its potential to reach transformative results (Harley, 2012; Prins, 2010). Harley (2012) has commented on the two most noted review articles by Hergenrather, Rhodes, Cowan, Bardhoshi, and Pula (2009) of 31 photovoice articles and Catalani and Minkler's (2010) review of 37 articles summarising that in most of the studies reviewed, there was little attempt to evaluate any long-term impact of the method on individuals and communities (Harley, 2012). These studies showed an overall lack of the 'bigger picture' of structural inequalities and available resources needed to enact social and policy change (Harley, 2012, p. 329). In the review article of Catalani and Minkler (2010), the photovoice projects culminated in vague descriptions of project evaluations and practices stating a lack of consistent reporting. Approximately 60% of the projects reported having an action plan or action component yielding three outcomes: enhanced community engagement in action or advocacy, improved understanding of community needs and assets and increased personal empowerment (Harley, 2012). Yet, the project outcomes overwhelmingly summarised to 'enhanced understanding' of social problems (Catalani & Minkler, 2010).

Tanjasiri et al. (2011) have also stated the potential to raise false hopes for change among participants, unless the project is already facilitated by policy activist or other external resources (Tanjasiri et al., 2011). In the Tanjasiri photovoice study, one of the few citing actual policy change, it was recognised that the youth had the opportunity to share their pictures with local policy-makers to support the successful passage of a tobacco vendor licensing law that was already under review. Tanjasiri et al. (2011) state that, as discussed by Wang (2006), involvement of policy-makers at the outset of a project could facilitate the changing of local policies or organisational practices (Tanjasiri, 2011). In most photovoice studies, it is not practice to organise with policy-makers in the beginning but rather later, during public exhibition or display (Catalani & Minkler, 2010).

In efforts for research to be community-based and participatory, it is often overlooked that Photovoice projects are similar to other 'parachute projects' or other one-time research interventions. Strack et al. (2004) argue that participation in a photovoice project will not lead to a complete state of empowerment. This complete state of empowerment would illustrate a meaningful shift in the modes of power and the establishment of new relationships to reduce inequalities and power differences in access to resources (Baum et al., 2006). Strack et al. (2004) further this statement that photovoice projects might have damaging consequences and the real and negative outcome of false hopes and disillusioned expectations by failing to inform policy or rally public concern in an effective way to incite change. There is a risk in certain studies that the outcome for participants is that they may feel 'more hopeless and unempowered than when they started the program' (Strack et al., 2004, p. 57). It is argued here that it is imperative that researchers select sites for photovoice project that have an already or ongoing commitment to policy change or further empowerment to ensure successful goals of the project (Catalani & Minkler, 2010; Strack et al., 2004; Tanjasiri et al., 2011).

Discussion

Photovoice as a micro-social movement?

This leads to a discussion and examination of resource mobilisation theory as positioned by Tarrow (1998) and McCarthy and Zald (1979), to question the underlying social structure and mobilisation potential that can be transformed into action on any level, big or small. As most photovoice projects work with marginalised groups who have been noted as 'powerless' (Booth & Booth, 2003), how then does change happen? How does one incite meaningful change when you have no power to incite that change, no political or policy influence? Tarrow (1998) argues that a combination of external factors will effect meaningful change with a clear statement that 'powerless actors' need support to bring about political change. Often, this requires interactions with power holders, third parties that concur with public opinion in order to enter the discussion and hope to enact social change (Della & Diani, 2006; McAdam, McCarthy, & Zald, 1996; Staggenborg, 2011). In summary, to enact change, especially in policy, the participants will need two things: public opinion and political alliances. When important social issues are brought forward for discussion, the goal is to try to raise public awareness and concern about certain issues. In doing so, the aim is to directly provoke structural and cultural changes in society by influencing people's attitudes and behaviours and address public opinion in order to make it an ally (Della & Diani, 2006; McAdam et al., 1996; Staggenborg, 2011). Tarrow (1998) argues that when anyone wanting to make change benefits from the support of public opinion, individuals or groups rallying for public change increase their legitimacy as political actors when in alliance with public opinion. Tarrow (1998) argues that while important, this needs to be politically supported under a system of organised political action that can sustain itself for an undetermined duration requiring resources and various forms of capital (McAdam et al., 1996). The integration of material, human, social and cultural resources together increases the chance that policy changes will occur (Diani & McAdam, 2003; Staggenborg, 2011).

Resource mobilisation and social change

As researchers, we need to look at the dimensions of the political and social environment that provide incentives for collective action and help shape success or failure (Della & Diani, 2006; McAdam et al., 1996; Staggenborg, 2011; Tarrow, 1998). The key point here is the access and maintenance of resources and how and to whom they are available. As mentioned, the groups selected by researchers for a photovoice project are typically marginalised groups: HIV/AIDS (Gosselink & Myllykangas, 2007; Mitchell, DeLange, Molestane, Stuart, & Buthelezi, 2005), cancer survivorship (López, Eng, Robinson, & Wang, 2005), lone mothers (Duffy, 2010), indigenous peoples (Castleden et al., 2008), mental illness (Erdner et al., 2009; Sitvast et al., 2010; Thompson et al., 2008), the homeless (Wang et al., 2000), just to cite a few. The question asked by Mitchell, 'why is finding the solution to a social issue always the responsibility of those most affected by the issue?' (2011, p. 14) is a question of resources, expectations and communication. It has been stated that mobilisation of resources external to the group is key to social and policy change. Especially, when the potential change fits into existing schemes or widening opportunities of change. Allies become important; the public or political figures who can repress or facilitate a project's goals or voice. A photovoice project essentially creates an interest group (Olson, 1965; Snow, Soule, & Kriesi, 2007) or a micro version of a social movement. In its most simplistic definition provided by the Blackwell Companion to Social Movements (2007), social movements are: a collective that gives voice to their grievances and well-being of themselves and others and would engage in collective action (Snow et al., 2007, p. 3). This potential collective change intersects within a spatial, historical and political context requiring an ecological perspective that recognises that it exists as part of a complex web of social relations. A major component of that web is the unequal distribution of resources among social groups as the result of durable patterns of resource inequality in the broader society that shapes the differential ability of individual resources between and within particular social groups (McAdam, Tarrow, & Tilly, 2001). These resources are limited not only to financial capital but also to actual human resources; labour, expertise, skills, leadership, emotional and physical ability (Della & Diani, 2006; McAdam et al., 1996; Snow et al., 2007; Staggenborg, 2011). There is a necessity to combine internal and external sources with the understanding that marginalised groups have had far less success mobilising for collective action

(Snow et al., 2007, p. 143). Photovoice recognises participants' input and control over agenda setting, facilitates communication and reflection concerning their surroundings and fosters the development of skills. As a needs assessment tool, Photovoice offers insight into a tangible point of view perspective of participants and what they feel is important. In some instances, these groups may experience empowerment and feel for the first time they are being listened to and their concerns taken seriously as noted by Akesson et al. (2014). At the same time, there is a real danger for researchers to manifest false hopes or make unrealistic promises that cannot be fulfilled in the extent and practice of the research, making it vital to not mislead or raise unrealistic expectations (Akesson et al., 2014).

Like many CBPR approaches, photovoice includes a standard and repeated component of social change. From www.photovoice.org the official mission is

> to build skills within disadvantaged and marginalized communities. To achieve this, we utilize innovative participatory photography and digital storytelling methods. These skills enable individuals to represent themselves and create tools for advocacy and communication. Through this, and *through developing partnerships*, we deliver positive social change. (www. photovoice.org, emphasis added)

The message highlights the advantages of photovoice while underlying the importance of partnerships in the social change process. In photovoice.org's statement of ethical practice, it states a concern for well-being: Section (2.1) states,

> managing expectations: it is important that a project doesn't unrealistically raise participant's expectations. From the outset participants need to know the timetable, the end point, and what the project is likely to mean for them in concrete terms. They should never be led to believe that their circumstances will be dramatically or immediately changed by being involved. (www.photovoice.org)

Adding to Section (4.3), support: 'once it is all over, there can be a sense of disappointment and frustration if nothing material has changed. It is important that the participants be well supported throughout the project' (www.photovoice.org). Though these overall issues are addressed at photovoice.org, there is still a general lack of this discussion in most photovoice projects. Part of this aspect of being 'well supported' would be an essential focus on communication of goals so that researcher and community members can align their ideas about expectations of social and policy change. Additionally, the overall photovoice goal is often to reach policy-makers who have the power to implement changes within that community (Wang & Burris, 1997). But what about the inability to develop partnerships, the unequal access or distribution of resources? As Akeeson et al. (2014) have asked, what are the ethical implications when meaningful change is complex, challenging and perhaps an impossibility? What are the ethical implications of employing methods that seek transformation where such transformation can in no way be guaranteed? (Akeeson et al., 2014).

Recommendations for further inquiry

The community where the photovoice project takes place is a useful point of departure for investigating the potential concerns of a photovoice project. The community, small or large-scale is a site of vast differences in access to material and symbolic resources amongst its members (McAdam et al., 1996). There is an implied tone in some CBPR projects that the marginalised have no power and that it must be conferred on them by someone from the outside (Banks, 2001). This suggests that an 'external change agent raises the consciousness of the marginalised population on the underlying causes of their (health) problem and through a collaborative process facilitates their capacity development to address the problem' (Cargo, Delormier, Lévesque, McComber, & Macaulay, 2011, p. 96). Each CBPR and photovoice study should be adjusted for the cultural and social context (Blackburn, 2000, p. 10) so that inappropriate impositions of a certain vision of power on those who may not actually perceive themselves as powerless do not occur (Thompson, 2008). Ideally, local people should be inviting researchers in, not the agencies of interest setting the agenda (McIntyre, 2003, p. 49). This was discussed by Cargo et al. (2011) in terms of the established mistrust generated from externally driven research and the self-determination movement of Aboriginals in a Kanien'kehaka (Mohawk) community near Montreal, Canada. This study illustrates an effective use of an 'inside job' where the community initiated control over the Kahnawake Schools Diabetes Prevention Project (KSDPP) study. With a range of leaders working in partnership such as the KSDPP Staff, a Community Advisory Board of members from health, social, political, spiritual, recreational, private and community sectors, academic researchers, community researchers, community affiliates and a supervisory board, this study illustrates that effective change relies on an understanding that 'community capacity is dynamic and develops in stages of readiness' (Cargo et al., 2011, p. 99). This willingness to partner in collaboration with varying aspects of the community shows the potential of reducing initiation of an 'external agent' and points to growth in effective strategies for social change.

Photovoice may be best utilised as a method as part of a comprehensive system that will unlikely stand alone to bring about policy change. If photovoice is to be used as a means of completing a community needs assessment, the group should be made to understand that the project has the potential to be *policy informing rather than policy changing*. There is good potential for photovoice to inform community and policy leaders about community issues but the direct path to social and policy change involves a variety of material, social and cultural factors. The vague evaluation of most photovoice projects should shift from a focus on policy change and 'reaching policy makers' and rely on the strengths of the method to avoid false hopes and disappointment (Catalani & Minkler, 2010). Photovoice goals should include a focus on empowerment as a long-term process with many steps, such as building self-esteem or participation in community organising efforts (Wallerstein & Bernstein, 1988). In the photovoice study conducted by Wallerstein and Bernstein (1988) with patients in an HIV treatment programme, the authors argue that patients do not have sole responsibility in creating a healthier environment,

> empowerment education with its dual focus on participatory reflection and action should be incorporated into the other prevention strategies of health promotion, disease prevention, and health protection. By becoming incorporated into current prevention approaches, empowerment education can enhance changes in personal growth, social support, community organizing, policy and environmental changes, and other indicators of increased control over one's life in society. (Wallerstein & Bernstein, 1988, p. 388)

Conclusion

Although photovoice is not without its limitations, it has great appeal as a method of engaging people in the political and social lives of their communities. Photovoice has been noted as a flexible tool for strengthening public health research through community participation including enhanced community involvement and individual empowerment (Catalani & Minkler, 2010, p. 448). The proposed shift in power, from the traditional researcher to the participants as co-learners, is noticeably its greatest and desirable strength. The shift in power should be recognised as a shift in viewpoint and authority in the image-making process without the unnecessary leap to responsibility to enact meaningful yet sometimes complicated social and policy change. I remind the reader that photovoice should be regarded as a tool for policy informing rather than changing. For further understanding of the utility of the photovoice method, new projects are needed that will take into account some of the suggestions made in this article. The article highlights current gaps in the research and poses several unanswered questions in the application and ethical practice of photovoice as a research methodology. I began this review inspired by the question posed by Mitchell, 'why is finding the solution to a social issue always the responsibility of those most affected by the issue?' (2011, p. 14). Perhaps, with further collaboration and engaged inquiry, we may work towards an answer void of false hopes for effective policy and social change.

Disclosure statement

No potential conflict of interest was reported by the author.

References

Akesson, B., D'Amico, M., Denov, M., Khan, F., Linds, W., & Mitchell, C. (2014). Stepping back as researchers: Addressing ethics in arts-based approaches to working with war-affected children in school and community settings. *Educational Research for Social Change (ERSC)*, 3(1), 75–89. Retrieved from http://ssrn.com/abstract=2476379

Armstrong, R., Hall, B., Doyle, J., & Waters, E. (2011) 'Scoping the scope' of a Cochrane review. *Journal of Public Health*, 33(1), 147–150. doi:10.1093/pubmed/fdr015

Baker, T., & Wang, C. (2006). Photovoice: Use of a participatory action research method to explore the chronic pain experience in older adults. *Qualitative Health Research*, 16(10), 1405–1413. doi:10.1177/1049732306294118

Banks, M. (2001). *Visual methods in social research*. London: Sage.

Baum, F., MacDougall, C., & Smith, D. (2006) Participatory action research. *Journal of Epidemiology and Community Health*, 60(10), 854–857. doi:10.1136/jech.2004.028662

Blackburn, J. (2000). Understanding Paulo Friere: Reflections on the origins, concepts, and possible pitfalls of his educational approach. *Community Development Journal*, 35(1), 3–15. doi:10.1093/cdj/35.1.3

Booth, T., & Booth, W. (2003). In the frame: Photovoice and mothers with learning difficulties. *Disability & Society*, 18(4), 431–432. doi:10.1080/0968759032000080986

Cargo, M. D., Delormier, T., Lévesque, L., McComber, A. M., & Macaulay, A. C. (2011). Community capacity as an 'inside job': Evolution of perceived ownership within a university-Aboriginal community partnership. *American Journal of Health Promotion*, 26(2), 96–100. doi:10.4278/ajhp.091229-ARB-403

Castleden, H., Garvin, T., & First Nation, H. (2008). Modifying photovoice for community-based participatory indigenous research. *Social Science & Medicine, 66*(6), 1393–1405. doi:10.1016/j. socscimed.2007.11.030

Catalani, C., & Minkler, M. (2010). Photovoice: A review of the literature in health and public health. *Health Education and Behavior, 37*(3), 424–451. doi:10.1177/1090198109342084

Chio, V. C. M., & Fandt, P. M. (2007). Photovoice in the diversity classroom: Engagement, voice, and the eye of the camera. *Journal of Management Education, 31*(4), 484–504. doi:10.1177/ 1052562906288124

Della, P. D., & Diani, M. (2006). *Social movements: An introduction.* Malden, MA: Blackwell.

Diani, M., & McAdam, D. (2003). *Social movements and networks: Relational approaches to collective action.* Oxford: Oxford University Press.

Duffy, L. (2010). Hidden heroines: Lone mothers assessing community health using photovoice. *Health Promotion Practice, 11*(6), 788–797. doi:10.1177/1524839908324779

Erdner, A., Andersson, L., Magnusson, A., & Lützén, K. (2009). Varying views of life among people with long-term mental illness. *Journal of Psychiatric & Mental Health Nursing, 16*(1), 54–60. doi:10.1111/j.1365-2850.2008.01329.x

Foster-Fishman, P., Nowell, B., Deacon, Z., Nievar, M. A., & McCann, P. (2005). Using methods that matter: The impact of reflection, dialogue, and voice. *American Journal of Community Psychology, 36*(3–4), 275. doi:10.1007/s10464-005-8626-y

Gosselink, C. A., & Myllykangas, S. A. (2007). The leisure experiences of older U.S. women living with HIV/AIDS. *Health Care for Women International, 28*(1), 3–20. doi:10.1080/ 07399330601001402

Guillemin, M., & Drew, S. (2010). Questions of process in participant-generated visual methodologies. *Visual Studies, 25*(2), 175–188. doi:10.1080/1472586X.2010.502676

Harley, A. (2012). Picturing reality: Power, ethics, and politics in using photovoice. *International Journal of Qualitative Methods, 11*(4), 320–339.

Harrison, B. (2002). Seeing health and illness worlds –Using visual methodologies in a sociology of health and illness: A methodological review. *Sociology of Health and Illness, 64*(6), 856–872. doi:10.1111/1467-9566.00322

Hergenrather, K. C., Rhodes, S. D., Cowan, C. A., Bardhoshi, G., & Pula, S. (2009). Photovoice as community-based participatory research: A qualitative review. *American Journal of Health Behavior, 33*(6), 686–698.

Jaggar, A. M. (2008). *Just methods: An interdisciplinary feminist reader.* Boulder, CO: Paradigm Publishers.

Killion, C. M., & Wang, C. C. (2000). Linking African American mothers across life stage and station through photovoice. *Journal of Health Care for the Poor and Underserved, 11*(3), 310–325. doi:10.1353/hpu.2010.0816

LeClerc, C. M., Wells, D. L., Craig, D., & Wilson, J. L. (2002). Falling short of the mark: Tales of life after hospital discharge. *Clinical Nursing Research, 11*(3), 242–263. doi:10.1177/ 10573802011003002

López, E. D. S., Eng, E., Randall-David, E., & Robinson, N. (2005). Quality-of-life concerns of African American breast cancer survivors within rural North Carolina: Blending the techniques of photovoice and grounded theory. *Qualitative Health Research, 15*(1), 99–115. doi:10.1177/ 1049732304270766

López, E. D. S., Eng, E., Robinson, N., & Wang, C. C. (2005). Photovoice as a community-based participatory research method. In B. Israel, E. Eng, A. J. Schulz, & E. A. Parker (Eds.), *Methods in community-based participatory research for health* (pp. 326–348). San Francisco, CA: Jossey-Bass.

McAdam, D., McCarthy, J. D., & Zald, M. N. (1996). *Comparative perspectives on social movements: Political opportunities, mobilizing structures, and cultural framings.* Cambridge: Cambridge University Press.

McAdam, D., Tarrow, S. G., & Tilly, C. (2001). *Dynamics of contention.* New York, NY: Cambridge University Press.

McCarthy, J. D., & Zald, M. N., (1979). *The dynamics of social movements: Resource mobilization, social control, and tactics.* Cambridge, MA: Winthrop Publishers.

McIntyre, A. (2003). Through the eyes of women: Photovoice and participatory research as tools for reimagining place. *Gender, Place & Culture, 10,* 47–66.

Mitchell, C. (2011). *Doing visual research.* London: Sage.

Mitchell, C., DeLange, N., Moletsane, R., Stuart, J., & Buthelezi, T. (2005). Giving a face to HIV and AIDS: On the uses of photo-voice by teachers and community health care workers working with youth in rural South Africa. *Qualitative Research in Psychology, 2*(3), 257–270. doi:10.1191/1478088705qp042oa

Moffitt, P., & Vollman, A. R. (2004). Designer's corner. Photovoice: Picturing the health of aboriginal women in a remote northern community. *Canadian Journal of Nursing Research, 36*(4), 189–201. Retrieved from http://www.ingentaconnect.com/content/mcgill/cjnr/2004/00000036/00000004/art00012?crawler=true

Olson, M. (1965). *The logic of collective action: Public goods and the theory of groups.* Cambridge, MA: Harvard University Press.

Pauwels, L. (2010). Visual sociology reframed: An analytical synthesis and discussion of visual methods in social and cultural research. *Sociological Methods & Research, 38*(4), 545–581. doi:10.1177/0049124110366233

Poudrier, J., & Mac-Lean, R. (2009). 'We've fallen into the cracks': Aboriginal women's experiences with breast cancer through photovoice. *Nursing Inquiry, 16*(4), 306–317. doi:10.1111/j.1440-1800.2009.00435.x

Prins, E. (2010). Participatory photography: A tool for empowerment or surveillance? *Action Research, 8*(4), 426–443. doi:10.1177/1476750310374502

Reason, P., & Bradbury, H. (2001). *Handbook of action research: Participative inquiry and practice.* London: SAGE.

Schneider, B. (2010). *Hearing (our) voices: Participatory research in mental health.* Toronto, ON: University of Toronto Press.

Sitvast, J. E., Abma, T. A., & Widdershoven, G. A. (2010). Facades of suffering: Clients' photo stories about mental illness. *Archives of Psychiatric Nursing, 24*(5), 349–361. doi:10.1016/j.apnu.2010.02.004

Snow, D. A., Soule, S. A., & Kriesi, H. (2007). *The Blackwell companion to social movements.* Malden, MA: Blackwell.

Staggenborg, S. (2011). *Social movements.* Don Mills, ON: Oxford University Press.

Stevens, C. A. (2006). Being healthy: Voices of adolescent women who are parenting. *Journal for Specialists in Pediatric Nursing, 11*(1), 28–40. doi:10.1111/j.1744-6155.2006.00041.x

Strack, R. W., Magill, C., & McDonagh, K. (2004). Engaging youth through Photovoice. *Health Promotion Practice, 5*(1), 49–58. doi:10.1177/1524839903258015

Tanjasiri, S., Lew, R., Kuratani, D., Wong, M., & Fu, L. (2011). Using photovoice to assess and promote environmental approaches to tobacco control in AAPI communities. *Health Promotion Practice, 12*(5), 654–665. doi:10.1177/1524839910369987

Tarrow, S. G. (1998). *Power in movement: Social movements and contentious politics.* Cambridge: Cambridge University Press.

Thompson, N. C., Hunter, E. E., Murray, L., Ninci, L., Rolfs, E. M., & Pallikkathayil, L. (2008). The experience of living with chronic mental illness: A photovoice study. *Perspectives in Psychiatric Care, 44*(1), 14–24. doi:10.1111/j.1744-6163.2008.00143.x

Wagner, J. C. (1979). *Images of information: Still photography in the social sciences.* Beverly Hills, CA: Sage.

Wallerstein, N., & Bernstein, E. (1988). Empowerment education: Freire's ideas adapted to health education. *Health Education Quarterly, 15*(4), 379–394. doi:10.1177/109019818801500402

Wang, C. (1999). Photovoice: A participatory action research strategy applied to women's health. *Journal of Women's Health, 8*(2), 185–192.

Wang, C. (2006). Youth participation in photovoice as a strategy for community change. *Journal of Community Practice, 14*(1), 147–161. doi:10.1300/J125v14n01_09

Wang, C., & Burris, M. (1994). Empowerment through photo novella: Portraits of participation. *Health Education Quarterly*, *21*(2), 171–186. doi:10.1177/109019819402100204

Wang, C., & Burris, M. (1997). Photovoice: Concept, methodology, and use for participatory needs assessment. *Health Education & Behavior*, *24*(3), 369–387. doi:10.1177/109019819702400309

Wang, C., Cash, J. L., & Powers, L. S. (2000). Who knows the streets as well as the homeless? Promoting personal and community action through photovoice. *Health Promotion Practice*, *1*(1), 81–89. doi:10.1177/152483990000100113

Wang, C., & Redwood-Jones, Y. A. (2001). Photovoice ethics: Perspectives from flint photovoice. *Health Education & Behavior*, *28*(5), 560–572. doi:10.1177/109019810102800504

Wang, C., Yi, W. K., Tao, Z. W., & Carovano, K. (1998). Photovoice as a participatory health promotion strategy. *Health Promotion International*, *13*(1), 75–86. doi:10.1093/heapro/13.1.75

Wilson, N., Dasho, S., Martin, A., Wallerstein, N., Wang, C., & Minkler, M. (2007). Engaging young adolescents in social action through photovoice. *The Journal of Early Adolescence*, *27*(2), 241–261. doi:10.1177/0272431606294834

Index

MSM *see* men who have sex with men
multiple sexual partnerships (MSPs) 200–1;
   health communication 201–2; mock dialogues
   and internal monologues 208–10; motivations
   and gender issues 201; photo vignettes 207–8,
   208; scripted photos 207, **207**, **211**; typologies
   210; unscripted photos **206**, 206–7, **209**
music and theatre 245

National AIDS Council 200, 216n2
New Orleans Police Department (NOPD) **230**
N'weti Health Communication 204

Ohler, Jason 17
OpenStreetMap 75, 76

PARCES movement 93–4
participant-empowered visual timelines, sexual
   behaviour: building rapport 192, 194;
   case-based analysis 187; community-based
   participatory research 180–1; data analysis
   187–8; identification of patterns **189**,
   189–91, **190**; in-depth interviews *see* in-depth
   interviews; life-history calendar 182; men
   who have sex with men 179–80; participatory
   interaction 193–4; personal relationship
   diaries 183, 185; recruitment 183; self-
   reflection 191–2; thematic analysis 187;
   traditional qualitative methods 180, 195
participation 5–6
participatory action research (PAR), in social
   change context 80–1; and 'Beyond Glue and
   Bazuco' project 84–5, **86**; dissemination
   practices 83–4, **91**, 91–3; reflexivity practices
   83, 86–91, **89**, **90**; sustainability and 'afterlife'
   84, 93–4
participatory action research process 236
participatory geographic information system
   (PGIS) 66
participatory mapping: in HIV prevention
   research *see* Kenyan youth, participatory
   mapping
participatory photography methodology 225
participatory video 5; stigma-reduction strategy
   see Stigma Assessment and Reduction of
   Impact project
participatory video (PV) 12–13
patient information sheets: for older children **120**;
   for younger children 118–19, **119**
peace education, digital storytelling and 17, 18
personal relationship diaries (PRDs) 183, 185
PGIS *see* participatory geographic information
   system
photo-based projective techniques
   (photo-based PT): advantages 211–13; focus
   group discussions 200; for health behaviour
   research 199–200; HIV health communication
   research 204–5, 214–15; limitations 213;

multiple sexual partnerships *see* multiple
   sexual partnerships; photographic visuals 203;
   psychoanalytic assumption 203; qualitative
   method 213; uniqueness 213–14
photo-elicitation strategy 224–5
photoPAR process 225; action-reflection
   process 230; antiracist feminist 239;
   co-researchers, engagement of 225–7;
   personal and cross-community communication
   227–9; photo-elicitation strategy 224–5;
   photonarratives 234–6, **235**; phototexts and
   collective storytelling 229–33, **231**, **233**
photovoice 3–4, 11–12, 279, 288; analysing
   photographic data in 28; community-based
   participatory research and 281; content
   analysis **32**, 32–4, **35**; ethical consideration
   29–30; false hopes and expectations 283–4;
   flow chart **30**; focus of photographs 33, **34**;
   goals 281, 287; limitations 40; methodology
   280; as micro-social movement 284–5;
   Minh's photograph 37–8, **38**; modifications
   to 30–1, 40; number of photographs **33**;
   overview of 26–7; participants 29, **29**, 40;
   participatory analysis 32–3, 38; policy
   change 282–3; practises 282; projects 284;
   recommendations for inquiry 286–7;
   resource mobilisation 285–6; social action
   and 283; social change and 285–6; Thái's
   photograph 37, **37**; Thuy's photograph 36–7;
   visual material interpretation 39; youth and
   community capacity *see* youth and community
   capacity
*Picturing Inclusion: Voices of Girls with
   Disabilities* 142
policy and community dialogue, digital tools
   for 132; arts-based workshops 134; children's
   daily realities 139–40; data analysis 134–5;
   data collectors 140–1; 'digital dialogue
   tool', development of 135; Kibera youth
   development project 138, **138**; *More Than
   Bricks and Mortar* **136**, 136–8, **137**, 141;
   overview of 131–2; with policy-making process
   140; researcher-led video production 132–3
policy poster process, in social research 273
Population Services International (PSI) 204
post-Katrina New Orleans, community-based
   health promotion in: African-American and
   Latino context 224, 225, **233**; challenges and
   limitations 236–9; co-researchers, engagement
   of 225–7; photonarratives 234–6, **235**;
   photoPAR process *see* photoPAR process;
   racial and economic inequalities in 223
PRDs *see* personal relationship diaries
process surveys 69–70, 72, **74**
PSI *see* Population Services International
PV *see* participatory video

qualitative generalisability 256